MICROVASCULAR ANASTOMOSES FOR CEREBRAL ISCHEMIA

MICROVASCULAR ANASTOMOSES FOR CEREBRAL ISCHEMIA

Jack M. Fein and
O. Howard Reichman, Editors

with 197 illustrations
including 12 four-color plates

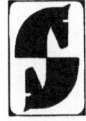

Springer-Verlag
New York Heidelberg Berlin

Dr. Jack M. Fein
Department of Neurosurgery
Albert Einstein College of Medicine
Montifiore Hospital Medical Center
Bronx, New York 10461

Dr. O. Howard Reichman
Division of Neurological Surgery
Loyola University Medical Center
Maywood, Illinois 60153

Library of Congress Cataloging in Publication Data

International Symposium on Microneurosurgical Anastomoses
    for Cerebral Ischemia, 2d, Chicago, Ill., 1974.
    Microvascular anastomoses for cerebral ischemia.

    Includes bibliographies and index.
    1. Cerebral ischemia—Surgery—Congresses.
2. Cerebral arteries—Surgery—Congresses.
3. Microsurgery—Congresses. 4. Cerebrovascular
disease—Surgery—Congresses. I. Fein, Jack M.
II. Reichman, Owen Howard, 1932-
RD594.I57 1974   617'.481   78-1977

© 1978 by Springer-Verlag New York Inc.
Softcover reprint of the hardcover 1st edition 1978

9 8 7 6 5 4 3 2 1

ISBN-13: 978-1-4612-9913-4   e-ISBN-13: 978-1-4612-9911-0
DOI: 10.1007/978-1-4612-9911-0

Foreword

We have witnessed a remarkable development during the past 10 years in the development of extra–intracranial anastomosis to revascularize the brain. Initially, the intention was to create a means of performing embolectomy in small cortical arteries after cardiac surgery. Gradually a plan was conceived to form an extra–intracranial bypass(10) to treat inaccessible lesions of the carotid and vertebral arteries as well as tumors and giant aneurysms that involved these arteries.

The basic techniques and principles of microvascular surgery, which had been refined over 30 years on peripheral arteries(1–7, 9) were applied in 1966 to the intracerebral arteries of dogs(4). The arterial patching and suturing were successful, while extra–intracranial long bypasses were a constant failure. This was attributed to the damage that was inevitably inflicted on the vasa vasorum of the autogenous graft during dissection(9). This situation posed a dilemma until eventually the idea of Pool and Potts(8) was adopted and an anastomosis was performed on a dog between the superficial temporal artery and a cortical branch. Because of the vessels' small size and the doubts regarding its capacity for improving the circulation, the procedure was performed with a certain amount of apprehension. It was a pleasant surprise, therefore, to discover that it was possible to attain a high rate of patency. If the middle cerebral artery was used and was isolated from its carotid inflow, an even higher rate was achieved. An important point to take into account when performing intracranial microvascular reconstructive surgery is the fact that exact knowledge of the arachnoidal anatomy in relation to the vessels ensures successful atraumatic dissection and preparation of the fine branches.

Although the basic technique was proven in the laboratory, the application of this procedure to the human brain was intentionally delayed because of the lack of well-defined indications and the uncertainty of a beneficial long-term result to the patient. It is advisable for the surgeon to consider each case individually, to study the collateral circulation, cerebral blood flow measurements, coaxial tomograms, and the general physical and mental condition of the patient in deciding on the best course of treatment. In order to make full use of the technical progress and advances that have been made, a formula for determining and defining valid indications for surgery is needed.

A decade has passed since the first research and investigations were undertaken, and this excellent monograph presents evidence that the evolution of this technique has taken a fruitful and effective course. The content is of a distinctive quality and features clear and precise accounts of various aspects of the procedure which will undoubtedly be of benefit in teaching other surgeons. It makes a major contribution to a field of microsurgery that continues to progress and develop toward a safer and more successful treatment of the patient.

REFERENCES

1. Buncke HJ, Schulz WP: Experimental digital amputation and reimplantation. Plast Reconstr Surg 36:62, 1965.
2. Cobbett, J: Presentation to the British Association of Plastic Surgeons. Dec. 2, 1965, London, England.
3. Crawford ES, et al: A technique permitting operation upon small arteries. Surg Forum 10:671, 1959
4. Donaghy RMP, Yasargil MG: *Microvascular Surgery*. St. Louis, Mosby, 1967
5. Hedberg SE: Suture, anastomosis of small vessels following relief of spasm by hydrostatic pressure dilatation. Ann Surg 155:51, 1962
6. Jacobson JH II, Suarez EL: Microsurgery in anastomosis of small vessels. Surg Forum 11:243, 1960
7. Lougheed WM, Khodadad B: A new clip for surgery of intracranial and small blood vessels. J Neurosurg 22:397, 1965
8. Pool JL, Potts G: *Aneurysms and Arteriovenous Malformations of the Brain*. New York, Hoeber, 1965
9. Smith JW: Microsurgery: Review of the literature and discussion of microtechniques. Plast Reconstr Surg 37:227, 1966
10. Woringer E, Kunlin J: Anastomose entre la carotide primitive et la carotide intra-cranienne ou la sylvienne par greffon selon la technique de la suture suspendue. Neurochirurgie (Paris) 9:181, 1963

M. Gazi Yasargil

Preface

The extracranial–intracranial bypass graft to augment collateral cerebral blood flow (CBF) represents a significant advance in the treatment of cerebrovascular insufficiency. Since its introduction in 1967, the original technique and its modifications have been utilized to treat approximately 2,000 patients with complete occlusion of the internal carotid artery or segmental occlusive disease of the intracranial arteries. The first such procedure was an anastomosis of the superficial temporal artery (STA) to a temporal cortical branch of the middle cerebral artery (MCA). Since then other cortical branches have been utilized. Occipital artery anastomoses with the angular artery and the posterior inferior cerebellar artery have been reported more recently. Alternate techniques using both branches of the superficial temporal artery, the radial artery, and short and long vein grafts have also been employed.

Developments in this area seemed to group themselves naturally into the seven major sections of this text. Laboratory research continues to extend our understanding of cerebral ischemia and provides the rationale for efforts to revascularize the brain. Although a true laboratory model for cerebral atherosclerosis has not been extensively utilized in investigation of cerebrovascular insufficiency, many of the hemodynamic changes associated with ischemia have been reproduced by various other techniques reported here.

The metabolic consequences of ischemia are described separately. This provides some insight into how brain energetics can be manipulated as a result of and in conjunction with the surgical augmentation of CBF. We have included a discussion of contemporary techniques of STA-MCA anastomosis to bridge the gap between innovative development and clinical application. While the indications for the procedure are becoming crystallized in patients with transient ischemic attacks, it was apparent that a good deal of work still needs to be done to select patients and to evaluate the results of this surgery in cases with mild to moderate neurologic deficit.

It is the opinion of some that this surgical approach is the optimal therapy for symptomatic patients with complete occlusion of the internal carotid artery or segmental occlusive disease of the intracranial internal carotid and middle cerebral arteries. If this is true, then a large group of patients with cerebrovascular insufficiency are the potential beneficiaries of a new therapy which may have a significant impact on the recurrence rate of strokes.

Jack M. Fein
O. Howard Reichman

Contents

Contents

Contents

xi

List of Contributors

R. E. ANDERSON, Department of Radiology, University of Utah College of Medicine, Salt Lake City, Utah.

G. AUSTIN, Section of Neurological Surgery, Loma Linda University School of Medicine, Loma Linda, California.

B. AZAR-KIA, Department of Radiology, Loyola University Medical Center, Maywood, Illinois.

C. M. BANNISTER, Department of Neurosurgery, The General Infirmary at Leeds, Yorkshire, England.

A. L. CARNEY, Department of Thoracic & Cardiovascular Surgery, La Grange Professional Center, La Grange, Illinois.

J. E. CASSIDY, Department of Medicine, Loyola University Medical Center, Maywood, Illinois.

N. L. CHATER, Department of Neurological Surgery, University of California Medical Center, San Francisco, California.

M. DUJOVNY, Department of Neurological Surgery, The University of Pittsburgh School of Medicine, Pittsburgh, Pennsylvania.

M. H. EPSTEIN, Department of Neurological Surgery, Johns Hopkins Hospital, Baltimore, Maryland.

J. M. FEIN, Department of Neurosurgery, Albert Einstein College of Medicine, Bronx, New York.

W. GEE, Department of Muscular Surgery, University of California School of Medicine, San Francisco, California.

O. GRATZL, Department of Neurosurgery, University of Munich, West Germany.

G. HAUGEN, Section of Neurological Surgery, Loma Linda University School of Medicine, Loma Linda, California.

W. HAYWARD, Section of Neurological Surgery, Loma Linda University School of Medicine, Loma Linda, California.

M. P. HEILBRUN, Division of Neurosurgery, University of Utah College of Medicine, Salt Lake City, Utah.

J. KARASAWA, Department of Neurological Surgery, Kitano Hospital, Osaka, Japan.

H. KIKUCHI, Department of Neurological Surgery, Kitano Hospital, Osaka, Japan.

D. LAFFIN, Section of Neurological Surgery, Loma Linda University School of Medicine, Loma Linda, California.

R. LAMOND, Department of Neurological Surgery, University of California Medical Center, San Francisco, California.

E. LICHTER, Section of Neurological Surgery, Loma Linda University School of Medicine, Loma Linda, California.

J. C. MAROON, Department of Neurological Surgery, University of Pittsburgh School of Medicine, Pittsburgh, Pennsylvania.

G. F. MOLINARI, Department of Neurology, George Washington University School of Medicine, Washington, D.C.

J. R. MOZINGO, Division of Neurological Surgery, University of Florida Health Center, Gainesville, Florida.

L. A. MUNDY, Department of Neurosurgery, The General Infirmary at Leeds, Yorkshire, England.

C. P. OSGOOD, Department of Neurological Surgery, University of Pittsburgh School of Medicine, Pittsburgh, Pennsylvania.

E. PALACIOS, Department of Radiology, Loyola University Medical Center, Maywood, Illinois.

E. PFENNINGER, Department of Neurosurgery, University of Zurich, Zurich, Switzerland.

C. B. POWELL, Division of Neurosurgery, University of Utah College of Medicine, Salt Lake City, Utah.

O. H. REICHMAN, Division of Neurosurgery, Loyola University Medical Center, Maywood, Illinois.

A. L. RHOTON, Jr., Division of Neurological Surgery, University of Florida Health Center, Gainesville, Florida.

T. S. ROBERTS, Division of Neurosurgery, University of Utah College of Medicine, Salt Lake City, Utah.

S. A. ROUHE, Section of Neurological Surgery, Loma Linda University School of Medicine, Loma Linda, California.

P. SCHMIEDEK, Department of Neurosurgery, University of Munich, Munich, West Germany.

W. SCHULER, Section of Neurological Surgery, Loma Linda University School of Medicine, Loma Linda, California.

H. STEINHOFF, Department of Neurosurgery, University of Munich, Munich, West Germany.

H. W. STEPHENS, Jr., Allentown, Pennsylvania.

J. R. THOMPSON, Loma Linda University School of Medicine, Loma Linda, California.

R. VASUDEVAN, Section of Neurological Surgery, Loma Linda University School of Medicine, Loma Linda, California.

A. C. WALTZ, Professor, Department of Neurology, Cerebrovascular Clinical Research Center, University Hospital, Minneapolis, Minnesota.

P. R. WEINSTEIN, Department of Neurological Surgery, University of California Medical Center, San Francisco, California.

C. J. WHANG, Division of Neurological Surgery, University of Florida Health Center, Gainesville, Florida.

M. G. YASARGIL, Neurochirurgische Universitatsklinik, Kantonsspital Zurich, Switzerland.

I

STRUCTURE AND FUNCTION

1

Anatomy and physiology
pertinent to stroke

Arthur C. Waltz

Microsurgical anastomosis of cerebral vessels can be technically successful: anastomosis can be made between cerebral arterial vessels or venous vessels, these can be kept patent, and blood can be made to flow through them. The question that arises relates to the value of such an anastomosis. An important goal in the treatment of patients with cerebrovascular disease is to prevent or minimize neurologic deficits by preserving or maximizing neuronal function. A most important aspect of this is going to be the prevention of atherosclerosis. No matter how effective preventive measures will become, however, there will always be some patients who will have atherosclerosis and some of these will have strokes. Therefore, we need to consider the treatment of stenoses caused by atherosclerosis, of embolization from atherosclerotic plaques, and of acute ischemic episodes and acute strokes in order to minimize neurologic deficits and maximize neuronal function.

Cerebrovascular anastomosis may be worthwhile, as many have stated, in patients who have continuing transient ischemic attacks associated with occlusion or inaccessible stenosis of a major vessel. Anastomosis also may be of value in the treatment of an acute ischemic episode. Reperfusion of an ischemic area within a few hours after a stroke has occurred may prevent the extension of a cerebral infarct or prevent irreversible impairment of neuronal function. Reperfusion may prevent neurons that are "paralyzed" or not functioning from actually dying.

Anatomy of Penetrating and Intracerebral Vessels

Rational treatment of stroke requires knowledge of anatomy and physiology. For example, all the blood vessels that supply the brain originate from the surface. The arterial vessels that penetrate the brain are all less than 70 μ in diameter, except for the lenticulostriate arteries and others at the base, virtually all of which are less than 50 μ in diameter. Moreover, there are no interarterial anastomoses in penetrating vessels until branches of approximately 20 to 30 μ in diameter are reached.(1,10)

The question of intracerebral arteriovenous shunts has arisen repeatedly. Small arterioles approximately 25 μ in diameter anastomosing with veins have been described.(6) If these exist in the brain, they must be extremely rare. Superimposition of vessels in histologic sections may give an appearance of arteriovenous anastomoses.(10) However, there may be "thoroughfare channels," in that capillaries that are about 10 μ in diameter may pass directly from arterioles to venules, but true arteriovenous shunts probably do not exist.(6,9)

The arterial vessels within the brain are the most important ones for the regulation of cerebral blood flow locally and regionally. In cats, which have a rete mirabile, there is a 39% loss of the pressure head from the aorta to the pial arteries, probably because of the rete(11); in monkeys and humans, the pressure head loss attributable to the surface vessels of the brain is only about 10 to 15%.(7) The major decrease in pressure from the aorta to cerebral veins occurs in the small vessels within the brain.(7,11) These are the vessels, then, that contribute the greatest amount of resistance to the flow of blood; and these are the regulatory vessels that control regional and local cerebral circulation. These vessels, unfortunately, cannot be seen by angiography, which is only capable of resolving vessel diameters greater than about 150 μ.

Mechanisms for Production of Transient Ischemic Attacks

The internal carotid artery in humans is potentially capable of carrying much more blood than it ordinarily does. It must be constricted to a cross-sectional diameter of less than 2 mm before a pressure gradient develops across the stenosis and before arterial blood flow, measured with an electromagnetic flow meter, decreases.(4,14) The percentage constriction is not nearly as important as the actual diameter. Similarly, the length of a stenosis has only a minor effect on a pressure gradient or a decrease of blood flow, and is not nearly as important as the cross-sectional diameter.(8)

Transient ischemic attacks (TIAs) can occur, however, with severe stenosis of a carotid artery or a large surface vessel of the brain. Associated factors, such as transient decreases of blood flow caused by cardiac arrhythmias or systemic hypotension, may play a role here. In the vertebrobasilar circulation,

TIAs as well as small infarcts may be caused by the extension of a thrombus into or next to a small penetrating arteriole. However, TIAs associated with carotid artery disease more frequently may be related to embolization from an atherosclerotic plaque.

The stereotyped signs and symptoms of TIAs must be explained by any proposed theory. If there is severe stenosis or occlusion of a major artery, stereotyped events may be related to decreased blood flow through tortuous collateral channels with high resistance to an area of brain previously supplied by a distal vessel that has itself become obstructed. This clinical picture results from a combination of proximal vascular disease, distal vascular disease, and transient decreases of cardiac output or systemic blood pressure. Stereotyped events may also follow embolization. The embolus is likely to go to the same location distally if it enters the circulation where there is relatively laminar or streamlined flow, as is usually true in the carotid artery.

Cerebral Blood Flow and Neuronal Function

Cerebral tissue can often survive and function despite markedly impaired perfusion. For example, in a study in which cerebral blood flow (CBF) was measured during clamping of the carotid artery for endarterectomy, CBF was found to decrease to less than 30 or even 20 ml/100 g/minute in a number of patients who did not have neurologic deficits after the surgical procedure.[16] More recently, it has been shown that EEG changes occur during endarterectomy at a CBF of about 20 ml/100 g/minute,[12] and that evoked potentials of the brains of animals become affected by ischemia only when blood flow decreases to approximately the same level.[3]

One of the major problems in studying the treatment of stroke is to determine when a neuron is functioning and when it is not. The measurements that we use, namely, the EEG, evoked potentials, and the neurologic examination, indicate that CBF can be reduced remarkably and function can still persist. CBF itself is not an index of neuronal function. However, in experimental models, ischemic regions of brain frequently are larger than infarcted regions.[17] There may be some cells that are ischemic and functioning, but there may be other cells that are ischemic, not functioning, and yet not dead. Perhaps it would be possible, by reperfusion, to restore flow to these areas and allow some of these cells to recover function. How long after the onset of ischemia one could hope for recovery of function, if it could occur, is still debatable: it may be weeks, but it may only be several hours.

Reperfusion of Ischemic Regions

There has been a great deal of discussion recently about the so-called "no reflow" phenomenon, a term that I prefer not to use. After some minutes of total cerebral ischemia, there may be difficulty reperfusing the brain.(2) With focal ischemia, such is not the case. If the middle cerebral artery is occluded in a squirrel monkey there may be very little flow through arteries and stagnation in veins on the surface of the brain at about 2 hours after occlusion.(15) Despite this, it is possible to reperfuse the brain and to restore blood flow to the same levels that were present before occlusion, or even to produce reactive hyperemia.(13) However, reperfusion depends upon maintenance of blood pressure. In rhesus monkeys the middle cerebral artery can be occluded for 2 to 4 hours, or even up to 24 hours, and yet the animal can recover without a neurologic deficit and without pathologic evidence of an infarct.(5) Reperfusion of ischemic brain is possible.

All of the things I have mentioned have relevance to the treatment of stroke, and specifically to treatment by vascular surgical procedures.

References

1. Alexander L, Putnam TJ: Pathological alterations of cerebral vascular patterns. Res Publ Assoc Res Nerv Ment Dis 18:471, 1938
2. Ames A III, Wright RL, Kowada M, et al: Cerebral ischemia. II. The no-reflow phenomenon. Amer J Pathol 52:437, 1968
3. Branston NM, Symon L, Crockard HA, et al: Relationship between the cortical evoked potential and local cortical blood flow following acute middle cerebral artery occlusion in the baboon. Exp Neurol 45:195, 1974
4. Brice JG, Dowsett DJ, Lowe RD: Hemodynamic effects of carotid artery stenosis. Br Med J 2:1363, 1964
5. Crowell RM, Olsson Y, Klatzo I, et al: Temporary occlusion of the middle cerebral artery in the monkey. Clinical and pathological observations. Stroke 1:439, 1970
6. Hasegawa T, Ravens JR, Toole JF: Precapillary arteriovenous anastomoses. "Thoroughfare channels" in the brain. Arch Neurol 16:217, 1967
7. Kanzow E, Dieckhoff D: On the location of the vascular resistance in the cerebral circulation. In Brock M, Fieschi C, Ingvar DH, et al (eds): Cerebral Blood Flow. Berlin, Springer, 1969, pp. 96–97
8. Kindt GW, Youmans JR: The effect of stricture length on critical arterial stenosis. Surg Gynecol Obstet 128:729, 1969
9. Ogata J, Feigin I: Arteriovenous communications in the human brain. J Neuropathol Exp Neurol 31:519, 1972
10. Saunders RL de CH, Bell MA: X-ray microscopy and histochemistry of the human cerebral blood vessels. J Neurosurg 35:128, 1971

11. Shapiro HM, Stromberg DD, Lee DR, et al: Dynamic pressures in the pial arterial microcirculation. AM J Physiol 221:279, 1971
12. Sharbrough FW, Messick JM, Sundt TM Jr: Correlation of continuous electroencephalograms with cerebral blood flow measurements during carotid endarterectomy. Stroke 4:674, 1973
13. Sundt TM Jr, Waltz AG: Cerebral ischemic and reactive hyperemia. Studies of cortical blood flow and microcirculation before, during and after temporary occlusion of middle cerebral artery of squirrel monkeys. Circ Res 28:426, 1971
14. Tindall GT, Odom GL, Cupp HB Jr, et al: Studies on carotid artery flow and pressure. Observations in 18 patients during graded occlusion of proximal carotid artery. J Neurosurg 19:917, 1962
15. Waltz AG, Sundt TM Jr: The microvasculature and microcirculation of the cerebral cortex after arterial occlusion. Brain 90:681, 1967
16. Waltz AG, Sundt TM Jr, Michenfelder JD: Cerebral blood flow during carotid endarterectomy. Circulation 45:1091, 1972
17. Yamaguchi T, Waltz AG, Okazaki H: Hyperemia and ischemia in experimental cerebral infarction. Correlation of histopathology and regional blood flow. Neurology (Minneap) 21:565, 1971

References

2

Canine cerebral ischemia

*Manuel Dujovny, Carroll P. Osgood,
Joseph C. Maroon, and Peter Jannetta*

Introduction

Clinical interest in microvascular neurosurgery is increasing, and a reliable canine cerebral ischemia preparation would seem desirable. Microvascular grafting procedures could subsequently be superimposed on this "stroke" model to test their efficacy.

We have recently studied two new canine cerebral ischemia techniques—only one of which proved successful. A review of various cerebral ischemia models is presented and our methods and results discussed.

Materials and Methods

Group A: Intracranial Isolation of the Circle of Willis

Seven mongrel dogs were selected, weighing from 15 to 30 kg (male and female). The dogs were anesthetized with intravenous (IV) pentobarbital sodium (25 mg/kg), and an endotracheal tube inserted. Each animal was given 8 mg decadron and 50 ml of 50% mannitol after intubation, and placed supine, with the head tilted 30° to the left and elevated 15°. A femoral artery catheter for constant arterial pressure monitoring was inserted. Animals that became significantly hypotensive (systolic pressure less than 50 mmHg) for 15 minutes or longer during the procedure were excluded.

A right craniotomy was performed via a vertical 3-inch incision, and the temporal muscle was split to expose the temporal calvarium. A 2 × 2 cm temporal craniectomy was extended as far as 0.3 mm medial to and beneath the fifth nerve, which is extradural at this point, and easily identified with the operating microscope at 6× magnification. This insures removal (curettage) of the thin bony partition between the pituitary area and middle fossa, and will permit retraction of the tentorial edge later.

The middle fossa dura was then opened with a medially curved 1.5-cm incision to expose the tentorial edge 3 mm anterior to the third nerve. The tentorium was elevated with a curved microspatula to reveal the internal carotid artery lateral to the optic chiasm. The artery was doubly clipped or ligated (8-0 nylon) and divided 1 mm below its bifurcation. Using × 16 magnification and microinstrumentation, the optic chiasm was depressed gently with a small cotton pledget. This gave good exposure of the opposite internal carotid, which was similarly divided. One or two 1-cm gelfoam squares were placed at the operative site, and the dura was loosely approximated with several 8-0 nylon sutures. The wound was closed in two layers using 4-0 cotton interrupted sutures.

Six dogs underwent basilar ligation at a second stage, occurring from 1 week to 4 months after the first procedure. The basilar artery was exposed through a small 4 × 8 mm oval clival craniotomy, using a high-speed air drill. A 5-mm midline dural opening was used to expose the basilar artery just above the take-off of the inferior cerebellar arteries, about 5 mm above the vertebral artery entrance. The basilar artery was both clipped and ligated (6-0 silk) to insure its complete occlusion, but was not actually divided. The seventh dog underwent basilar occlusion acutely, 1 hour following division of both internal carotids.

These seven dogs were anesthetized and sacrificed 4 weeks post–basilar ligation by hemodilution using normal saline solution, and subsequently perfused with 10% formalin. The right common carotid artery was then hand-injected with 40 ml of micronized barium sulfate, and an anterior–posterior (A-P) and lateral angiogram obtained. Then 50 ml of latex compound was injected into the same common carotid, and the cranium removed and soaked in 10% formalin for several days.

Group B: Occlusion of Brachiocephalic-Subclavian Arterial Flow

Fifty large mongrel dogs weighing between 16 and 26 kg were selected and divided into six subgroups. Anesthesia consisted of IV sodium pentobarbital, 25 mg/kg. All animals continued to breathe spontaneously following pentobarbital injection. An endotracheal tube was inserted and the Harvard respirator and O_2 flow were adjusted to maintain blood gases and pH within physiologic limits. Blood gases and pH were checked every 30 minutes. Intravenous fluids consisted of normal saline solution (1.5 liters average infusion).

Bitemporal stainless steel EEG electrodes were inserted just above each zygoma, and a "ground" lead attached to the upper lip. An EEG tracing was recorded continuously on a Grass polygraph, as was blood pressure, via a femoral artery cannula and Statham strain gauge. The EKG tracing was likewise recorded on the polygraph and the head temperature was registered separately on a Yellowspring probe inserted nasally to a depth of 6 cm.

From a right lateral decubitus position, the left forelimb was extended anteriorly to facilitate exposure. A left thoracotomy was made at the first intercostal space, a rib spreader was inserted, and the left subclavian artery identified. It and its major branches (vertebral, costocervical, mammary, omocervical, and axillary) were individually tied and divided so that the distal trunk of the left subclavian could be excised. The left phrenic nerve was carefully identified and its continued integrity checked with a nerve stimulator.

Subsequently, the right brachiocephalic trunk and its main branches—both carotids, vertebral, costocervical, mammary, omocervical, and axillary arteries—were ligated and divided in this order in the 12 dogs of subgroup B_1. The chest was then closed in four layers over a small chest tube, which was connected to an underwater seal. Position of the chest tube was checked periodically to maintain good fluctuations in the chest bottle.

In six animals (subgroup B_2) the basilar artery was exposed following the same approach described for group A. Electromagnetic flow studies (Caroline Model 311) were obtained on the basilar artery, before and after ligation of the brachiocephalic-subclavian vessels (as described in subgroup B_1), and during stimulation of the brachial plexus. Hence, only the left common carotid remained to meet cephalic perfusion requirements. After chest closure, a small 5-cm cervical incision was made and the lower left common carotid identified and isolated. A Selverstone clamp was placed around the carotid, and its hub brought out through the partially closed cervical incision. When each animal was normally alert and active 24 hours postsurgery, the Selverstone clamp was screwed down.

Another six animals (subgroup B_4) underwent identical anesthesia and first interspace thoracotomy, except that the left internal mammary artery was microanastomosed to the proximal left common carotid prior to occlusion of the remaining, right-sided brachiocephalic arteries. Electromagnetic flow studies were performed on the left mammary and left carotid before and after anastomosis to supply cerebral perfusion.

Eight more dogs (subgroup B_5) had an identical thoracotomy, with occlusion of the entire brachiocephalic subclavian outflow, with the exception of the left vertebral which was left open. Electromagnetic flow studies were performed on the left vertebral artery before and after ligature of the other brachiocephalic-subclavian vessels.

A left mammary–left vertebral anastomosis was performed on 12 dogs in subgroup B_6. The left costocervical, omocervical, and axillary arteries were doubly ligated and divided; and the proximal vertebral and distal mammary were clamped with small bulldogs and divided prior to this anastomosis. The adventitia was stripped back about 4 mm from the vertebral and mammary transection sites. The arterial lumina were irrigated with a mixture of heparin and xylocaine following adventitia removal (1000 units heparin and 5 ml of 1% xylocaine in 100 ml normal saline), and the largest internal diameter of both mammary and vertebral arteries measured with a special ruled probe.

A 2 × 6 cm strip of rubber dam was placed beneath the proximal vertebral artery lumen and the distal mammary end was brought over from the chest wall. The anastomosis was done at × 10 to × 16 magnification using the Zeiss operating microscope. From 9 to 12 9-0 nylon everting mattress sutures were generally required. Following anastomosis, the suture line was wrapped in gelfoam and gently compressed with a surrounding strip of rubber dam. The clamps were then released. After 15 minutes, the rubber dam was removed and the right brachiocephalic trunk and its branches ligated, at which point cerebral perfusion depended upon the mammary-vertebral anastomosis. An electromagnetic flow study was obtained, repeated during brachial plexus stimulation, and similar chest closure was performed.

The brain of each of the 24 dogs dying from total brachiocephalic occlusion (subgroups B_1, B_2, and B_3) was carefully removed, weighed on blotting paper, and immersed in formalin. Five animals with one vertebral artery left open expired from 1 to 2 days following surgery. An autopsy study was performed on each case; the chest was reopened to exclude significant hemopneumothorax; and the brain removed, weighed, and immersed in formalin.

The three one-vertebral survivors, six mammary-carotid survivors, and four mammary-vertebral survivors were reanesthetized 1 month postsurgery. The lower cervical carotid or vertebral artery was exposed and cannulated in a retrograde fashion with an 18-gauge cannula, and hand-injected for angiography. Immediately following angiography, these 13 survivors were sacrificed by saline hemodilution and formalin perfusion. The chests were reopened in the mammary-carotid group, so that the anastomosis site could be excised. The brains were also carefully removed and immersed in formalin.

Results

Group A

All seven dogs survived. Four of the seven had a unilateral third nerve palsy, which cleared in all but one dog. Three of the seven revealed a transient hemiparesis, as manifested by circling toward the right side for the first several postoperative days. One dog developed a neurotropic corneal infection which caused severe scarring, but healed after a 10-day course of topical antibiotics. The seven dogs otherwise appeared neurologically normal thereafter, and were observed for 3 weeks prior to sacrifice.

We were frankly surprised that these dogs survived complete occlusion of the three major intracranial vessels feeding the circle of Willis, and sought to identify the remaining, obviously effective intracranial anastomotic arteries. The angiograms were difficult to interpret due to the small size of these vessels, and careful microscopic dissection of the entire circle of Willis proved to be a more accurate means of identifying these arteries. These proved to be of rather significant size (0.2 mm) and constant location, comprised of an ophthalmic and ethmoidal artery on each side, both joining the proximal anterior cerebral artery. In addition to these four well-developed extra- to intracranial collaterals, a few much smaller and variable dural to cerebral arterial anastomoses were found over each olfactory nerve, and around the pituitary gland. There is also normally a small (0.05 mm) dural to basilar arterial twig, but in all our dogs this tiny artery had been transected at the time of basilar ligation, and so was no longer present.

Contrary to the otherwise excellent descriptions of De La Torre et al,(8) we did not find any superior dural to pial anastomotic arterial connections, neither over the cerebrum nor cerebellum.

Group B

All 18 dogs in subgroups B_1 and B_2 died of respiratory failure, though all were breathing spontaneously and adequately following induction of anesthesia. Respiratory support was continued for at least 3 hours after arterial shutoff in all 18 animals. Sixteen dogs showed at least some spontaneous respiratory activity following these ligations, and, in fourteen, the respiratory pattern was initially very deep and rapid. However, this hyperventilation lasted only a few minutes in each case, giving way to shallow, less frequent, progressively ataxic respirations. Two dogs simply became apneic following the occlusion of the last vessel (Tables 2.1 and 2.2).

EEG was satisfactorily recorded in 17 of the 18 B_1 and B_2 dogs.

Table 2.1 Subgroup B_1: Brachiocephalic subclavian vessels transected

No.	Blood Pressure		Respiration		Decerebration	Decrease in Temperature(C)	EEG	
	Start	Max Rise	Hyperpnea	Apnea			Slow Wave	Isoelectric
1.	120/180	230/145	2 minutes	20 minutes	Flaccidity	—	—	—
2.	150/90	250/150	None	1 minute	Flaccidity	8	30 seconds	2 hours
3.	150/100	260/180	None	$2^{5}/_{12}$ hours	Rigidity	3	30 seconds	$2^{1}/_{3}$ hours
4.	125/100	225/100	3 minutes	1 hour	Ridigity	7	5 minutes	7 minutes
5.	150/90	250/150	None	1 minute	Flaccidity	8	3 minutes	40 minutes
6.	150/100	260/170	3 minutes	8 hours	Rigidity	8	2 minutes	4 hours
7.	140/100	250/145	3 minutes	6 hours	Rigidity	3.5	30 seconds	8 minutes
8.	140/100	265/135	5 minutes	45 minutes	Rigidity	4	30 seconds	45 minutes
9.	140/100	265/175	1 minute	32 minutes	Rigidity	3	20 seconds	27 minutes
10.	175/125	250/175	30 minutes	4 hours	Rigidity	2.5	15 seconds	10 minutes
11.	140/80	250/175	15 minutes	$1^{1}/_{2}$ hour	Rigidity	1.5	1 minute	7 minutes
12.	150/100	250/150	3 minutes	$5^{1}/_{2}$ hours	Rigidity	9	20 seconds	45 minutes

Table 2.2 Subgroup B_2: Brachiocephalic subclavian vessels transected (basilar flow measurement)

No.	Blood Pressure		Respiration		Decerebration	Decrease in Temperature(C)	EEG	
	Start	Max Rise	Hyperpnea	Apnea			Slow Wave	Isoelectric
1.	130/90	230/150	3 minutes	40 minutes	Rigidity	7	40 seconds	$1^{1}/_{4}$ hour
2.	140/80	250/140	2 minutes	20 minutes	Rigidity	5	4 minutes	25 minutes
3.	120/70	260/140	1 minute	5 minutes	Ridigity	8	2 minutes	40 minutes
4.	110/70	240/150	$4^{1}/_{12}$ minutes	3 hours	Rigidity	4	3 minutes	2 hours
5.	130/70	260/140	1 minute	15 minutes	Rigidity	6	40 seconds	30 minutes
6.	140/80	275/130	2 minutes	20 minutes	Rigidity	7	80 seconds	20 minutes

It slowed significantly following brachiocephalic shutoff in each case, and became faster when the left brachial plexus was stimulated. These 17 animals later developed flat, "isoelectric" EEG recordings prior to death, at a time when cardiac function remained good (as manifested by hypertension), and assumed decerebrate postures following last vessel shutoff. Pressor responses were most impressive, and recurred in all 18 dogs (Table 2.1). Nose temperatures had decreased an average of 5.7C by the time of expiration.

In subgroup B_3, all six dogs regained consciousness promptly, and appeared physically and neurologically normal 24 hours later. Occlusion of the one remaining brachiocephalic vessel at that time (the left common carotid) produced immediate unconsciousness with urination and defecation. Hyperventilation developed within the first minute (Table 2.3), and eventually gave way to ataxic and progressively inadequate respiratory efforts. Decerebration developed in all six dogs and death occurred in the first 4 hours.

In subgroup B_4, all six dogs protected by a mammary-carotid anastomosis regained consciousness and appeared neurologically normal. Pressor responses were significant during surgery, when the last remaining brachiocephalic vessels were occluded. However, the pressure responses in subgroup B_4 were not as marked as those in subgroups B_1 and B_2. The differences, however, just missed statistical significance ($P = 0.05$) because of wide intergroup pressure variations (Table 2.4). Angiograms taken 1 month postsurgery revealed patency of all six mammary-carotid anastomoses, with relatively little narrowing at the anastomosis lines.

In subgroup B_5, all eight dogs with an unoccluded left vertebral artery regained consciousness postoperatively, and only two were unable to stand and walk 24 hours postsurgery. Their functional neurologic status at this time, however, was noticeably worse compared to that of the virtually normal dogs in subgroups B_3 and B_4. Dogs with one remaining vertebral artery were much more ataxic and considerably less active than dogs in subgroups B_3 and B_4. Five of these eight dogs died of progressive neurologic dysfunction within 72 hours of surgery (Table 2.5). Evaluation of blood pressure and EEG recordings during surgery did not reveal any particular prognostic patterns for the survivors as compared to the nonsurvivors.

Dogs with a left mammary–left vertebral anastomosis fared less well. Although all 12 of these dogs regained consciousness initially, and the majority were able to stand and walk, their mortality for the first two postoperative weeks was 66% (Table 2.6). Their functional neurological status was noticeably worse compared to the virtually normal postoperative status of the mammary-carotid dogs. Morbidity was likewise increased and the average checksheet score was 9.6. Only one dog succumbed

Table 2.3 Subgroup B₃: Brachiocephalic subclavian vessels transected (except left carotid artery—Selverstone occlusion) (after 24 hours)

No.	Blood Pressure		Respiration			Decerebration	Decrease in Temperature(C)	EEG	
	Start	Max Rise	Hyperpnea	Apnea				Slow Wave	Isoelectric
1.	140/90	245/150	1 minute	30 minutes		Rigidity	—	30 seconds	30 minutes
2.	150/80	260/120	30 seconds	2 hours		Rigidity	—	20 seconds	3¹/₁₂ hours
3.	110/70	220/130	30 seconds	1 hour		Rigidity	—	20 seconds	30 minutes
4.	145/80	230/140	45 seconds	1½ hours		Rigidity	—	1 minute	1 hour
5.	150/100	270/130	1 minute	2 hours		Rigidity	—	1 minute	1¹/₁₂ hours
6.	110/80	260/150	50 seconds	1 hour		Rigidity	—	1 minute	40 minutes

Table 2.4 Subgroup B₄: Mammary-carotid anastomosis (other vessels transected)

No.	Blood Pressure		Respiration			Decerebration	Decrease in Temperature(C)	EEG	
	Start	Max Rise	Hyperpnea	Apnea				Slow Wave	Isoelectric
1.	150/100	155/95	None	None		None	None	Remains Normal	
2.	150/100	230/140	None	None		None	None	Remains Normal	
3.	150/100	200/150	None	None		None	None	Remains Normal	
4.	150/75	260/165	None	None		None	None	Remains Normal	
5.	125/80	180/100	None	None		None	None	Remains Normal	
6.	160/110	180/130	None	None		None	None	Remains Normal	

Table 2.5 Subgroup B$_5$: Brachiocephalic vessels transected (except left vertebral artery)

No.	Blood Pressure		Respiration			Decrease in Temperature(C)	EEG		Died (postoperative day)
	Start	Max Rise	Hyperpnea	Apnea	Decerebration		Slow Wave	Isoelectric	
1.	140/90	160/110	None	None	None	Normal	Yes	No	2 days
2.	150/100	160/100	None	None	None	Normal	Yes	No	1 day
3.	150/100	170/100	None	None	None	Normal	No	No	Sacrificed
4.	140/90	170/100	None	None	None	Normal	No	No	3 days
5.	150/90	180/100	None	None	None	Normal	Yes	No	2 days
6.	140/80	160/100	None	None	None	Normal	No	No	Sacrificed
7.	155/90	170/100	None	None	None	Normal	Yes	No	1 day
8.	140/80	160/100	None	None	None	Normal	No	No	Sacrificed

Table 2.6 Subgroup B$_6$: Mammary-vertebral Anastomosis (other vessels transected)

No.	Blood Pressure		Respiration			Decrease in Temperature(C)	EEG Slow Wave	Died (postoperative day)
	Start	Max Rise	Hyperpnea	Apnea	Decerebration			
1.	130/90	150/110	None	None	None	Normal	Yes	Survived
2.	140/90	170/100	None	None	3 days	Normal	Yes	3 days
3.	120/80	160/100	None	None	2 days	Normal	Yes	2 days
4.	125/80	180/100	None	None	6 days	Normal	Yes	6 days
5.	140/80	175/120	None	None	4 days	Normal	No	4 days
6.	150/90	210/130	None	None	None	Normal	No	Survived
7.	130/70	150/80	None	None	None	Normal	No	Survived
8.	120/80	160/90	None	None	2 days	Normal	Yes	2 days
9.	140/90	180/100	None	None	None	Normal	Yes	Survived
10.	160/100	200/110	None	None	2 days	Normal	Yes	2 days
11.	140/90	190/110	None	None	1 day	Normal	Yes	1 day
12.	130/80	180/100	None	None	10 days	Normal	Yes	10 days

during the first 24 hours, the others having delayed mortality occurring after 2 to 10 days. Only two of these animals had a nonpatent anastomosis (ie, thrombosed). Two of the eight non-surviving vertebral-mammary dogs had a peculiar pattern of weakness on their first postoperative day. This consisted of a complete inability to extend their forepaws, so that they walked (and ran) on their flexed forepaw knuckles as if the forepaws were flippers or paddles. Both of these dogs died during the second postoperative day of progressive neurologic dysfunction. The anastomosis site was grossly patent at autopsy. Section of each formalin-immersed brain revealed bilateral, symmetric hemorrhagic infarctions at the vertex and over the parasagittal cortex. Electromagnetic flow studies were performed and indicated an average baseline left common carotid flow of 201 ml/minute, which could increase to 275 ml/minutes (all other vessels occluded). Mean flow at baseline conditions for the left vertebral artery was 20 ml/minute, which, in 60% of the dogs, could increase by only an average of 24 ml/minutes (all other vessels occluded); but in the other 40% could increase to 100 ml/minute. Baseline mean internal mammary flow was 98 ml/minute, and could increase to 150 ml/minute (all other vessels occluded). Baseline flow of the basilar artery averaged 7 ml/minute and could increase to 30 ml/minute. Mammary-carotid flow averaged only 18 ml/minute. Most of the animals tested showed significant decreases in vertebral flow (to less than 10 ml/minute) during brachial plexus stimulation. Left carotid flow did not change during brachial plexus stimulation, but basilar flow decreased or reversed in most of the cases (four of the six animals).

Neuropathologic study of the dogs with mammary-carotid anastomoses showed the brains to be normal; but evaluation of the dogs with one vertebral artery open, mammary-vertebral anastomoses, and acute ischemia revealed signs of diffuse hypoxic cortical and cerebellar damage, even in the 33% surviving (one vertebral artery or mammary-vertebral anastomosis). The cerebellum was most severely affected, with widespread damage to the Purkinje cells. Edema, necrosis, and hypoxic changes were noted in the Purkinje cell layer. The cerebral cortex showed diffuse hypoxic changes, ranging from mild to frank necrosis in three dogs. The temporal lobes showed more severe hypoxic changes in the parahippocampal cortex than in Sommer's sector. The midbrain, medulla, and pons were generally without neuropathologic abnormalities.

Discussion

About 70% of human cerebrovascular stenotic or occlusive pathology occurs in arteries of the neck or chest.(3,9,10,11,19) Such atherosclerotic pathology is difficult, if not impossible, to reproduce in animal models. At present, experimental recourse must be taken to surgical reduction or interruption of brachiocephalic blood flow if the more common patterns of human atherosclerotic cerebrovascular disease are to even be crudely simulated in the laboratory.

Extracranial-intracranial artery bypass grafts and anastomoses are recognized, if not fully evaluated, therapeutic modalities for some of these more advanced clinical situations of cerebrovascular insufficiency.(2,4,6,10,12,21) For research projects examining new or improved extraanatomic bypass techniques, it is important that a dependable cerebral ischemia model be available for subsequent evaluation of these anastomoses. Not only should this ischemia model be consistently effective (i.e., a demonstrable degree of cerebral ischemia must always result), but it must be as atraumatic as possible. To keep the surgical production of cerebral ischemia relatively atraumatic, an expeditious anatomic approach similar to that used for potential clinical bypass grafts must be employed. Thus, the development of improved surgical bypass techniques might eventually be of potential benefit to some patients with symptoms of cerebrovascular insufficiency.

Although the dog remains the standard surgical laboratory animal, its extensive collateral circulation makes complete interruption of cerebral blood flow quite difficult. Numerous techniques for producing canine cerebral ischemia have been developed and are summarized in Table 2.7.

Marshall's(16) method is similar to ours in that major thoracic arteries are ligated, i.e., the brachiocephalic trunk, subclavian, mammaries, and upper five intercostals. However, ligation of these intercostal arteries involves a more extensive thoracic dissection at the fourth or fifth intercostal space. A first intercostal space exposure such as we used permits the lung apex to be more easily and gently retracted and all major divisions of the subclavian and brachiocephalic trunks may be readily exposed and divided. This achieves more complete interruption of cervical and thoracic muscular collaterals, and several vessels are conveniently available should a graft or anastomosis project be contemplated.

Guyton(13) used bilateral lower cervical incisions to interrupt both subclavian, axillary, mammary, costocervical, omocervical, vertebral, and carotid arteries. This approach has the advantage, as does ours, of a more complete division of potential cervical-thoracic collaterals. However, it necessitates two separate incisions and very difficult neck dissections. The probability of hemorrhage from the veins near and around the brachial plexus is substantial, as is the intracranial change of pneumothorax. Intracranial occlusion of the basilar and both internal carotid arteries, as in our group A animals, does not produce significant cerebral ischemia because of the ophthalmic, ethomoidal, and other collaterals.

Table 2.7 Surgical ischemia models in dogs

Method	Result
Ligate common carotids and vertebrals in neck.*	40% dogs die within 24 hours.
Tie common carotids and branches in neck. Clip basilar.(18)	Immediate apnea and decerebration.
Occlude both mammaries, brachiocephalic, left subclavian, and upper five intercostals. Marked hypertension. Some fluorescein did appear in cerebral circulation in majority of dogs after IV injection.(16)	50% survive 10 minutes of venous occlusion. None survive more than 15 minutes of occlusion.
Staged occlusion both subclavian, carotid, vertebral, mammary, costocervical, and omocervical arteries via bilateral neck incisions. Problems with excessive blood loss. Marked rise in blood pressure.(13)	Apnea in 66% within 45 seconds to 8 minutes.
Staged occlusion occipital basilar arteries. Then common carotids.(18)	Dog faints when remaining carotid shut off.
Occlude brachiocephalic, left subclavian, aorta, and vena cava.(15)	Survive up to 10 minutes intact; 66% die after 14 minutes in decerebrate state. Animals survive with hypertension.
Staged and acute intracranial occlusion of internal carotids and basilar at circle of Willis.	Survive.
Divide brachiocephalic and subclavian arteries; and both carotids, vertebrals, mammaries, costocervicals, and axillaries. Marked hypertension in all. Frequent hyperventilation and decerebration.	100% mortality from respiratory failure.

*Includes review of literature prior to 1935.

White's(20) method of basilar occlusion and bilateral carotid system division produces immediate apnea and decerebration, but requires a potentially dangerous craniotomy and two difficult, lengthy neck dissections.

Comparatively, our small thoracotomy approach is technically much easier and faster to perform. All of these arterial occlusion methods, however, have the advantage of not interfering with cardiopulmonary function significantly. In fact, marked systemic arterial hypertension usually accompanies these methods. This cannot be said of methods such as ventricular fibrillation,(7) or occlusions of the aorta or great veins.(4,5,15,22) In addition, these methods and those using cervical tourniquets(14) or increased intracranial pressure are not suitable for surgical ischemia models using grafts or anastomoses to circumvent imposed ischemia.(17)

Our model does not achieve total cerebral ischemia because a considerable period of time is required for complete flattening of the EEG. Some blood flow undoubtedly persists through the anterior spinal-basilar artery system, but it is not enough to sustain brain stem function very long.

It is evident that the internal mammary artery can meet acute canine cerebral perfusion requirements when anastomosed to the thoracic left carotid artery. All dogs with a mammary-carotid anastomosis appeared virtually normal both physically and neurologically postoperatively. Dogs with one thoracic vertebral artery left open had a 50% postoperative mortality; and those surviving had significant initial morbidity in terms of ataxia and reduced activity. The delayed nature of this mortality is quite striking, and we feel it may be related to collateral shunting or "stealing" of blood from the vertebral system into the rest of the neck and forelimb.

Electromagnetic flow studies of the vertebral artery showed relatively low maximal flow rates in 60% of the dogs tested (below 40 ml/minute); 80% of the animals tested showed significant decrease in vertebral flow (to less than 10 ml/minute or reverse flow) during brachial plexus stimulation. These findings are similar to those reported by Anazawa et al.(1) Left carotid flow did not change during brachial plexus stimulation.

Mammary-vertebral anastomosis was less successful technically (84% patency versus 100% patency for the mammary-carotid group). The increased mortality and morbidity in these dogs compared to those with one vertebral artery left open but not surgically traumatized, is probably related to the inevitable narrowing accompanying end-to-end anastomosis of vessels this size, and also to the thromboses mentioned. Mammary artery flow is certainly not the limiting factor, as evidenced by the excellent postoperative status of the mammary-carotid group. Rather, the vertebral artery per se seems to be the limiting factor, and can meet cerebral perfusion requirements by itself only 50% of the time.

Occlusion of the remaining carotid or vertebral artery, very low in the neck, 1 month postanastomosis, surprisingly produced no mortality. Evidently, considerable development of collateral circulation has occurred by this time. Possible sources of collateral cerebral circulation for these dogs would be the anterior spinal-basilar artery complex or the muscular and cutaneous arteries. Basilar flow can increase considerably in conditions of cerebral ischemia. We have also found a 3-fold rise in basilar flow (average baseline flow, 7 ml/minute; average maximum, 30 ml/minute) following occlusion of all major thoracic, brachiocephalic, and subclavian arteries. However, substantial neurologic morbidity did occur and was almost certainly related to the further reduction in cerebral perfusion produced by the Selverstone clamp. The effort-related decerebration or spasticity noted initially in six dogs whose remaining arteries were occluded may have represented transient ischemia of the brain stem.

This is the first reported experimental or clinical series of mammary-carotid or mammary-vertebral anastomoses. Functional evaluation of these anastomoses would indicate the mammary-carotid anastomosis to be superior to the mammary-vertebral anastomosis.

ACKNOWLEDGMENTS

Special thanks to Vender Knowles Weir, PhD, and Thadeus Stasiak, BS, for their technical assistance.

REFERENCES

1. Anazawa W, Shigeno K, Toole JF, et al: The effect of body position and forelimb exercise on cephalic blood flow. Stroke 2:168, 1971
2. Andreyev LA: Functional changes in the brain of the dog after reduction of cerebral blood supply. Arch Neurol Psychiat 34:481, 1935
3. Blaisdell W: Extracranial arterial surgery in the treatment of stroke. In McDowell FH, Brennan RW (eds): Eighth Princeton Conference. Cerebral Vascular Diseases. New York, Grune, 1972, pp 3–15
4. Boyd, RJ, Connolly JE: Total cerebral ischemia in the dog. Arch Surg 84:434, 1962
5. Brockman SK, Jude JR: The tolerance of the dog brain to total arrest of circulation. Bull Johns Hopkins Hosp 106:74, 1960
6. Crawford ES, DeBakey ME, Morris GC Jr, et al: Surgical treatment of occlusion of the innominate, common carotid, and subclavian arteries. A 10-year experience. Surgery 65:17, 1969
7. Crowell JW, Sharpe GP, Lambright RL, et al: The mechanism of death after resuscitation following acute circulatory failure. Surgery 38:696, 1955
8. De La Torre E, Netsky M, Meschan I: Intracranial and extracranial circulations in the dog. Anatomic and angiographic studies. Am J Anat 105:343, 1959
9. Deweese JA, May AG, Lipchik EO, et al: Anatomic and hemodynamic correlations in carotid artery stenosis. Stroke 1:149, 1970
10. Eklof B, Schwartz SI: Effects of subclavian steal and compromised cephalic blood flow on cerebral circulation. Surgery 68:431, 1970
11. Field WS: Selection of stroke patients for arterial reconstructive surgery. Am Surg 125:527, 1973

12. Gillespie JA: Extracranial Cerebrovascular Disease and Its Management. London, Butterworths, 1969

13. Guyton AC: Acute hypertension in dogs with cerebral ischemia. Am J Physiol 154:45, 1948

14. Kabat H, Dennis C, Baker AB: Recovery of function following arrest of the brain circulation. Am J Physiol 132:737, 1941

15. Kaupp HA, Lazarus RE, Wetzel N, et al: The role of cerebral edema in ischemic cerebral neuropathy after arrest in dog and monkeys and its treatment with hypertonic urea. Surgery 48:404, 1960

16. Marshall SB, Owens JC, Swan H: Temporary circulatory occlusion to the brain of the hypothermic dog. Arch Surg 72:98, 1956

17. Neely WA, Youmans JR: Anoxia of ischemic brain without damage. JAMA 183:1085, 1963

18. Roberts TDM: Method for repeatable acute occlusion of the blood supply to the brain of the conscious dog. J Physiol 142:248, 1958

19. Vitek JJ, Halsey JH Jr, McDowell HA: Occlusion of all four extracranial vessels with minimal clinical symptomatology. Case report. Stroke 3:462, 1972

20. White RJ, Donald DE: Basilar-artery ligation and cerebral ischemia in dog. Arch Surg 84:470, 1962

21. Wylie EF, Ehrenfeld WK: Extracranial Occlusive Cerebrovascular Disease. Diagnosis and Treatment. Philadelphia, Saunders, 1969

22. Yashon D, Wagner FC, White RJ, et al: Intracranial pressure during circulatory arrest. Brain Res 31:139, 1971

3

Anatomical studies of the posterior circulation relevant to occipital artery bypass

Philip R. Weinstein, Norman L. Chater, and Roderick Lamond

Introduction

With the advent of microsurgical techniques, extra- to intracranial arterial anastomosis has become technically feasible for the treatment of inoperable or inaccessible intra- or subcranial occlusive cerebrovascular disease.(1) Patency rates for end-to-side superficial temporal to middle cerebral artery anastomosis are acceptable at 90%, morbidity rates are 2%, and collateral augmentation has been documented angiographically as well as with clinical and experimental cerebral blood flow studies. (2,4,6,7,11,12) The value of such procedures for preventing completed stroke in patients suffering transient ischemic attacks will be demonstrated only when a large randomized study has been performed. Previous work in our laboratory has shown that a cortical branch of the middle cerebral artery at least 1 mm in diameter could be found under a 4-cm craniectomy centered 6 cm above the external auditory meatus, in 90% of 50 brains dissected.(5) The purpose of the current study was to determine if the occipital artery could be used for anastomosis, with suitable cerebellar or cerebral cortical branches, in patients with vertebrobasilar occlusive disease.

Although stenosis or thrombosis of the vertebral and basilar arteries is thought to be relatively uncommon, it has in fact been found in 30% of patients studied angiographically for cerebrovascular disease.(8,9) Thus, it remains a potentially serious condition in which transient symptoms may persist or progress to fixed deficit or death if there is no response to anticoagulation therapy.(3,10)

A case in point is that of a 47-year-old man who recovered from his first attack of a right Wallenberg's syndrome only to have a recurrence 3 weeks later after anticoagulants were stopped because of hematemesis. Arteriograms showed bilateral vertebral artery occlusion in the high cervical area. The patient deteriorated and died 4 days later despite the presence of collateral flow from the posterior communicating artery, seen angiographically. It is possible that surgical augmentation of collateral blood flow could prevent brain stem infarction in such patients.

Methods

In order to determine whether posterior circulation extra- to intracranial arterial anastomosis would be anatomically possible, 60 brains were dissected in search of adequate recipient vessels, and three cadavers were examined to verify occipital artery size and location as well as for correlation of donor and recipient vessel relationships with skull landmarks. Fifty normal vertebral arteriograms and 20 normal external carotid arteriograms were also reviewed to determine the likelihood of finding recipient and donor vessels of adequate size and location.

The following possible recipient vessel sites were selected for study according to the requirements that they be superficially located to avoid brain retraction, that they be close to 1 mm in diameter to assure patency, and that they be distal enough so that temporary occlusion would be tolerated without danger of infarction:

1. The tonsillohemispheric branch of the posterior inferior cerebrellar artery (PICA) (4-cm craniectomy centered 2 cm lateral to midline and 3 cm inferior to inion)
2. The lateral hemispheric branch of the superior cerebellar artery (SCA) (4-cm craniectomy centered 3 cm posterior and 2 cm superior to mastoid process tip)
3. The calcarine or parietooccipital branch of the posterior cerebral artery (PCA) (4-cm craniectomy centered 3 cm lateral to midline and 3 cm superior to inion)

Results

The occipital artery requires a more painstaking microdissection than does the superficial temporal, since it lies within or deep to the fascia of the occipital muscles. It has been used successfully for middle cerebral anastomosis in three cases where an adequate temporal vessel was not available.(13) It was found to be of adequate diameter in 16 of 20 normal external carotid arteriograms. Length was sufficient to reach the PICA branch in all of these and to reach the PCA in two-thirds.

Table 3.1 Availability of Recipient Vessels (%) for Extra- to Intracranial Anastomosis to the Posterior Circulation. Detailed Results of Brain Dissections and Review of Normal Arteriograms

	Vessel		
	PICA	SCA	PCA
Craniectomy Site	Paramedian posterior fossa	Lateral posterior fossa	Paramedian above inion
Brain Dissection			
Right	46/58 (83%)	17/49 (36%)	21/44 (48%)
Left	52/60 (87%)	21/49 (43%)	16/46 (35%)
Total	98/118 (83%)	38/96 (40%)	37/90 (41%)
Arteriograms			
Right	22/50 (44%)	6/50 (12%)	21/50 (42%)
Left	33/50 (66%)	7/50 (14%)	23/50 (46%)
Total	55/100 (55%)	13/100 (13%)	44/100 (44%)

A suitable branch of the caudal loop of either the right or left PICA was found in 51 of the 60 brains dissected. However, such vessels could be identified at only 55 of 100 possible sites on 50 normal vertebral arteriograms. At least one SCA yielded a suitable branch in only 50% of the dissected brains and one could be found angiographically at only 13% of the possible sites. An ideally situated branch of either PCA was found on 32% of the occipital pole dissections without retraction. With minimal retraction a vessel was available in 40% of the brains, side unspecified (Table 3.1). Such a branch was visualized angiographically at 44% of the possible sites.

Summary

Our results indicate that in four-fifths of patients in whom an occipital artery may be present, a recipient branch of the PICA might be available for anastomosis in 85%, a branch of the SCA in 40%, and a branch of the PCA in 40%.

REFERENCES

1. Austin GM (ed): Microsurgical Anastomosis for Cerebral Ischemia. Springfield, Ill. Thomas, 1974
2. Austin G, Laffin D, Hayward W: Cerebral blood flow and pressure in patients undergoing STA-MCA anastomosis. Presented at the Second International Symposium on Microneurosurgical Anastomoses, Chicago, June 1974

3. Bradshaw P, McQuaid P: The syndrome of vertebro-basilar insufficiency. J Med 128:279, 1963

4. Chater N, Peerless SJ: The early effects of neurosurgical microvascular bypass operations on problems of cerebrovascular occlusive disease. Presented at the American Academy of Neurology Meeting, San Francisco, April 1974

5. Chater N, Spetzler R: Anatomical studies of the cerebral cortical vasculature of microvascular surgical significance. Presented at the Symposium on Microneurosurgery, Kyoto, Japan, October 14–15, 1973

6. Crowell RM, Olsson Y: Effect of extracranial-intracranial vascular bypass graft on experimental acute stroke in dogs. J Neurosurg 38:26, 1973

7. Fein JM, Molinari G: Experimental augmentation of regional cerebral blood flow by microvascular anastomosis. J Neurosurg 41:421, 1974

8. Hass WK, Fields WS, North RR, et al: Joint study of extracranial arterial occlusion. JAMA 203:961, 1968

9. Meyer JS, Sheehan S, Bauer RB: An arteriographic study of cerebrovascular disease in man. Arch Neurol 2:37, 1960

10. Moscow NP, Newton TH: Angiographic implications in diagnosis and prognosis of basilar artery occlusion. Am J Roentgenol Radium Ther Nucl Med 119:597, 1973

11. Schmiedek P, Steinhoff H, Gratzl O. Current status of regional blood flow measurement in revascularization microsurgery of the brain. Presented at the Second International Symposium on Microneurosurgical Anastomoses, Chicago, June 1974

12. Spetzler RF, Chater N: Superficial temporal artery–middle cerebral artery blood flow measurements. Presented at the American Association of Neurological Surgeons Meeting, St. Louis, April 1974

13. Spetzler RF, Chater N: Occipital middle cerebral artery anastomosis for cerebral arterial occlusive disease. Surg Neurol 2:235, 1974

4

Comparison of blood flow and patency in arterial and vein grafts to the basilar artery

A. L. Rhoton, Jr., J. Robert Mozingo, and C. J. Whang

Cerebral revascularization procedures have been limited largely to the carotid circulation in man, although revascularization of the vertebrobasilar system has been done in animals (3,4) and more recently in man.(1) Previous studies of anastomotic grafts to the basilar system in animals have demonstrated that they may remain patent for a year or longer,(3,4) but few studies have been done to evaluate the physiologic results of these surgical approaches. The following reports quantitative measurements of blood flow in a basal state and the effects of physiologic variables on flow, and compares flow and patency rates obtained by two experimental methods aimed at reestablishing flow in the canine basilar artery.

Methods and Materials

Blood flows obtained by lingual artery–basilar artery anastomosis were compared with those obtained by saphenous vein bypass graft from the carotid to the basilar artery in two groups of ten dogs. All blood flow measurements were recorded with an electromagnetic blood flow meter (Statham 2202).

Lingual Artery–Basilar Artery Anastomosis

Ten healthy mongrel dogs weighing 17 to 22 kg were anesthetized with sodium pentothal (25 mg/kg) IV and maintained with an endotracheally delivered methoxyflurane/oxygen mixture. Ventilation was adjusted to maintain normocarbia during the procedure. With the animal in the supine position, using sterile

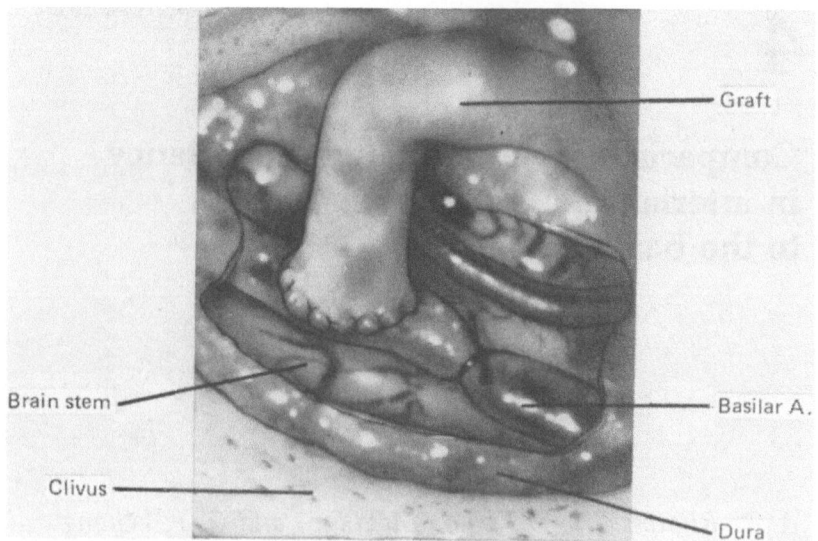

Fig. 4.1. Surgical magnification view (× 16) of completed lingual artery–basilar artery anastomosis. Basilar artery is permanently ligated at vertebrobasilar junction. Anastomosis performed with interrupted 10-0 nylon sutures. (From Rhoton et al: Stroke 6:445, 1975)

technique, a 6-cm right paramedian incision was made at the mandibular angle. After the carotid sheath was separated from the midline structures, the hypoglossal nerve was identified and a 5- to 6-cm segment of subjacent lingual artery was mobilized just distal to its origin from the external carotid artery. Blood flow was measured in the intact lingual artery. All branches of the lingual artery were ligated and divided. The trachea and esophagus were retracted medially. The paired longus colli muscles were separated to expose the clivus (basioccipital bone) from the tympanic bullae superiorly to the condylar notches inferiorly. The pharyngeal cavity was not entered with this approach. The remainder of the operative procedure was performed using surgical magnification of × 16 and × 25.

A 9 × 12 mm clival craniectomy was made with a dental drill. A temporary clip was applied at the origin of the lingual artery. The distal end of the lingual artery was sectioned and the lumen was irrigated with a heparin-saline solution. The dura was opened and reflected laterally. The basilar artery was thus exposed, freed from overlying arachnoid, and permanently ligated with 7-0 silk at the vertebrobasilar junction. A temporary ligature was applied approximately 5 to 6 mm distally. A 1- to 1.5-mm elliptical arteriotomy was made in the ventral wall of the basilar artery between the ligatures. An end-to-side lingual artery–basilar artery anastomosis requiring 12 to 16 interrupted sutures of 10-0 nylon was done (Fig. 4.1). The distal temporary ligature was removed from the basilar artery and retrograde filling of the graft initially confirmed anastomotic patency. The clip from the proximal lingual artery was removed. Blood flow through the lingual-basilar arterial anastomosis was recorded during normocarbia. The wound was closed in layers. Antibiotics were given for the next 7 days.

Chapter 4: Blood Flow and Patency in Arterial and Vein Grafts

Carotid-Basilar Saphenous Vein Bypass

In this group of ten healthy mongrel dogs weighing between 17 and 23 kg, the anesthesia and operative approach to the basilar artery was identical to that described above. A 6- to 7-cm segment of autogenous medial saphenous vein with a 0.8- to 1.5-mm external diameter was dissected from the hind limb. Side branches were ligated with 6-0 silk or surgical clips. A 1.27-mm (external diameter) silastic tube was passed through the lumen of the vein and the cannulized vein was placed in heparin-saline solution. The carotid artery was dissected free at the bifurcation. A segment of basilar artery was isolated between two ligatures. A small arteriotomy was made in the basilar artery and the proximal end of the vein was anastomosed to the basilar artery in an end-to-side fashion with 12 to 16 interrupted sutures of 10-0 nylon.

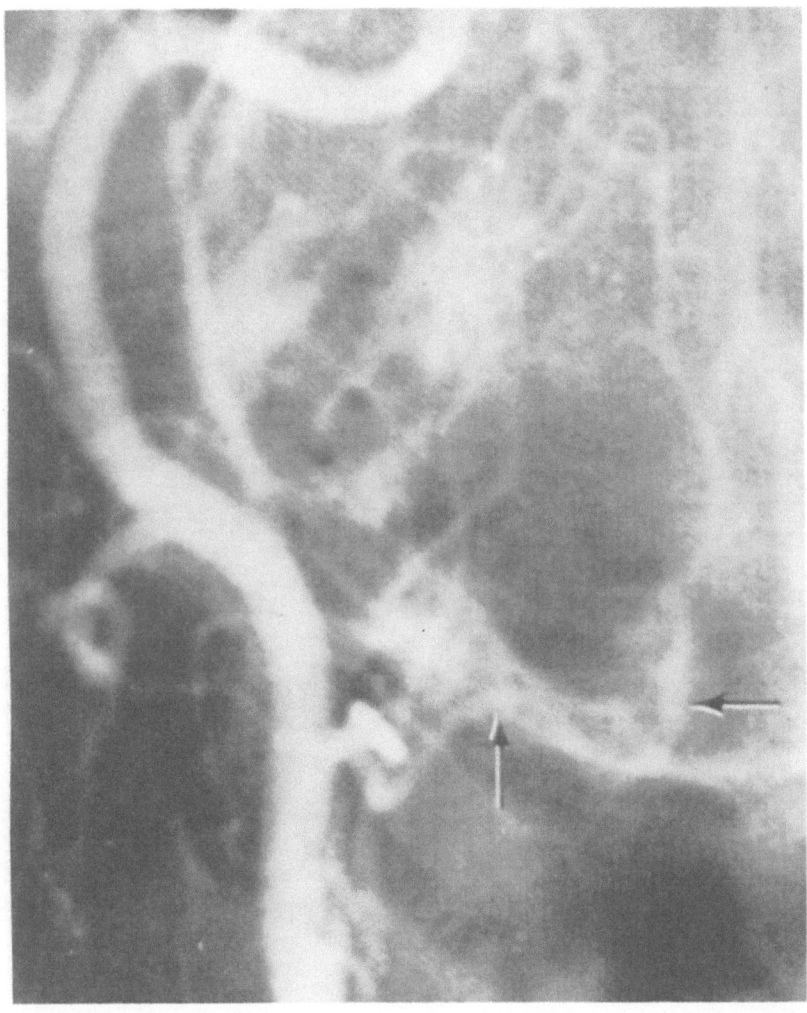

Fig. 4.2. Right carotid angiogram representative of lingual artery (↑) to basilar artery (←) grafts patent angiographically at 1 week postoperatively. (From Rhoton et al: Stroke 6:445, 1975)

Methods and Materials

A segment of the previously isolated common carotid artery was then temporarily occluded and a small arteriotomy was made. The lumen of the carotid artery was irrigated with heparin-saline solution. The distal end of the vein graft was anastomosed to the carotid artery in an end-to-side fashion with 10 to 14 sutures of 10-0 nylon. The temporary ligature in the basilar artery distal to the anastomosis was removed to initially confirm anastomotic patency. The two temporary clips on the carotid artery were then removed. After completion of the anastomosis blood flow in the vein graft was measured at normocarbia.

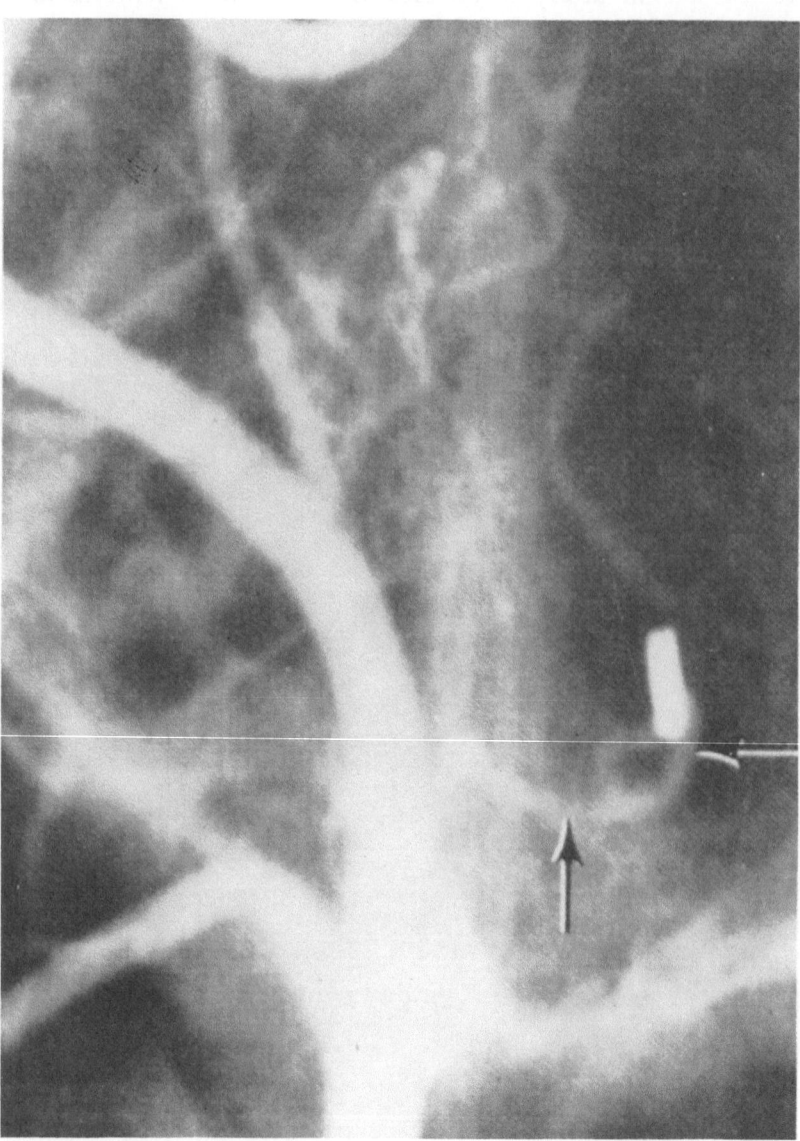

Fig. 4.3. Right carotid angiogram representative of lingual artery (↑) to basilar artery (←) grafts patent at 6 weeks postoperatively. (From Rhoton et al: Stroke 6:445, 1975)

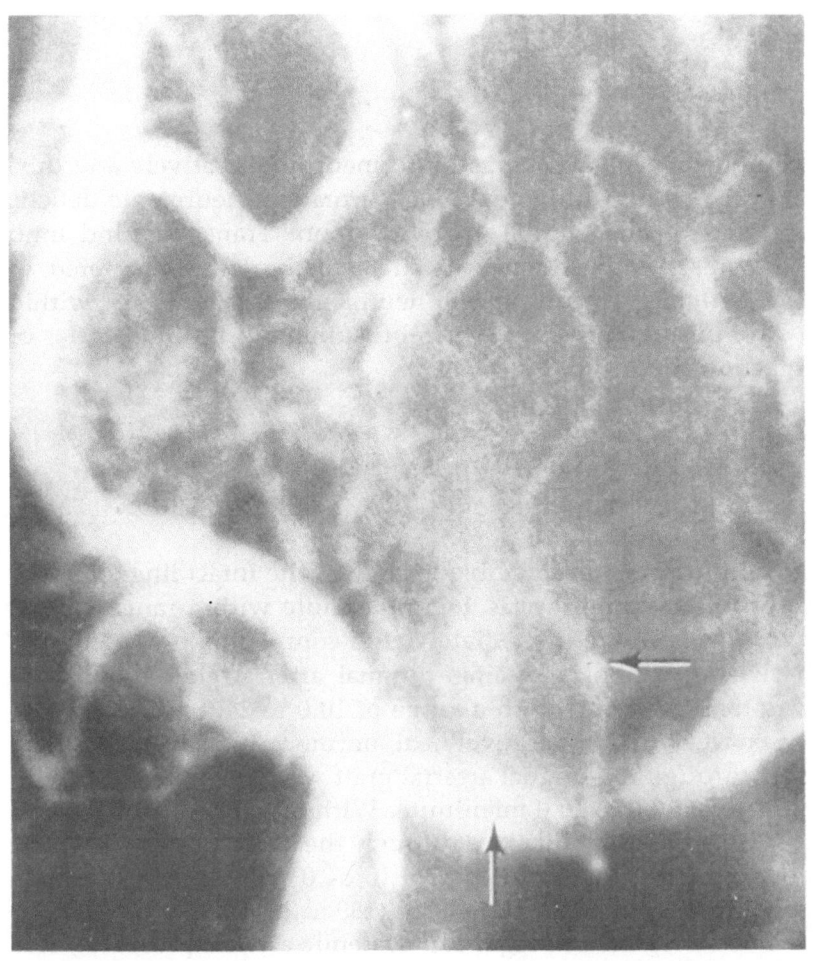

Fig. 4.4. Right carotid angiogram representative of saphenous vein (↑) bypass grafts between common carotid and basilar (←) arteries patent at 6 weeks postoperatively. (From Rhoton et al: Stroke 6:445, 1975)

Follow-up

All animals underwent common carotid angiography using Conray-60 to evaluate angiographic evidence of graft patency 1 (Fig. 4.2) and 6 (Fig. 4.3 and 4.4) weeks after surgery. After the second angiographic evaluation, the wound was reopened for blood flow measurements. Blood flow response to hypercarbia and hypertension was assessed. $PaCO_2$ was altered by changing ventilatory rate and hypertension was induced by intravenous ephedrine (2.5 mg). Blood pressure was monitored from a catheter placed through the left femoral artery into the abdominal aorta. All animals were then sacrificed by a saline-formalin perfusion technique for histologic examination of the brain and graft.

Results

Neurologic Deficits

Neurologic evaluation was performed preoperatively and during each postoperative day. No permanent neurologic deficits occurred in any animal operated upon. Transient hind limb paraparesis and tendency to circle to the left were noted in three animals. These transient neurologic deficits cleared within 3 days postoperatively. No cerebrospinal fluid (CSF) fistulas or infections occurred.

Blood Flow with Lingual-Basilar Anastomosis

At normocarbia, average blood flow in the intact lingual artery prior to anastomosis was 16.5 ml/minute with a range of 11.0 to 21.0 ml/minute. Immediately after completion of the lingual-basilar anastomosis, average lingual arterial graft blood flow was 15.6 ml/minute with a range of 10.0 to 24.0 ml/minute.

Six weeks postoperatively, at normocarbia, average blood flow through the lingual arterial graft was 13.0 ml/minute with a range of 10.0 to 16.0 ml/minute. With hypercarbia ($PaCO_2$, 62 to 78), average blood flow through the arterial graft was 27.8 ml/minute with a range of 17.0 to 54.0 ml/minute; and, with ephedrine-induced hypertension (180 to 200 mmHg, from baseline of 110 to 120 mmHg mean systemic arterial pressure), was 26.2 ml/minute with a range of 18.0 to 36.0 ml/minute (Table 4.1).

Blood Flow with Vein Graft

At normocarbia, average blood flow in the carotid-basilar vein bypass graft was 15.5 ml/minute with a range of 10.0 to 20.0 ml/minute. Six weeks postoperatively, at normocarbia, average blood flow was 11.5 ml/minute with a range of 10.0 to 13.0 ml/minute. With hypercarbia ($PaCO_2$, 72 to 76), blood flow averaged 23.5 ml/minute with a range of 18 to 28.0 ml/minute and, with induced hypertension, was 24.0 ml/minute with a range of 22.0 to 26.0 ml/minute (Table 1).

Angiographic and Histologic Patency

Carotid angiography, done 1 and 6 weeks postoperatively, revealed patency in only 80% of the grafts at 1 week and in only 60% at 6 weeks. At 1 week postoperatively, angiography re-

Table 4.1. Graft blood flow (ml/minute) immediately following anastomosis and 6 weeks later

	Immediate	6 Weeks
Arterial		
Normocarbia	15.6	13.0
Hypercarbia	—	27.8
Hypertension	—	26.2
Venous		
Normocarbia	15.5	11.5
Hypercarbia	—	23.5
Hypertension	—	24.0

vealed arterial and venous anastomosis patency rates of 90 and 70%, respectively; at 6 weeks the rates were 70 and 50%, respectively. These patency rates were obtained even though all grafts were patent by flow and histologic determinations. This failure of angiography represents a limitation of the radiographic resolution in millimeter-size vessels.

Patency by Electromagnetic Flow Technique

Blood flow in the arterial and venous grafts was measured in all animals after completion of the anastomosis. All grafts were found to be patent. Blood flow was measured again at 6 weeks after surgery and all of the grafts were patent at that time.

Discussion

Using an electromagnetic blood flow meter we have measured blood flow quantitatively through arterial and venous grafts between carotid and basilar arteries in the dog. We have been unable to find references documenting blood flow measurements through the canine lingual artery. Average blood flow through the intact lingual artery in this study was 16.5 ml/minute. Average normal blood flow of the basilar artery in dogs has been recorded as 9.5 ml/minute.(2)

The arterial and venous grafts carried more than enough blood to maintain a normal flow rate through the basilar system of the dogs and hypercarbia and hypertension produced significant increases in flow in both types of graft, but a greater increase in blood flow with hypercarbia and hypertension was found in the arterial grafts than in the venous grafts. Immediately after anastomosis, average flow through the venous grafts was 15.5 ml/minute (range, 10 to 20 ml/minute), and through the arterial anastomosis was 15.6 ml/minute (range, 10 to 24 ml/minute). Six weeks later, average flow through the venous graft was 11.5 ml/minute, and through the arterial graft was 13.0 ml/minute. With induced hypertension, flow increased in the arterial grafts to an average of 26.2 ml/minute and in the venous grafts to 24.0 ml/minute. Hypercarbia increased arterial graft flow to an average of 27.8 ml/minute and venous graft flow to 23.5 ml/minute.

The grafts in all surviving animals were patent by blood flow measurements and by histologic examination at 6 weeks postoperatively, even though patency could not consistently be determined by angiography. This discrepancy in patency rate between angiography and flow meter technique reflects a limitation of the radiographic resolution in these small arteries. Khodadad(3) found angiographically that patency rate was greater in arterial grafts compared to venous grafts, both acutely and long-term. Our results agree with his angiographic findings. At 6 weeks postoperatively, all grafts were patent by blood flow measurements, whereas angiography disclosed a patency rate of only 70%.

ACKNOWLEDGMENT

Supported by the National Institutes of Health Grant No. 10978-02; Veterans Administration Hospital, Gainesville, Florida; and the Heart Association of Broward County Florida.

REFERENCES

1. Ausman J: Occipital to cerebellar artery anastomosis for brain stem infarction from vertebral basilar occlusive disease. Presented at the Joint Meeting on Stroke and Cerebral Circulation, Dallas, Texas, February 27–28, 1976
2. Fukuyama GS, Himwich WA: Canine basilar arterial flow and effects of common carotid occlusion. Am J Physiol 219:525, 1970
3. Khodadad G: Sublingual and lingual-basilar artery anastomoses and carotid-basilar bypass grafts. Surg Neurol 1:175, 1973
4. Reichman OH: Continued patency of canine lingual-basilar system. Stroke 3:586, 1972

5

The endothelial surface of arteries
A scanning electron microscopic
examination of normal
and anastomosed vessels

Carys M. Bannister, L. A. Mundy, and Janice E. Mundy

The scanning electron microscope (SEM) has proved to be a valuable tool for the examination of the surfaces of biologic material. Shimamoto et al(7) were among the first to use it for the investigation of arterial endothelium. They found that the endothelial surface was folded longitudinally, and thought that the folds were formed by endothelial cells standing one behind another in a file. Collatz and Garbarsch(3,4) demonstrated endothelial folds in their SEM studies of arteries, but concluded that the folds were due to endothelial cells covering ridges in the internal elastic lamina.

In a project designed to study the effects of growth on anastomoses performed on the common carotid arteries of immature rats, we found, using the scanning electron microscope, that the endothelial folds in the arteries without stenosed anastomoses were essentially normal, but in the few arteries with stenosed anastomoses the endothelial fold pattern was grossly distorted.(2) Intrigued by these findings, we undertook an investigation to attempt to discover the reason for the distortion of the fold pattern in the vessels with stenosed anastomoses.

Two groups of rat common carotid arteries were examined. In the first group, no operative procedures were conducted prior to the SEM studies; but in the second group various procedures were performed before the microscopic examination was undertaken (details of these procedures will be given later). The arteries in both groups were fixed in 2.5% buffered glutaraldehyde, dehydrated in graded acetone solutions, and coated with gold–palladium in a vacuum evaporator before being examined and photographed with a Cambridge 600 Stereoscan.

We found that in undistended arteries the endothelial folds ran a wavy longitudinal course along the length of the vessels

Fig. 5.1. A scanning electron micrograph of an undistended rat common carotid artery, showing longitudinal endothelial folds running a wavy course along the length of the vessel. Bar = 200 μ.

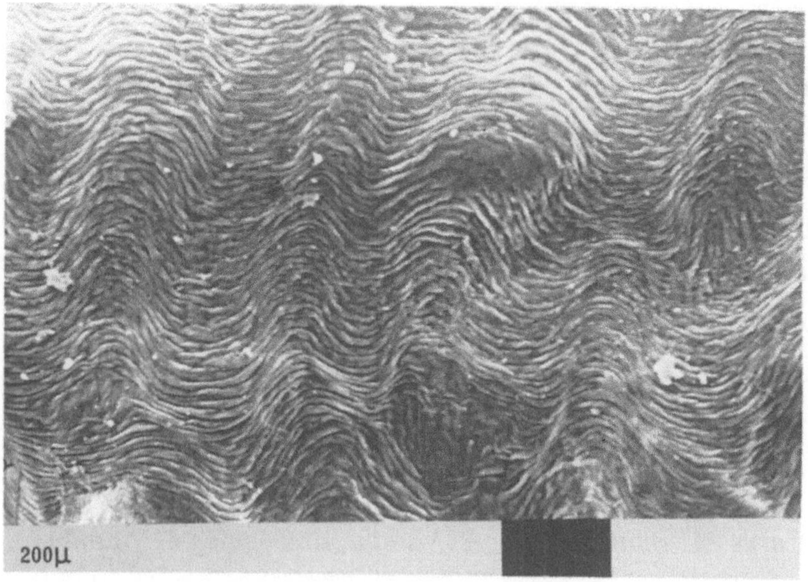

200μ

(Fig. 5.1). If the endothelial surface is stained with silver salts before fixation, silver is deposited in the intercellular substance to outline individual cells. Figure 5.2 shows that two or three endothelial cells are involved in the formation of each fold in undistended arteries.

Initially, we tried to study the relationship of the endothelial cells to the underlying internal elastic lamina by stripping away the endothelium(1), but examination with the transmission electron microscope of vessels so treated showed that in the majority of cases the internal elastic lamina had been damaged. As illustrated by Sheppard(6), the endothelium alone is more satisfactorily removed by immersing the arteries in 0.1m EDTA.

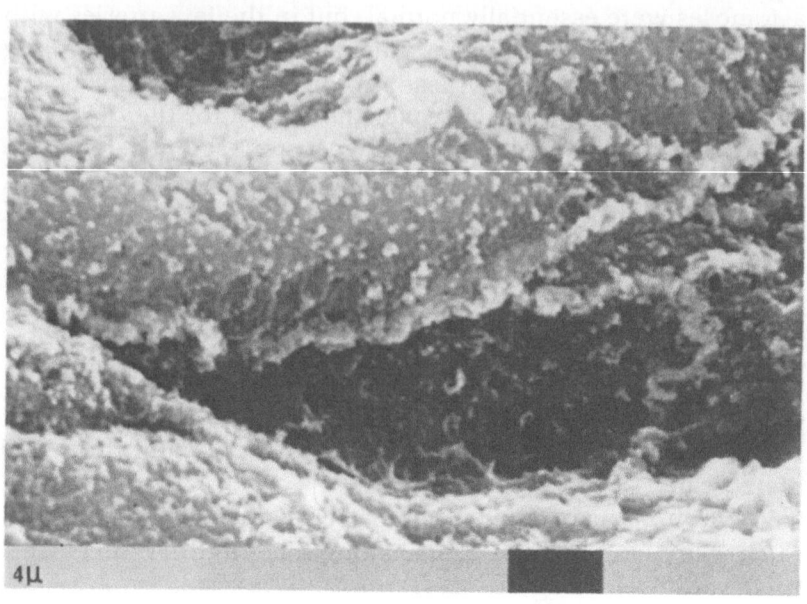

Fig. 5.2. A scanning electron micrograph of an undistended rat common carotid artery. The endothelial surface has been stained with silver salts. Silver has deposited in the intercellular substance to outline the endothelial cells covering one of the endothelial folds. Bar = 4 μ.

4μ

Chapter 5: Endothelial Surface of Arteries

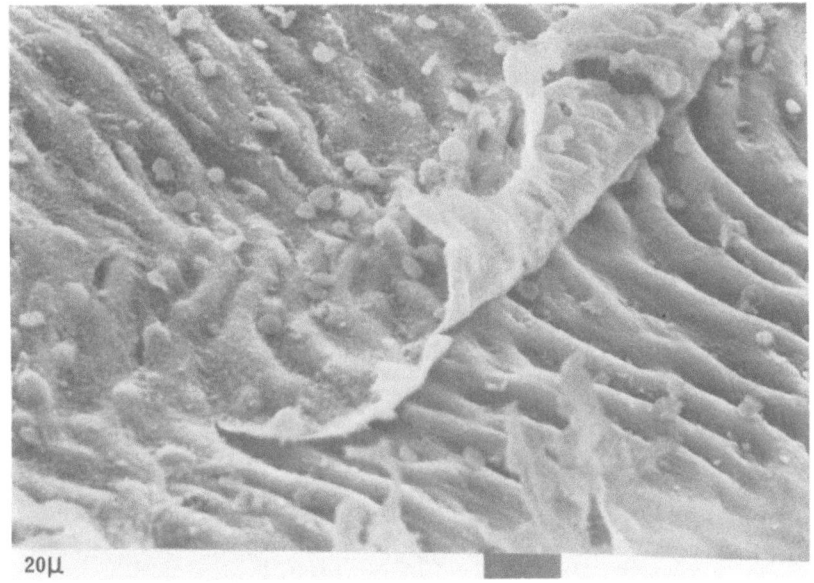

20μ

Fig. 5.3. A scanning electron micrograph of an undistended rat common carotid artery. The artery has been immersed in EDTA for 20 minutes. The endothelium has ruptured and separated from the internal elastic layer, exposing a part of it. The internal elastic layer is seen to be longitudinally ridged in an exactly similar manner to the intact endothelium. Bar = 20 μ.

Figure 5.3 shows an artery which was immersed in EDTA for 20 minutes. Its endothelium has ruptured in one location to expose the internal elastic lamina. The uncovered internal elastic lamina is seen to be longitudinally folded in exactly the same manner as is the intact endothelium. This finding confirms the opinion of Collatz and Garbarsch(3,4) and Sunga et al(8) that the endothelial folds are due to endothelial cells covering ridges in the underlying internal elastic lamina.

Distended arteries were found to have endothelial folds that were flatter, broader, and straighter than those of undistended vessels (Fig. 5.4). This broadening and flattening of the folds

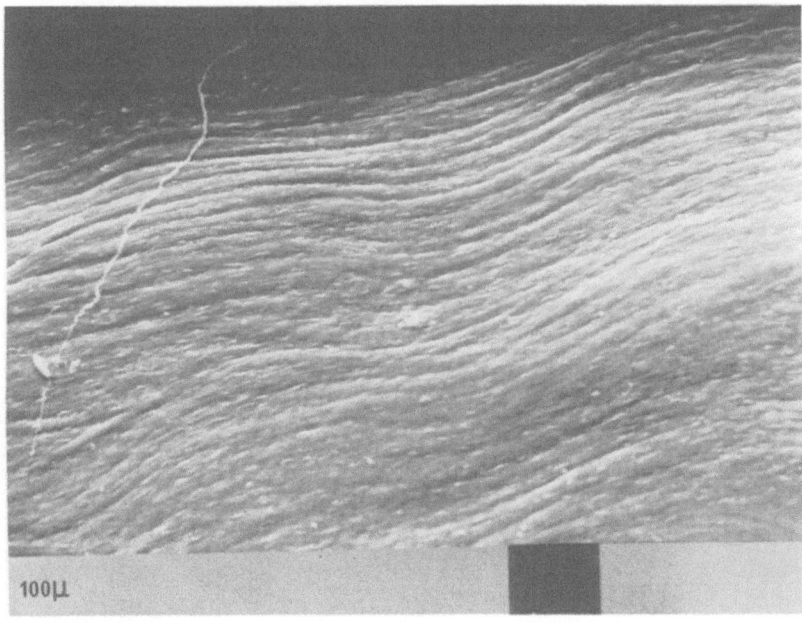

100μ

Fig. 5.4. A scanning electron micrograph of a distended rat common carotid artery. The endothelial folds are flatter, broader, and straighter than those of undistended arteries. Bar = 100 μ.

Endothelial Surface of Arteries

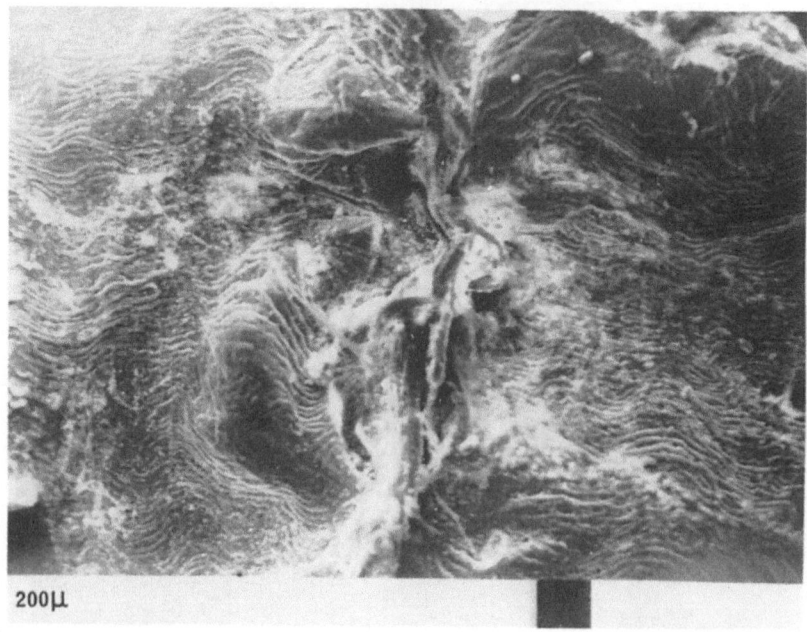

Fig. 5.5. A scanning electron micrograph of the common carotid artery of a rat showing the suture line of a satisfactory end-to-end anastomosis. The endothelial folds run longitudinally right up to the site of the anastomosis. Bar = 200 μ.

200μ

with distension suggests that one of their functions is to allow the vessels to dilate without damage to the endothelium and the immediate underlying layers.

In the second group of vessels, we examined common carotid arteries of rats which had end-to-end and end-to-side anastomoses performed on them while the animals were still growing. The SEM findings were similar for both kinds of anastomosis. In the vessels without stenosed anastomoses the endothelial folds ran longitudinally up to the site of anastomosis (Fig. 5.5). These appearances were quite different than those seen in the

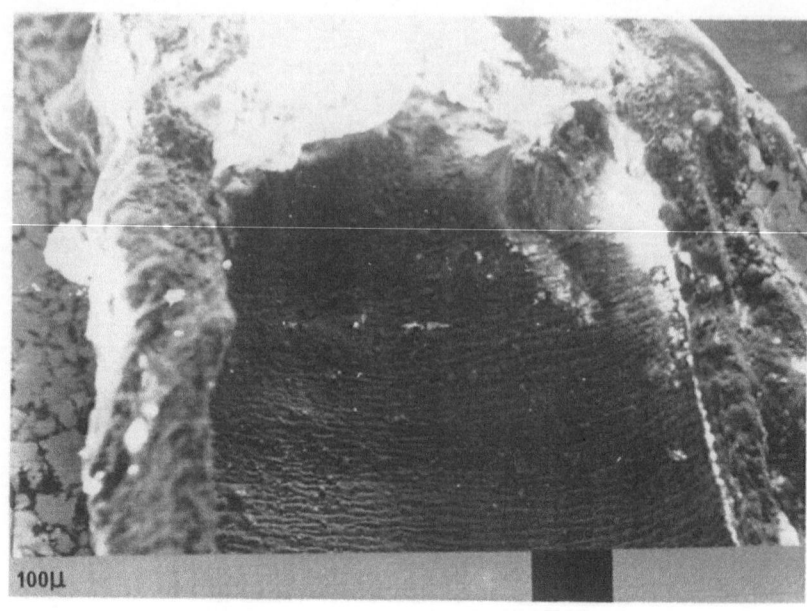

Fig. 5.6. A scanning electron micrograph of the common carotid artery of a rat in which an end-to-end anastomosis has resulted in stenosis. Transverse endothelial folds are seen running around the circumference of the vessel. Bar = 100 μ.

100μ

Chapter 5: Endothelial Surface of Arteries

vessels with stenosed anastomoses, where the folds were broader and flatter and ran transversely around the circumference of the arteries (Fig. 5.6).

We wondered whether division of the artery before anastomosis was in itself capable of altering the endothelial fold pattern, an alteration which in the course of healing reverted to normal, provided stenosis of the anastomosis did not occur. We therefore performed a series of anastomoses in the common carotid arteries of rats and examined them 1, 2, and 4 hours and 1, 3, and 4 weeks after operation. None of the vessels in this series developed stenosed anastomoses; and in all vessels longitudinal folds were found running up to the sites of anastomosis. No alteration of the normal endothelial fold pattern, therefore, occurs during the healing period following division and satisfactory anastomosis of arteries.

Flaherty and his colleagues(5) have shown that if a segment of the dog's aorta is excised, opened, and sutured so that it is rotated through 90°, and if it is then reinserted into the aorta, it take only 10 days for the endothelial cells of the segment to become reoriented along the long axis of the aorta. In Flaherty's opinion the reorientation of the cells is due to hemodynamic forces acting on the endothelial surface. It is possible that the stenosis of the anastomotic sites in our vessels caused sufficient alteration of the hemodynamic forces within them to change the orientation of the endothelial folds. To test this theory, we placed encircling sutures in the walls of a number of arteries and tied them tight enough to produce marked constriction. When we examined these vessels 4 weeks later, we found that not only had their endothelial folds retained their longitudinal

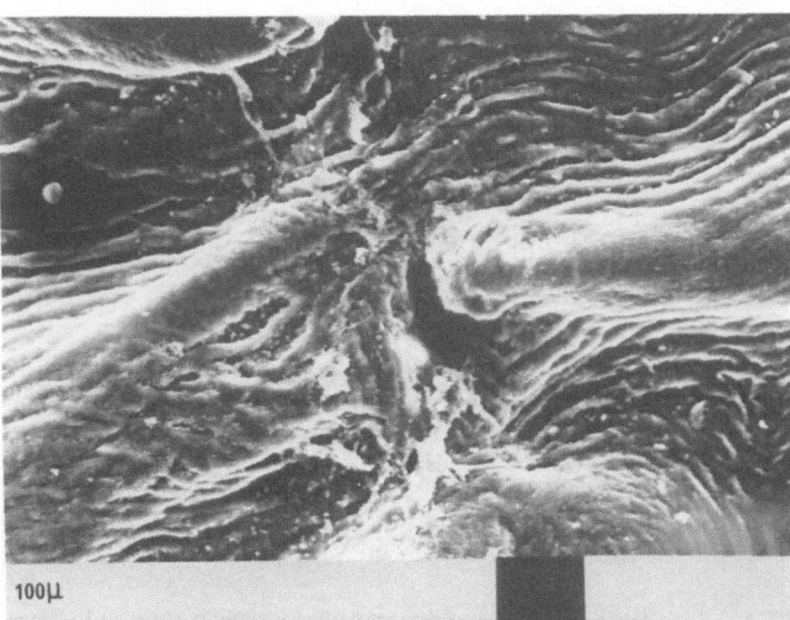

100μ

Fig. 5.7. A scanning electron micrograph of the common carotid artery of a rat 4 weeks after an encircling suture was placed in the wall of the artery to produce a constriction. Longitudinally running endothelial folds cross the site of the constriction. Bar = 100 μ.

direction right up to the constriction, but also in many cases the longitudinal folds actually crossed the site of constriction (Fig. 5.7). Naturally occurring turbulence does not alter the normal endothelial fold pattern either, as we found when we examined the mouths of intercostal arteries at their points of origin in rat aortas. The endothelial folds ran longitudinally up to the mouths of the branch arteries and then dipped smoothly into them without any distortion of the endothelial fold pattern in the adjacent part of the aorta (Fig. 5.8). The results of the encircling suture experiments and the appearances of endothelial folds around the mouths of branch arteries make it unlikely that disturbance of the normal hemodynamic forces or turbulence plays a major part in the production of the altered fold pattern seen in the arteries with stenosed anastomoses.

The arteries with stenosed anastomoses had thick, opaque walls and diameters which were significantly smaller than those of the vessels with satisfactory anastomoses. To investigate these changes further, some of the arteries that had previously been examined under the scanning electron microscope were stained by Mallory's method, which colors collagen blue. It was thus possible to compare the amounts of collagen present in arteries which had had no operative procedures performed, with that present in those which had been anastomosed. The unoperated arteries were found to have collagen only in their adventitial layers (Fig. 5.9) and those with satisfactory anastomoses had, in addition, small amounts of collagen in their muscle layers (Fig. 5.10), but the arteries with stenosed anastomoses had extensive amounts of collagen throughout the thickness of their walls (Fig. 5.11).

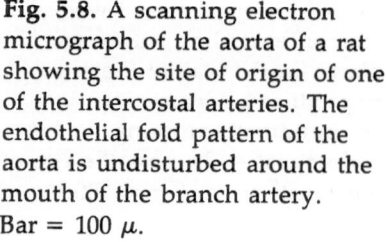

Fig. 5.8. A scanning electron micrograph of the aorta of a rat showing the site of origin of one of the intercostal arteries. The endothelial fold pattern of the aorta is undisturbed around the mouth of the branch artery. Bar = 100 μ.

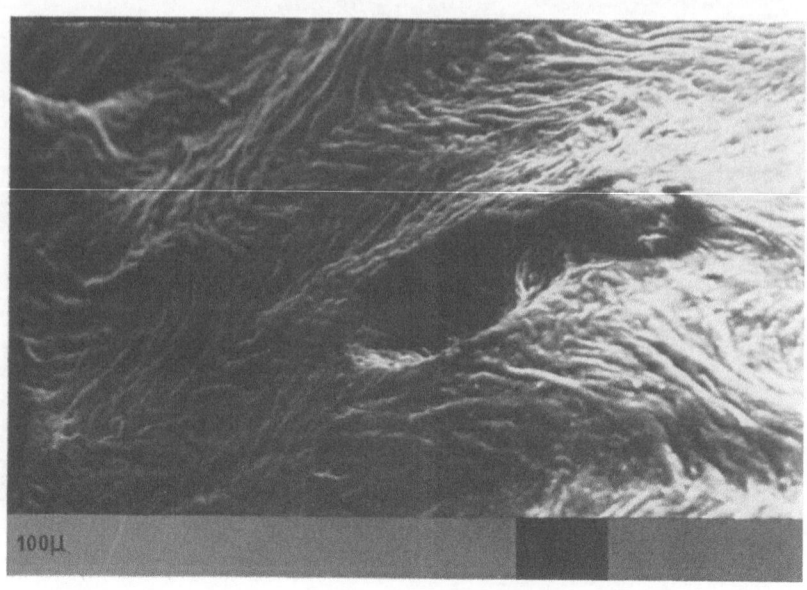

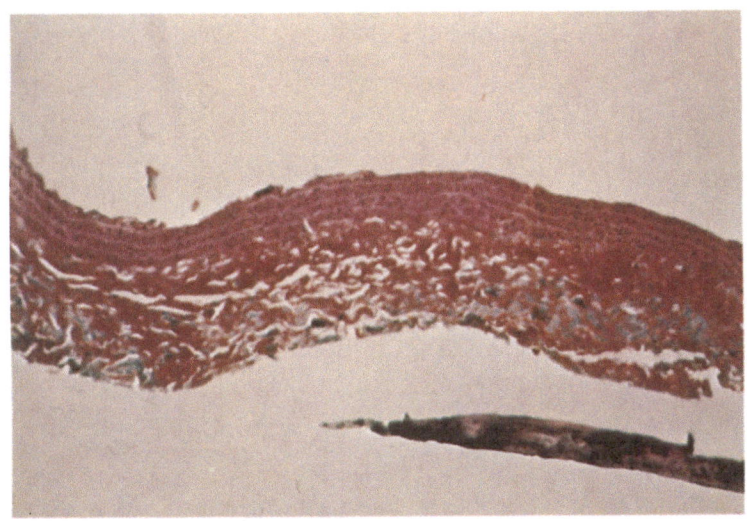

Fig. 5.9. A longitudinal section of a rat common carotid artery. Collagen, colored blue, is present only in the adventitial layer. Mallory's stain.

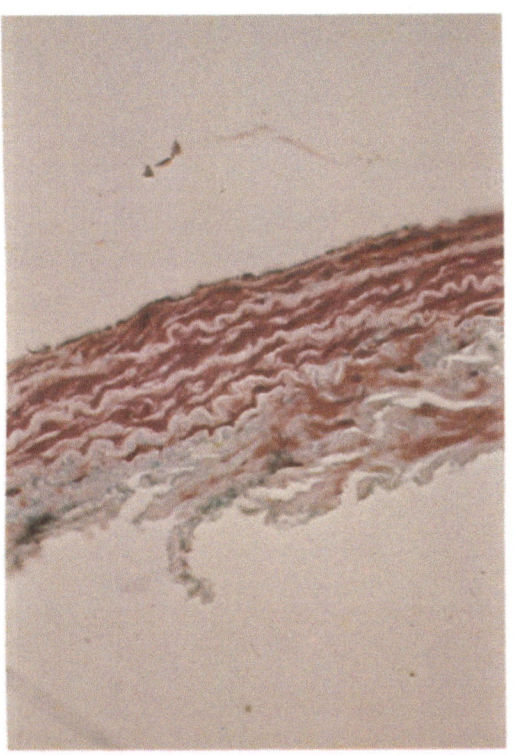

Fig. 5.10. A longitudinal section of the common carotid artery of a rat in which a satisfactory anastomosis has been performed. Small amounts of collagen, colored blue, are present in the muscle layers. Mallory's stain.

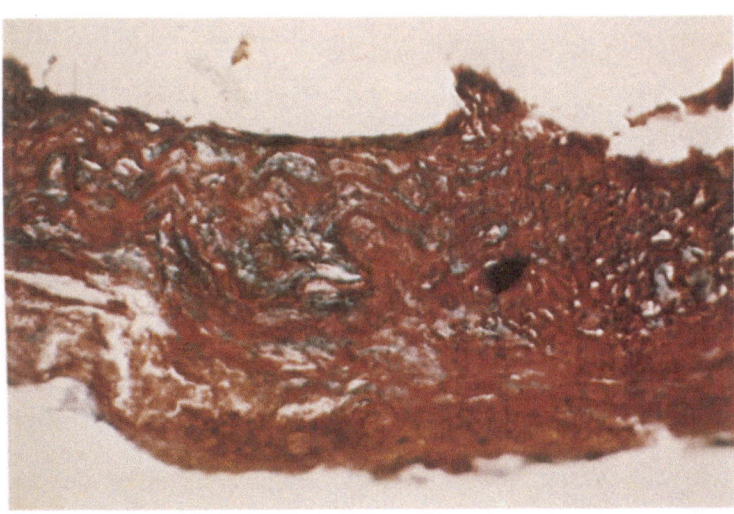

Fig. 5.11. A longitudinal section of the common carotid artery of a rat in which the anastomosis has resulted in a stenosis. Large amounts of collagen, colored blue, are present throughout all the layers of the vessel. Mallory's stain.

Conclusions

Our findings are that the endothelial folds of arteries are formed by endothelial cells covering longitudinal ridges in the internal elastic lamina. We have not found any evidence that the endothelial fold pattern is significantly altered by disturbances of the hemodynamic forces acting within the vessels. The endothelial fold pattern is not disturbed by either cutting or anastomosing together the ends of an artery, provided no stenosis occurs. An anastomosis resulting in a stenosis is accompanied by fibrosis throughout the wall of the artery and a profound alteration of the endothelial fold pattern. The underlying cause of these changes is most likely to be ischemic damage to the wall of the artery at the time of dissection and anastomosis. It is probable that fibrosis in the wall of the artery binds the endothelium to the subendothelial layers, and this results in the endothelium having a transverse instead of a longitudinal fold pattern. It is conceivable that endothelium with a transverse fold pattern is particularly vulnerable to damage that could lead to late thrombosis and the development of atheroma, both known to occur in some arteries that have been anastomosed. The most important finding is that gentle handling of an artery during dissection and anastomosis, with preservation of the blood supply to the vessel wall, leads to a satisfactory anastomotic site and little or no disturbance of the normal endothelial fold pattern.

REFERENCES

1. Bannister CM, Mundy LA, Mundy JE: A scanning electron microscopy study of the endothelial folds in normal and anastomosed common carotid arteries in albino rats. Br J Exp Pathol 56:329, 1975
2. Bannister CM, Mundy LA, Mundy JE: Anastomoses of small arteries in growing animals. In Austin GM (ed): Microneurosurgical Anastomoses for Cerebral Ischemia. Springfield, Ill, Thomas, 1976
3. Collatz C, Garbarsch CA: Scanning electron microscopic (SEM) study on the endothelium of the normal rabbit aorta. Angiologia 9:15, 1972
4. Collatz C, Garbarsch CA: Repair of arterial tissue. A scanning electron microscopic (SEM) study and light microscopic study on the endothelium of the rabbit thoracic aorta following simple dilatation injury. Virchows Arch [Pathol Anat] 360:93, 1973
5. Flaherty JT, Pierce JE, Ferrans VJ, et al: Endothelial nuclear patterns in the canine arterial tree with particular reference to haemodynamic events. Circ Res 30:23, 1972
6. Sheppard BL: Platelet adhesions in the rabbit abdominal aorta following the removal of the endothelium with EDTA. Proc R Soc Lond [Biol] 182:103, 1972

7. Shimamoto T, Yamashita Y, Sunga T: Scanning electron microscopic observations of endothelial surfaces of heart and blood vessels. Proc Jpn Acad 45:507, 1969
8. Sunga T, Shimamoto T, Nelson E: Correlated scanning and transmission electron microscopy of arterial endothelium. In Scanning Electron Microscopy, Part III. Chicago, IIT RI, 1973, pp. 459–463

6

The experimental effects
of prostaglandin E_1
on small vessel patency

Roderick G. Lamond and Norman L. Chater

Introduction

In the hands of skilled microsurgeons a patency rate close to 90% can be expected in the surgical anastomosis of 1.0-mm vessels. Considering today's instruments and techniques, however, if microsurgery is to progress to areas of new application (such as an occipital artery–posterior fossa bypass) several factors need to be overcome, one of the more important ones being consistent patency rates in vessels of 0.5-mm diameter.(1)

The response of the blood to vessel wall injury is the mechanism of thrombosis (or hemostasis, which is the same reaction). It was shown as early as the 1880s that arterial thrombi were initially composed of aggregated platelets and were not blood clots.(50)

Whenever a needle or suture is drawn through a vessel wall, collagen is exposed to the blood constituents within the lumen. Blood platelets, when exposed to a variety of stimuli (including ADP, collagen, serotonin, and thrombin), contract, evolving from their normal disc shape to a rounded form with multiple pseudopods (Figs. 6.1 and 6.2). This phenomenon of structural change is carried out by a protein fraction called thrombosthenin, and when contraction occurs a number of intracellular substances are released from the storage granules into the surrounding medium.(2,4,5,8,12,15,23,72) One of these substances is ADP which, either alone or in conjunction with other stimuli (such as collagen), induces adhesion of the platelets to each other and aggregation of blood platelets with eventual stabilization of the aggregates by the formation of fibrin.(60-62) After 24 hours platelets are apparently replaced by fibrin.(50) The complex relationship between platelet aggregation and blood coagulation involves platelet membrane phospholipoprotein

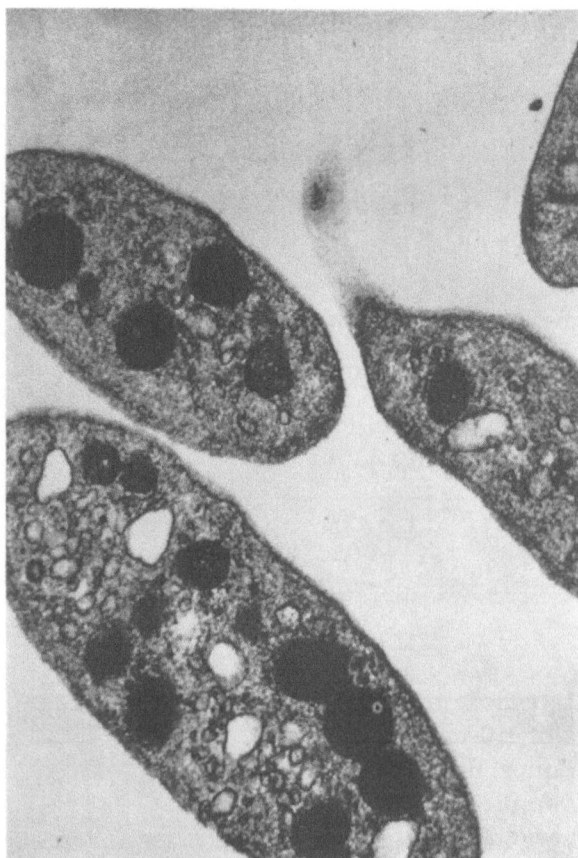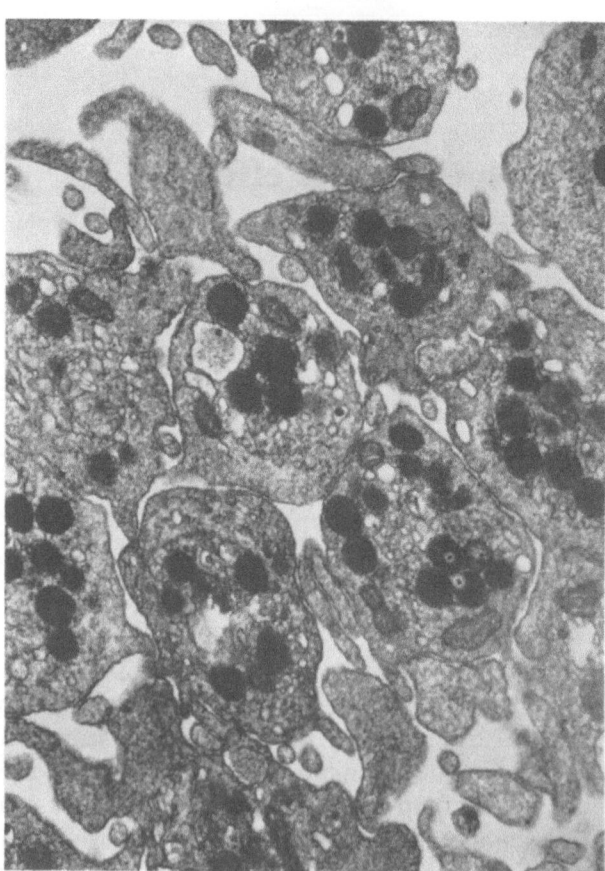

Fig. 6.1. Electron micrographs showing normal disc-shaped platelets (left) and platelets having undergone structural change and aggregation (right). × 20,000.

(or platelet factor III) and its interactions between factors IX and VIII and between factors X and V. We are concerned with the initial chain of events involving platelet stimulation and structural change followed by the release reaction leading to adhesion and finally aggregation.

A number of compounds have been described that inhibit platelet aggregation.(3,6,12,13,46,49) In in vitro studies to date, prostaglandin E_1 has been found to be the most potent inhibitor.(18,21,22,27,30,36,39)

The prostaglandins in general are a family of closely related, unsaturated hydroxy fatty acids containing a cyclopentane ring. They have now been identified in many tissues of the body and are most probably to be found in all body tissues, organs, and secretions.(16,24,26,28,29,34,57) They were discovered independently in 1933 by Goldblatt in human seminal fluid and by von Euler in sheep vesicular gland extracts. These substances were given the name prostaglandin by von Euler, who believed they were a product of the prostate gland, and the misnomer has remained. Identification of the actual structures and elucidation of these substances were later carried out by von Euler's student, Sune Bergström, who determined that they were 20-carbon compounds derived from the parent compound, prostanoic acid.(7) It is now known that there are six "primary" naturally occurring prostaglandins: PGE_1, E_2, E_3, $F_{1\alpha}$, $F_{2\alpha}$, $F_{3\alpha}$, and at least nine more "secondary" members which are obtained by chemical or biologic modification.

There are few classes of compounds that have so many different actions(68–70) on cells, tissues, and organs. All classes of smooth muscle(66) and all endocrine target tissues are affected by prostaglandins. Their high biologic activity with very small doses, combined with their wide range of effects,(64) indicate the potential importance of prostaglandins in therapy. A very strict specificity is exhibited by each individual prostaglandin structure; hence, few generalizations can be made about the group.

It is now clear that many prostaglandin effects are associated with an increase in adenylcyclase activity and an increase in intracellular cyclic-AMP.(48,59) The prostaglandin E compounds are enzymically formed in platelets.(16,19,47,58)

Prostaglandin E_1 (PGE_1) was first reported to inhibit platelet aggregation in the presence of ADP by Kloeze in 1967.(36-38) Butcher then reported the stimulation of human platelet aden-

Fig. 6.2. Scanning electron micrograph showing platelet structural change and illustrating pseudopod formation and adherence to vessel wall endothelium. $\times$ 20,000.

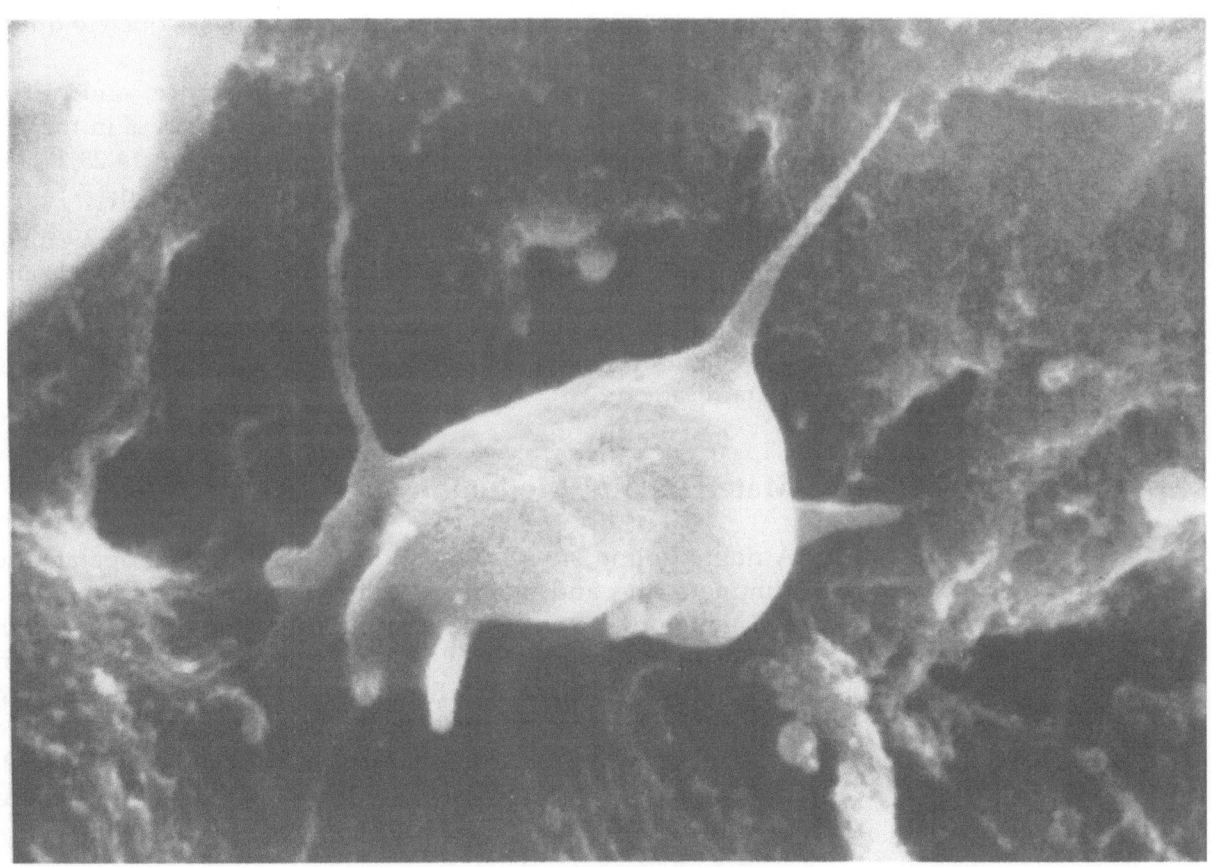

Fig. 6.3. Theoretical scheme of events showing prostaglandin E_1 acting on platelet adenylcyclase to bring about an increase in platelet cyclic-AMP and subsequent inhibition of platelet aggregation.

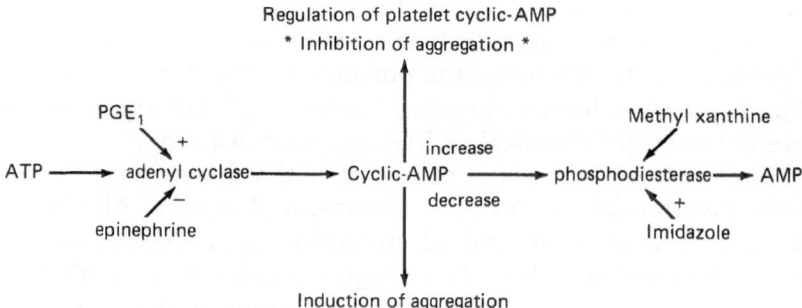

ylcyclase by PGE_1.(16) Wolfe and Schulman in 1969 then confirmed the stimulatory effects of PGE_1 on platelet adenylcyclase.(20,72) PGE_1 inhibition of platelet aggregation(67) is related to its activation of adenylcyclase, resulting in an increase in cyclic-AMP levels. Platelet adenylcyclase activity is apparently very sensitive to low concentrations of PGE_1 (Fig. 6.3).

There have been other attempts to increase patency rates in microvascular surgery and prevent thrombus formation.(40) Dipyridamole(46) provided only fair results. Pluronic F68(11,35) was used successfully as an adjunct in a study of 1.0-mm vessels but the Food and Drug Administration has banned this chemical. Studies using magnesium sulfate(3,46) are promising, but the use of $MgSO_4$ on cranial vessels and tissues is open to question.

Since PGE_1 is a naturally occurring substance, and in the light of in vivo experiments claiming some success in the inhibition of platelet aggregation using PGE_1(6,10,14,25,27,41-44,52,55,56) the following hypothesis was developed:

If prostaglandin E_1 inhibits collagen-induced platelet aggregation, and if the response of blood to injury in both larger vessels and the microcirculation is the formation of intravascular platelet aggregates, it follows that by interrupting the normal hemostatic response to insult, PGE_1 may increase patency rates in small vessel microsurgery.

Materials and Methods

A double-blind study was conducted by a single operator to eliminate bias and maintain technical factors and errors at a constant minimum. A 3-month training period was undertaken before the experiment was begun. The injected test solution containing prostaglandin E_1[1] was made by mixing 20.0 mg PGE_1 with 2.0 ml 95% ethanol and 18.0 ml sodium carbonate (0.2 mg/ml) in water to make a 1 mg/ml solution at a pH of 7.0. The control solution was lactated Ringer's. The solutions were

[1]Prostaglandin E_1 obtained from the Upjohn Co., Kalamazoo, Michigan.

prepared by a second party and stored in identical containers. Young hooded Norwegian rats were used in this study along with the basic microsurgical instruments. The animals were anesthetized with Nembutal (sodium pentobarbital). After shaving the surgical field, the femoral arteries and veins (0.4- to 0.7-mm diameter) along with the superficial epigastric vessels were dissected free. A femoral vessel was clamped with the Acland microvascular clamp, transected, and anastomosed with a 4-mm–3/8 circle 70-μ needle (7V43) and 18-μ (equivalent to 11-0) nylon suture[2] (Fig. 6.4 to 6.6, p. 51). Immediately after the anastomosis was completed and the clamps removed, 0.05 ml of either solution A (the control) or solution B (0.5 ml = 50 μg PGE$_1$) was injected into the anastomosed femoral vessel via a 30-gauge needle inserted in the superficial epigastric vessel.(54) Only six veins were operated on in each of the two groups; the great majority of procedures were confined to the femoral artery. A total of 41 operations were performed using solution A and a total of 39 were performed using solution B. The superficial epigastric vessel was cauterized, hemostasis was assured, and the wound was closed. Vessels were checked for patency 4 days to 1 month (usually 7 days) postanastomosis by reopening the surgical wound and observing blood flow distal to the site of anastomosis. The Zeiss operating microscope was used for all procedures.

Acland clearly described the adverse effects which can occur postanastomosis:(2) "The lumen at and distal to the suture line is seen to fill up progressively with a yellowish translucent substance until all flow ceases." It is this particular phenomenon of hemostasis, ie, platelet aggregation, toward which we have focused our attention (Fig. 6.7, p. 52). The platelet plug was seen to wash away with perfusion through the superficial epigastric vessel using either solution A or B (Fig. 6.8 and 6.9, p. 52).

Results

Twenty-four of the 41 anastomoses perfused with solution A (58.3%) remained patent postoperatively. Twenty-nine of the 39 anastomoses perfused with solution B (74.3%) remained patent postoperatively. The results are tabulated in Table 6.1.

Discussion

The outcome of this experiment, when subjected to the binomial test, is significant at the 5% level.

Ethanol is a part of the stock solution of PGE$_1$ now used by most laboratories. It can be argued that ethanol is responsible

[2]Nylon suture produced by the S&T Company, Munich, West Germany.

Table 6.1. Patency rates in 80 microvascular anastomoses.

	Group A (Control)	Group B (PGE₁ Solution)
Number of anastomoses performed	41	39
Number of patent vessels 1 week postoperatively	24	29
Percentage patent	58.3	74.3

The data are divided into two groups, based on the test solution perfused into the vessel immediately after operation.

for effective vasodilation and that it may be deleterious to tissues. The solution, however, is infused intraarterially, and whether a specific portion of the solution is affecting the results is secondary to the results themselves.

Although the rats were shaved and sterile suture material was used, the instruments were not sterile nor was the operating microscope draped. The closed wound was treated with tincture of iodine, but the animals were returned to their communal cage postoperatively. The possibility of infection is undoubtedly a factor to be considered in the patency rate.

Furthermore, there are species differences in platelet reactions and prostaglandin activity and these must be considered when studying this model in terms of its clinical application. There are reported differences in response to PGE_1 in man and in dogs and cats.(28,31-33,45,71)

The clinical application of prostaglandin E_1 in microsurgery requires that two important pharmacologic properties of the drug be kept in mind: (1) the marked hypotensive activity of PGE_1 requires the dose to be as low as possible; and (2) the rapid breakdown of PGE_1 in the lungs requires a continuous supply to achieve any therapeutic effect.

The effects of infused PGE_1 in human subjects have been observed.(8,9,17) Some of the adverse clinical reactions to very small quantities (0.2 $\mu g/kg$) include facial flushing, headache, abdominal cramps, thoracic oppression, nausea, vomiting, systolic and diastolic hypotension, and tachycardia. The effects are long lasting (15 minutes after infusion). The spasmolytic properties of PGE_1 in cerebral vasospasm after subarachnoid bleeding in man were assessed by Steiner et al.(65) The effects observed were minimal; however, extremely small doses were injected through the internal carotid artery. They observed no adverse effects, but documented improvement in one case.

An attractive feature of PGE_1 is the fact that it is indigenous to the brain. It does increase the patency rate in 0.5-mm vessels to 74.3%, as opposed to the 58.3% patency rate which is expected without such adjunctive therapy. The fact that PGE_1 did not prove to be effective to a level of greater significance may induce further search for more effective means of improving

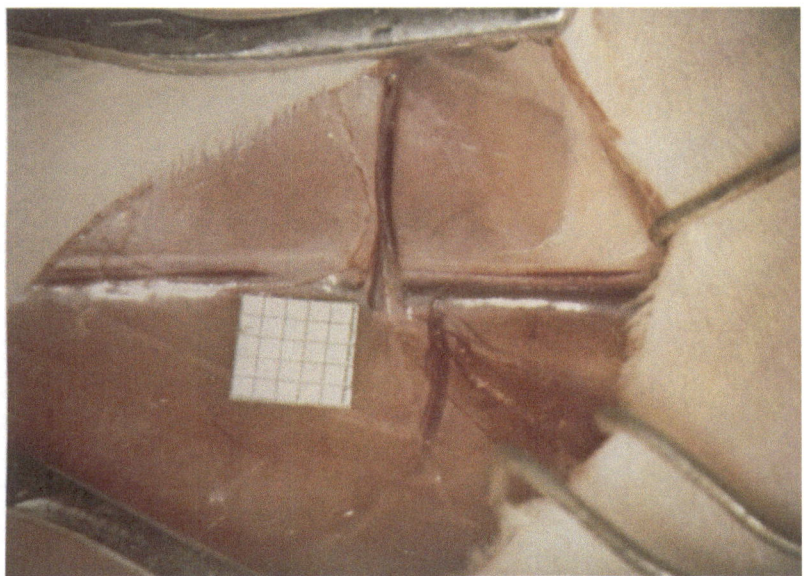

Fig. 6.4. Photograph of the operative field showing the exposed femoral neurovascular bundle and the superficial epigastric vessels branching in a perpendicular course toward the top. A millimeter rule (1 square equals 1 mm) is shown.

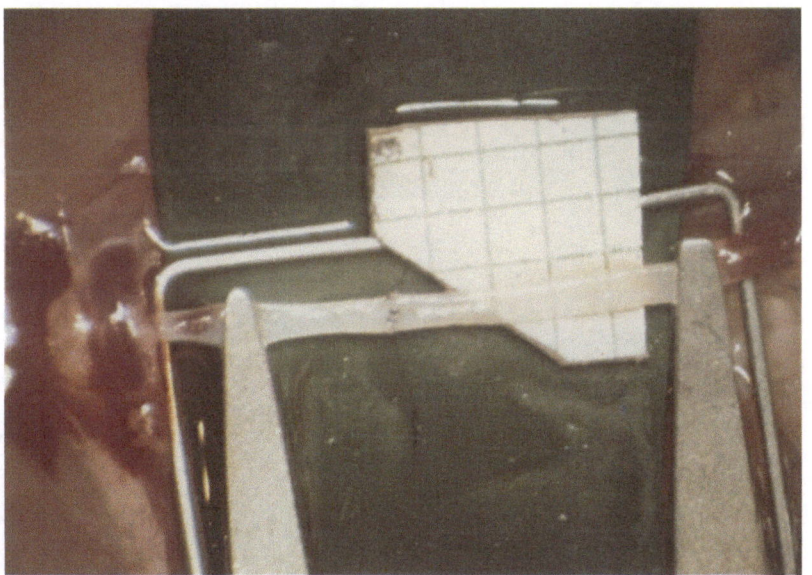

Fig. 6.5. Photograph of an isolated femoral artery after end-to-end anastomosis with microvascular clamp in place.

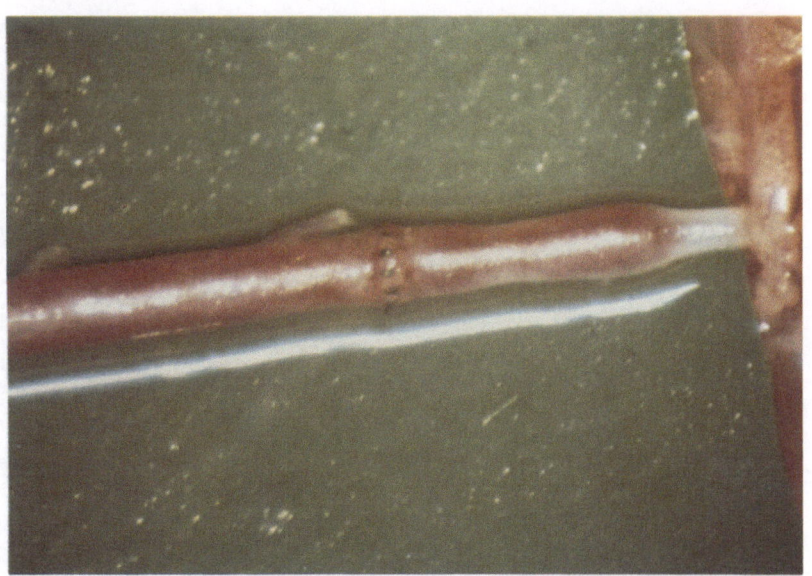

Fig. 6.6. Vessel seen in Figure 5 with anastomosis completed and clamps removed. Temporary vasospasm at site of clamp can be seen at right.

Fig. 6.7. Postanastomosis photograph showing the yellowish, translucent, jellylike platelet plug forming distal to (to the right of) the anastomosis. This aggregate of platelets adhering to the vessel wall formed in response to a multitude of stimuli, including collagen and ADP. It has the potential to act as a matrix for fibrin deposition, leading to occlusive thrombus formation and cessation of blood flow distal to the anastomosis.

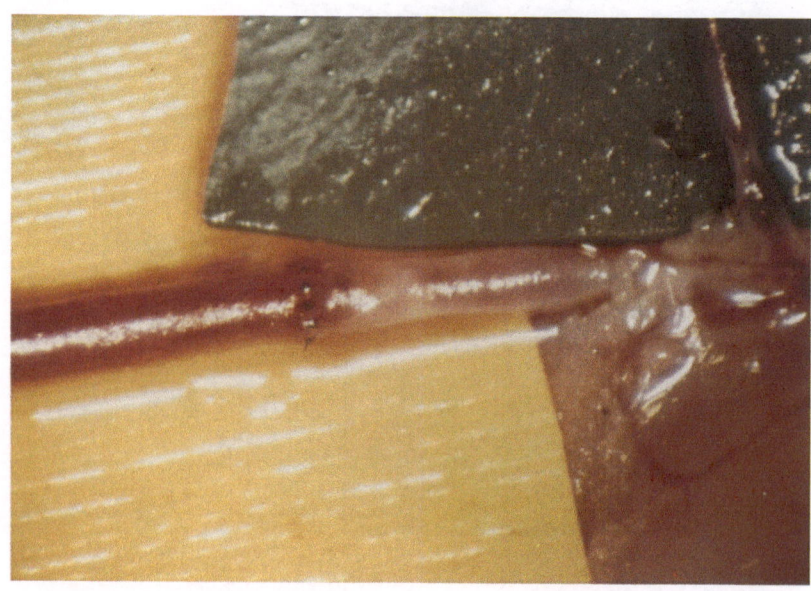

Fig. 6.8. Dissolution of thrombus after infusion through the superficial epigastric artery.

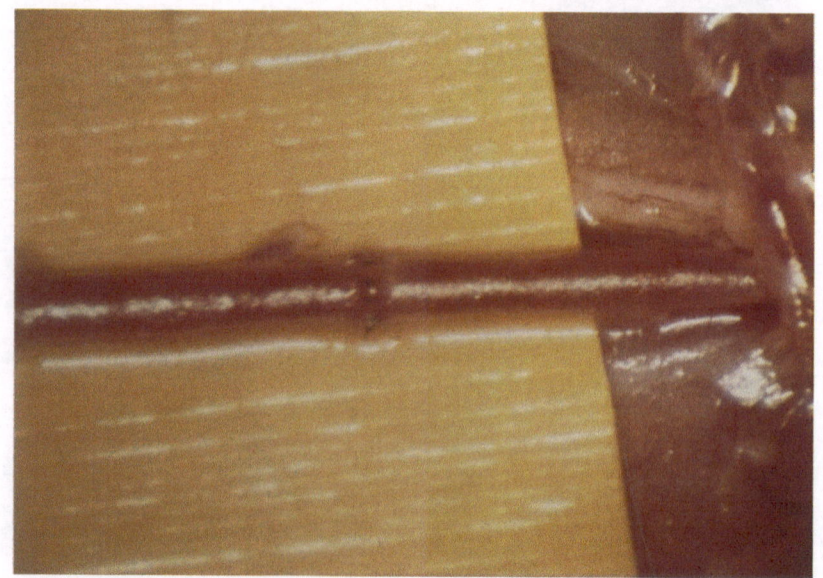

Fig. 6.9. Vessels being observed for patency 1 week postanastomosis.

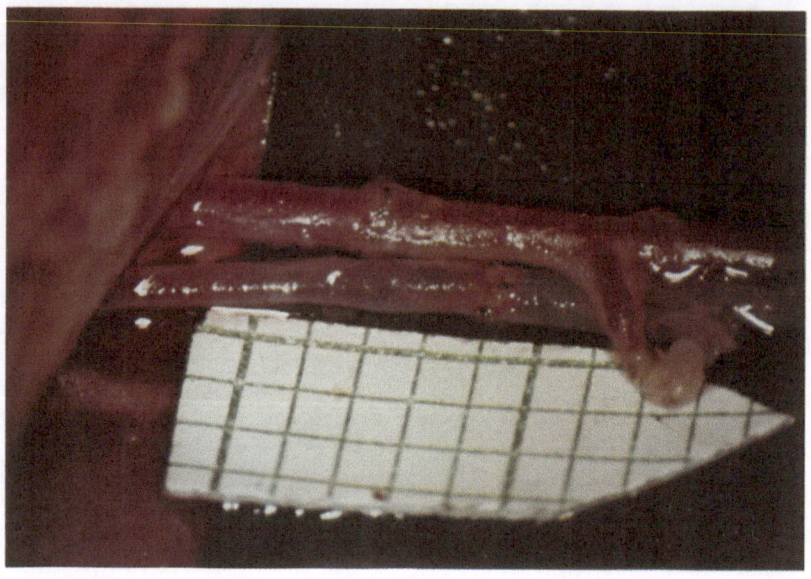

patency rates in small vessel microsurgery. To this end, aspirin and sulfinpyrazone(49,50,51,63) have provided impressive initial results as inhibitors of platelet aggregation. Arfors et al,(5) using laser-induced endothelial injury techniques, reported dextran 70 to have a pronounced inhibitory effect on platelet activity.

Summary

Spurred by the literature on prostaglandin E_1 (PGE_1) and its role in the inhibition of platelet aggregation, a double-blind study was undertaken to determine the effectiveness of PGE_1 for increasing patency rates in small vessel surgery. Using microscopic techniques, small rat vessels (femoral and superficial epigastric arteries less than 0.6 mm in diameter and veins less than 1.0 mm in diameter) were anastomosed using either an end-to-end or end-to-side technique. Postanastomosis, either PGE_1 or Ringer's solution was perfused into the repaired vessel to reduce thrombus formation and improve patency rates. One week postoperatively, the ratio of patent vessels to the total perfused with PGE_1 was 29/39, compared with 24/41 in the control group ($P < 0.05$). Despite these favorable results, the observed side-effects of PGE_1 in human subjects warrant further search for biochemical adjuncts to provide consistently higher patency rates in small vessel microsurgery.

REFERENCES

1. Acland R. Signs of patency in small vessel anastomosis. Surgery 72:744, 1972
2. Acland R. Thrombus formation in microvascular surgery. Surgery 73:766, 1973
3. Acland R: Prevention of thrombus in microvascular surgery by the use of magnesium sulphate. Br J Plast Surg 25:292, 1972
4. Arfors KE: Counteraction of platelet activity at sites of laser-induced endothelial trauma. Br Med J 4:430, 1968
5. Arfors KE, Dahl DP, Engeset J, et al: In vivo quantitation of platelet activity using biolaser-induced endothelial injury. 5th European Conference on Microcirculation. Bibl Anat 10:502, 1969
6. Ball G, Brereton G, Ireland D, et al: Effect of prostaglandin E_1 alone and in combination with theophylline or aspirin on collagen-induced platelet aggregation and on platelet nucleotides including adenosine 3,5-cyclic monophosphate. Biochem J 120:709, 1970
7. Bergström S: Isolation structure and action of the prostaglandins. In Nobel Symposium 2, Prostaglandins. S, Sammuelson B (eds): Bergström 1967, p. 21 Stockholm.
8. Bergström S, Carlson LA, Ekelund L, et al: Cardiovascular and metabolic response to infusions of prostaglandin E_1 and to simultaneous infusions of noradrenaline and prostaglandin E_1 in man. Acta Physiol Scand 64:332, 1965

9. Bergström S, Duner H, von Euler US, et al: Observations on the effects of infusion of prostaglandin E_1 in man. Acta Physiol Scand 45:145, 1959

10. Berman HJ, Tangen O, Ausprunk D: Prostaglandin E_1 inhibition of aggregation of hamster platelets. 5th European Conference on Microcirculation. Bib Anat 10:507, 1969

11. Born GVR: Observations on the rapid morphological reaction of platelets to aggregating agents. Ser Haemetol 3(4):114, 1970

12. Born GVR: Platelets in thrombogenesis. Mechanism and inhibition of platelet aggregation. Ann Coll Surg Engl 36:200, 1965

13. Boullin DJ, Green AR, Price KS: The mechanism of ADP-induced platelet aggregation binding to platelet receptors and inhibition of binding and aggregation by prostaglandin E_1. J Physiol 221:415, 1972

14. Bousser M: Effects of combined prostaglandin E_1 and aspirin on experimental arterial thrombosis in rabbits. Biomedicine 19:90, 1973

15. Brodie GN, Baeuziger N, Chase L: The effects of thrombin on adenyl cyclase activity and a membrane protein from human platelets. Clin Invest 51:81, 1972

16. Butcher RW: Prostaglandins and cyclic-AMP. In Greengard P, Costa E (eds): Advances in Biochemical Psychopharmacology, Vol. 3. 1970, p. 173

17. Carlson LA, Ekelund L, Orö L: Clinical and metabolic effects of different doses of prostaglandin E_1 in Man. Acta Med Scand 183:423, 1968

18. Carlson LA, Irion E, Orö L: Effect of infusion of prostaglandin E_1 on the aggregation of blood platelets in man. Life Sci 7:85, 1968

19. Clausen J, Srivastava KC: The synthesis of prostaglandins in human platelets. Lipids 7(4):246, 1972

20. Droller MJ, Wolfe S: Thrombin-induced increase in intracellular cyclic 3'5'-adenosine monophosphate in human platelets. J Clin Invest 51:3094, 1972

21. Elkeles RS, Hampton JR, Harrison MJ: Prostaglandin E_1 and human platelets. Lancet 2:111, 1969

22. Emmons PR, Hampton JR, Harrison MJ, et al: Effect of prostaglandin E_1 on platelet behavior in vitro and in vivo. Br Med J 2:468, 1967

23. Evans G, Mustard J: Platelet-surface reaction and thrombosis. Surgery 64:273, 1968

24. Glenn E, Wilks J, Bowman B: Platelets, prostaglandins, red cells, sedimentation rates, serum and tissue proteins and non-steroidal anti-inflammatory drugs. Proc Soc Exp Biol Med 141:879, 1972

25. Grottenlos J, Hornstra G: The influence of prostaglandin E_1 on experimental platelet aggregation in rats. In Jones JR (ed): Proceedings of the 2nd International Symposium on Atherosclerosis, Chicago, 1969. New York Heidelberg Berlin, Springer-Verlag, 1970

26. Hinman J: The prostaglandins. Bioscience 17:779, 1967

27. Hornstra G: Degree and duration of prostaglandin E_1-induced inhibition of platelet aggregation in the rat. Eur Pharmacol 15:343, 1971

28. Horton EW: Hypothesis on physiological roles of prostaglandins. Physiol Rev 49:122, 1969

29. Horton EW: The prostaglandins. In Staey RS, Robson JM (eds): Recent Advances in Pharmacology, 4th ed. p.186

30. Irion E, Blomback M: Prostaglandins in platelet aggregation. Scand J Clin Lab Invest 24:141, 1969

31. Jorgensen H, Sondergaard J: Vascular responses to prostaglandin E₁. Acta Derm Vener. (Stockh) 53:203, 1973

32. Kaegi H, Pineo G, Shimizu A, et al: Arterio-venous shunt thrombosis, prevention by sulfinpyrayone. N Engl J Med 290:304, 1974

33. Kaley G, Weiner R: Microcirculatory studies with prostaglandin E₁. In Ramwell PW, Shaw JE (eds): Prostaglandin Symposium of the Worchester Foundation for Experimental Biology. New York, Wiley Inter-science, 1968

33. Karim SMM (ed): Prostaglandin; Progress in Research. New York, Wiley Inter-science, 1972, p 240

34. Ketchum LD, Wennen WW, Masters FW, and Robinson DW: Experimental use of pluronic F68 in microvascular surgery. Plast Reconst Surg 53:288, 1974

35. Kloeze J: Influence of prostaglandins on platelet adhesives and platelet aggregation. In Bergström S, Sammuelson B(eds): Nobel Symposium 2, Prostaglandins. Stockholm, 1967, p241

36. Kloeze J: Relationship between chemical structure and platelet aggregation activity of prostaglandins. Biochem Biophys Acta 187:285, 1969

37. Kloeze J: Influence of prostaglandins on ADP-induced platelet aggregation. Netherlands Society for Physiology and Pharmacology Meeting, April 6, 1967

38. Kloeze J: Influence of Prostaglandins E₁ and E₂ on coagulation of rat blood. Experientia 26:307, 1970

39. Kluge TH, et al: Thrombosis prophylaxis with dextran and warfarin in vascular operations. Surg Gynecol Obstet 135:941, 1972

40. Lee J, et al: Prostaglandins as therapeutic agents. Arch Intern Med 131:294, 1973

41. Marquis N, Becker J, Vigdahl R: Platelet aggregation and epinepherine-induced decrease in cyclic-AMP synthesis. Biochem and Biophys Res Commun 39:783, 1970

42. Marquis N, Vigdahl R, Tavorina P: Biochemical role of prostaglandin E₁ in the inhibition of platelet aggregation. Second International Symposium on Atherosclerosis, Chicago, 1969

43. Marquis N, Vigdahl R, Tavorina P: Platelet aggregation regulation by cyclic-AMP and prostaglandin E₁. Biochem Biophys Res Commun 36:965, 1969

44. Mattila S, Fogarty T: Heterologous vascular grafts as small vessel substitutes. Annales, Chir Gynaecol Fenn 62:234, 1973

45. Mayer J, Hammond G: Dipyridamole and aspirin tested against an experimental model of thrombosis. Ann Surg 178:108, 1973

46. Mills D, Smith J: The control of platelet responsiveness by agents that influence cyclic-AMP metabolism. Ann NY Acad Sci 201:391, 1972

47. Mills D, Smith J: The influence of platelet aggregation of drugs that affect the accumulation of adenosine 3',5'cyclic monophosphate in platelets. Biochem J 121:185, 1971

48. Mustard J: Platelets, drugs, and Thrombosis. CMAJ 108:443, 1973

49. Mustard J, Packham M: Thromboembolism. A manifestation of the response of blood injury. Circulation 42:1, 1970

50. Mustard JF, Rowsell HC, Smythe HA: The effect of sulfinpyrazone on platelet economy and thrombosis formation in rabbits. Blood 29:859, 1967

References

51. Nakano T: Effects of prostaglandins E_1, A_1, F_2 on the coronary and peripheral circulation. Proc Soc Exp Biol Med 127:1160, 1968

52. Nomoto H, Buncke HJ, Chater NL: Improved patency rates in microvascular surgery when using magnesium sulfate and a silicone rubber vascular cuff. Plast Reconstr Surg 54:157, 1974

53. O'Brien J, Henderson P, Bennett RC, Crock GW: Microvascular surgical techniques. Med J Aust 1:722, 1970

54. O'Brien J, Tulevski V, Etherington M, Madgwick T: Platelet function studies before and after operation and the effect of post-operative thrombosis. J Lab Clin Med 83:342 1974

55. Pelofsky S, Jacobson E, Fisher R: Effects of prostaglandin E_1 on experimental cerebral vasospasm. J Neurosurg 36:634, 1972

56. Pickles V: Prostaglandins. Nature 224:221, 1969

57. Salzman E: Cyclic AMP and platelet function. N Engl J Med 286:358, 1972

58. Salzman E, Levine L: Cyclic 3',5'-adenosine monophosphate in human blood platelets. J Clin Invest 50:131, 1971

59. Silver MF, et al: Human blood prostaglandins. Formation during clotting. Prostaglandins 1:429, 1972

60. Smith E, McMorrow J, Covino B, et al: Studies on the vasodilator action of prostaglandin E_1. In Ramwell PW, Shaw JE (eds): Prostaglandin Symposium of the Worchester Foundation for Experimental Biology. New York, Wiley Inter-science 1968, p 259

61. Smith J, Ingerman C, Kocsis JJ, Silver MJ: Formation of prostaglandins during the aggregation of human blood platelets. J Clin Invest 52:965, 1973

62. Smythe H, Ogryzlo MA, Murphy EA, et al: The effect of sulfinpyrazone on platelet economy and blood coagulation in man. Can Med Assoc J 92:818, 1965

63. Sondergaard J, Helin P, Jorgensen H: Human cutaneous inflammation induced by prostaglandin E_1. J Pathol 109:239, 1973

64. Steiner L, Forster D, Bergvall U, et al: Effect of prostaglandin E_1 on cerebral circulatory disturbances following subarachnoid haemorrhage in man. Neuroradiology 4:409, 1972

65. Tuttle R, Skelly M: Interactions of prostaglandin E_1 and ouabain on Contractility of isolated rabbit atria and intracellular cation concentration. In Ramwell S, Shaw JE (eds): Prostaglandin Symposium of the Worchester Foundation for Experimental Biology. New York, Wiley Inter-science 1968, p 309

66. Van Crevald S, Pascha CN: Influence of the prostaglandins E_1 and E_2 on aggregation of blood platelets. Nature 218:316, 1968

67. Van Crevald S, Pascha CN: Abnormality in the aggregation of blood platelets in various morbid conditions and the influence of prostaglandins upon this abnormality. Thromb Diath Haemorrh 20:180, 1968

68. Vigdahl R, Marquis N, Tavormina P: Platelet aggregation, Adenyl Cyclase, Prostaglandin E_1 and Calcium. Biochem Biophys Res Commun 37:409, 1969

69. Viguera M, Sunahara F: Microcirculatory effects of prostaglandins. Can J Physiol Pharmacol 47:627, 1969

70. Weeks J, Sekhar N, Ducharme D: Relative activity of prostaglandins E_1, A_1, E_2, and A_2 on lipolysis, platelet aggregation, smooth muscle and the cardiovascular system. J Pharm Pharmacol 21:103, 1969

71. Wolfe S, Shulman N: Adenyl cyclase activity in human platelets. Biochem Biophys Res Commun 35:266, 1969

II

METABOLISM

7

Oxidative metabolism in cerebral ischemia

Jack M. Fein

The metabolic requirements for normal cerebral function include a continuous supply of glucose and oxygen. Microvascular neurosurgeons are now called upon to treat focal vascular obstructions which impede both the flow of these nutrients and the removal of metabolic waste products. These obstructive lesions threaten the balance between nutrient supply and demand. This deficit in the nutrients vital for energy metabolism may ultimately determine the ability of nervous tissue to recover from ischemic infarction. However, it should be recognized that other enzyme systems important in neurotransmitter synthesis, such as tyrosine and tryptophane hydroxylase(6) as well as monoamine oxidase, also utilize oxygen. A reduction in their activity may be related to the suppression of electrophysiologic activity seen in stroke. Our present understanding of these relationships is based on developments in oxygen-transport physiology, cellular biochemistry, and intact animal experiments which simulate clinical conditions during ischemia and anoxia.

In order to deal with the changes in oxygen metabolism resulting from focal cerebral ischemia and the effect of extracranial–intracranial (EC–IC) bypass procedures, a review of the more important aspects of oxygen transport and intermediary metabolism in the normal brain will first be presented.

Oxygen Transport and Delivery

Changes in arterial pH may determine the degree of dissociation of the oxyhemoglobin complex (the Bohr effect), but the delivery of oxygen to brain tissue from the blood is largely determined by physical diffusion. Within brain tissue the distribution of oxygen is dependent on the gradient of oxygen tensions. It is highest at a capillary and lowest at a point furthest from the capillary. Krogh(16) and Kety(14) developed a model for understanding the diffusion and distribution of oxygen within the brain by assuming a cylindric core of tissue with a capillary at its center. This allows an approximate calculation of tissue Po_2 values, if the values for intercapillary distances, capillary Po_2, and the oxygen consumption rate of the tissue are known. Thews(34) determined the diffusion constant and was able to make quantitative measurements of oxygen tension in brain.

According to these calculations, tissue hypoxia should occur at a venous Po_2 of 19 mmHg. This figure correlated with the empirically observed findings of Opitz.(25) Bander and Kiese(2) measured the oxygen consumption of isolated mitochondria and observed a fall at Po_2 values of 10 mmHg, thereby defining anoxia in terms of a "critical" mitochondrial Po_2. Using sensitive fluorometric techniques, Chance et al(5) determined that oxygen desaturation of cytochrome oxidase within mitochondria does not occur until the Po_2 tension falls to 1 to 2 mmHg. These latter in vitro experiments suggest a much lower critical oxygen tension for mitochondria. The general agreement among these studies is evident, however, since the higher values of tissue Po_2 measured by Bander and Kiese(2) are needed to maintain the diffusion gradient and insure the lower values at the cellular level.

Rate of Glycolysis

In all animal cells other than erythrocytes, oxidative metabolism provides the high-energy phosphates adenosine triphosphate (ATP) and (in muscle and brain) creatine phosphate for energy-requiring processes, such as biosynthesis and membrane transport. In the nervous system, approximately 70% of the ATP produced is involved in membrane-transport functions. In tissue-slice experiments(27) both ouabain administration and calcium deprivation selectively blocked active ion transport across membranes and significantly reduced the level of cellular oxygen metabolism. High-energy phosphates are provided by glycolysis in the cytoplasm and by oxidative phosphorylation within the mitochondria; however, only two ATP molecules are produced by glycolysis, whereas the number approaches the ideal of 36 by oxidative phosphorylation.

Since glycolysis comprises the first steps in energy transduction, certain noteworthy features should be emphasized. Although glycolysis is a ubiquitous feature of animal cells, there are several unique features of glycolysis in the brain. The only substrate that is utilized in significant quantities in the brain

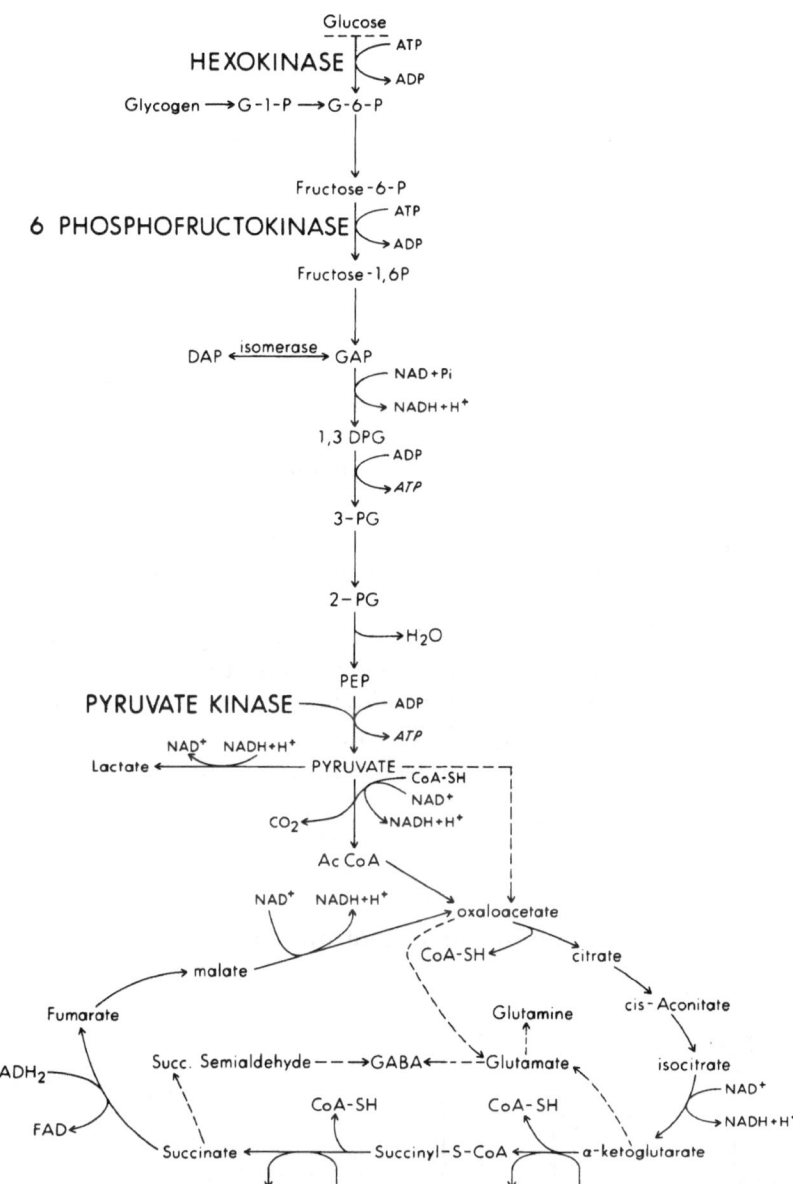

Fig. 7.1. Glycolysis and the tricarbcylic acid (TCA) cycle. The rate of glycolysis is controlled by the activities of hexokinase, 6 phosphofructokinase, and pyruvate kinase. These enzyme activities are in turn responsive to the levels of energy containing substrates as well as pH.

is glucose. In all other tissues a significant quantity of C^{14} glucose is stored as glycogen, which may be converted to lactate and CO_2 subsequent to glycogenolysis; however, only an insignificant amount of glycogen is found in nervous tissue. Labelled carbon also appears in glutamine, aspartic acid, GABA, and to a similar extent in alanine and glycine, within 1 minute of its administration.

The main events in glycolysis are summarized in Figure 7.1. Since most of the steps in the conversion of glucose to pyruvate or lactate are easily reversible processes, particular note should be made of the three enzymatic steps involving hexokinase, 6-phosphofructokinase (PFK) and pyruvate kinase, where the rate

Rate of Glycolysis

Fig. 7.2. Reducing equivalents provided by the TCA cycle may be utilized either for oxidative phosphorylation or equivalent processes such as accumulation of calcium ions. At the three points indicated adequate energy is available for phosphorylation of ADP.

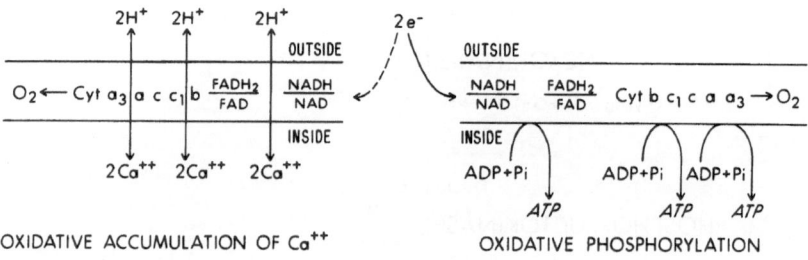

of glycolysis may be influenced. Brain hexokinase has been shown to have some controlling effect on the rate of glycolysis by virtue of its proximity to sources of ATP. The enzyme is inhibited by its product, so that the overall rate of glucose phosphorylation is tempered by the intracellular concentration of glucose-6-phosphate.

6-phosphofructokinase (PFK), which catalyzes the conversion of fructose-6-phosphate to fructose 1,6-diphosphate at the expense of ATP, is an allosteric enzyme with several subunits. It has very complex kinetic parameters. The positive allosteric modulators, which stimulate enzyme activity, are the substrate fructose-6-phosphate, the product fructose 1,6-diphosphate, NH^+_4, ADP, Pi, and AMP. The negative modulators are high concentrations of ATP, long-chain fatty acids, and citrate, as well as phosphocreatine, glyceraldehyde phosphate, and phosphoenol pyruvate. This complex dependence speaks for the efficiency of the system in energy conservation. Thus, when there is a large store of high-energy bonds in ATP, citrate, or fatty acids, the rate of glycolysis is controlled by the allosteric deac-

Fig. 7.3. The NAD/NADH systems on either side of the mitochondrial membranes are distinct. Reducing equivalents may be interchanged through the α-ketoglutarate-malate shuttle systems as indicated.

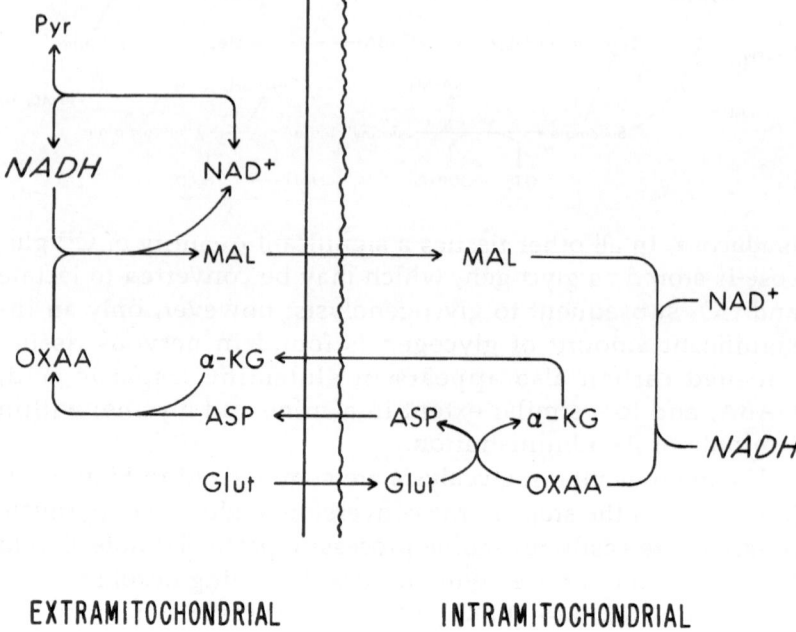

EXTRAMITOCHONDRIAL   INTRAMITOCHONDRIAL

Chapter 7: Oxidative Metabolism in Cerebral Ischemia

tivation of 6-phosphofructokinase. PFK is also inhibited by a relatively acid pH and is activated by alkalosis. This may provide an important mechanism for the control of intracellular pH in hypo- and hypercapnia.

Pyruvate kinase catalyzes the conversion of phosphoenolypyruvate and ADP to pyruvate and ATP. This is also an allosteric enzyme which requires potassium and, like PFK, is inhibited by elevated concentrations of ATP and long-chain fatty acids. Alanine and acetyl-CoA are also inhibitors. Fructose 1,6-diphosphate and phosphoenolypyruvate are both positive modulators at elevated concentrations. It is apparent, therefore, that the rate of glycolysis may be influenced by several factors at these crucial enzymatic steps. Under maximal stimulation, the rate of glycolysis can be increased five- to seven-fold, but glycolysis alone is still able to satisfy only about 30% of the energy requirements of the tissue.

Electron-Transport Systems

Under aerobic conditions pyruvate formed by glycolysis enters the tricarboxylic acid (TCA) cycle. The production of acetyl-CoA, α-ketoglutarate, succinyl-CoA, fumarate, and oxaloacetate in the TCA cycle (see Fig. 7.1) provides reducing equivalents (as hydrogen or electrons) for the mitochondrial electron-transport chain. These reducing equivalents are then passed along the electron-transport chain on the inner mitochondrial membrane via an ordered series of pyridine nucleotides (NADH/NAD$^+$), flavoprotein coenzymes (FADH/FAD$^+$), and cytochromes (CYT b, c, c_1, $a + a_3$). Each of these coenzymes exist in both an oxidized and reduced form in a proportion determined by their equilibrium potential, the availability of oxidizeable substrates, and the concentration of available oxygen. The progression of these reducing equivalents along the transport chain depends on the presence of adequate amounts of oxygen, which functions as the terminal electron acceptor (see Fig. 7.2).

The intact mitochondrial membrane is impermeable to the pyridine nucleotides. Therefore the NAD/NADH in the electron-transport chain is distinct from the NAD/NADH in the cytoplasm. Reducing equivalents are not directly interchangeable between the two systems. However, the α-ketoglutarate and malate/oxaloacetate shuttle system are used for this exchange, as indicated in Figure 7.3. An equilibrium is recognized between the cytoplasmic NADH/NAD redox couple and the concentration of intracellular lactate and pyruvate. This is expressed as:

$$\frac{NADH}{NAD^+} = \frac{Lac}{Pyr} \cdot \frac{K}{(H+)}$$

Lactate and pyruvate are in free communication with the extracellular fluid and CSF, and elevations of the extracellular lactate/pyruvate ratio may be an indication of the redox state of the tissue, with the qualification that the equilibrium reaction is pH-dependent. These relationships become important, since local acidosis due to hypercapnia may change the Lac/Pyr ratio in the absence of a change in the cortical redox state.(30)

Oxidative Phosphorylation

At each of the three points indicated in Figure 7.2, the oxidation-reduction potential changes are large enough to provide the necessary energy for ATP synthesis. The specific mechanism by which electron transport results in the production of ATP (oxidative phosphorylation) generates lively discussion, and it is still unsettled. Three postulates appear to be most reasonable: (1) *chemical coupling*, which requires the existence of a high-energy intermediate and is similar to substrate-level phosphorylation; (2) *conformational coupling*, which presupposes that the alteration in the inner mitochondrial membrane that is observed during phosphorylation is either responsible for or intimately involved in phosphorylation; and (3) *chemiosmotic coupling*, which presents the thesis that the mitochondria generate hydrogen gradients (chemiosmotic gradient) due to substrate oxidation and that this gradient then serves as the driving force for the reversal of the membrane-bound ATPase of the mitochondria. While the consensus is now in favor of the chemiosmotic coupling hypothesis, there is growing evidence to indicate that all three mechanisms contribute to the overall picture.

Electron transport may be coupled to the production of high-energy phosphates, which is influenced in turn by the ADP concentration. Electron transport may also be uncoupled for such alternative processes (see Figure 2) as the accumulation of divalent cations such as Ca^{2+}(19) or for energy-linked conformation changes of mitochondrial membranes. For every pair of electrons passing from NADH to oxygen, six Ca^{2+} ions may be accumulated from the medium. Uncoupling may also be induced pharamocologically by chemicals, such as dinitrophenol, triethyltin, and salicylates. Likewise, when the ionophorous antibiotics Valinomycin and Gramicidin cause accumulation of monovalent cations, such as K^+, in the mitochondria, oxidation and phosphorylation are uncoupled(24) as a function of the concentration of the ionophore. At high concentrations in the presence of K^+ and Pi, the mitochondria no longer phosphorylate ADP. Whenever uncoupling occurs, the rate of cellular respiration may be increased, but the free energy trapped in the glucose molecule is liberated as heat rather than chemical energy. It has been suggested that after anoxic cell injury there is uncoupling of oxidative phosphorylation.(22)

A more immediate consequence of anoxia is that electrons cannot be transferred from cytochrome $a–a_3$, so that this system becomes more reduced. Because of the buffering effect of this carrier system, the flavoprotein and NAD systems will not be reduced until the cytochromes have been reduced. Less ATP will be generated by the mitochondria, and Pi and AMP will increase. Soon a rise in ADP and a fall in ATP will activate PFK and PK to produce an increase in the rate of glycolysis. Eventually the redox couple of the system with the highest negative electromotive force, namely NADH/NAD, also becomes more reduced, and reducing equivalents generated by the TCA cycle will no longer be accommodated by the electron-transport chain.

Cerebral Ischemia

Much information on the metabolic consequences of anoxia and ischemia has been derived from analysis of acutely excised samples of brain tissue.(20,29,31) Tissue hypoxia activates glycolysis, resulting in increased production of lactic acid. The tissue acidosis that follows may produce an initial hyperemia. But if it is prolonged or severe, the acidosis alone may lead to cell edema and secondary capillary obstruction.

When gradual arterial hypoxemia is produced, significant changes in tissue lactate appear at Po_2 of 40 to 45 mmHg. Phosphocreatine is sensitive to pH change and is decomposed first. Then ATP, ADP, and AMP levels change as the Po_2 drops from 35 to 25 mmHg. Since the circulation is maintained, lactate does not accumulate in large quantities.

In ischemia secondary to systemic hypotension, however, the lactoacidosis is detectable as blood pressure is reduced, but it is still within the range of autoregulation. When hypotension is induced by hemorrhage,(31) elevated lactate/pyruvate ratios are already found at perfusion pressures in the range of 40 to 85 mmHg. Changes in the level of the energy metabolites phosphocreatine, ATP, ADP, and AMP, however, are not found until a mean blood pressure of 30 to 35 mmHg is achieved. When cerebral perfusion pressure is decreased by increasing intracranial pressure, the critical perfusion pressure for changes in labile phosphates was somewhat lower (24–30 mmHg), with correspondingly smaller changes in tissue lactate.(28) All of these changes can be delayed by agents such as barbiturates and 2% Halothane, which tend to depress the rate of oxidative metabolism more than the rate of cerebral blood flow. Therefore, these agents are said to play a protective role in ischemic and anoxic brain insults.

Normally the rate of nutrient supply to the brain is closely regulated by the rate of nutrient consumption.(13) With increased electrophysiologic activity, an increase in metabolic activity will evoke a hyperemia, while suppression of functional activity results in a decrease in blood flow. Therefore, a subnormal blood flow rate does not imply the presence of ischemia if it occurs in response to an appropriate metabolic cue.

Ischemia is therefore defined as a state in which the nutrient supply is insufficient for the metabolic requirements of the tissue at that moment. In the intact animal, nutrient supply can be estimated either from the blood flow rate or from the level of oxygen availability.(12) The rates of oxygen and glucose consumption have traditionally been measured in excised tissue slices. Until recently, it has not been possible to measure either local oxygen or glucose consumption rates in vivo.

A recent modification of oxygen polarography(9) allows one to estimate the rate of oxygen extraction from cortical tissue by assuming a steady state with regard to ambient brain tissue oxygen pressure just prior to the measurement. The cortical redox state can be determined by measuring the level of NADH, which is a sensitive indicator of cellular hypoxia.(5) In the cerebral cortex, 99.3% of the NADH fluorescence is derived from mitochondrial NADH, and 0.7% is derived from the cytoplasmic NADH. These techniques allow one to estimate the oxygen supply and oxygen consumption, and to determine the presence of ischemia in terms of the metabolic balance.

Focal Ischemic Insufficiency

The microvascular neurosurgeon is especially concerned with the treatment of regional ischemia produced by segmental arterial obstruction. In contrast to global ischemia, focal ischemic infarction implies a specific distribution of electrophysiologic,(35) biochemical,(32) and pathological gradients(21) from the central necrotic area to the peripheral periischemic zones. The changes in high-energy phosphate levels following middle cerebral artery (MCA) occlusion are slower and less pronounced (30% of control after 3 hours) than after global ischemia (25% of control after 4 minutes).(32) It is estimated that a cerebral ATP content of 25% of control is the minimal requirement for survival of brain tissue after reinstitution of flow.

The development of microvascular anastomosis as a means of augmenting focal cerebral blood flow (CBF) raises several theoretical and practical questions: (1) Is there a topographic distribution of changes in oxidative metabolism that develops after focal ischemia? (2) Are the nutritional needs of the tissue different within and around the area of ischemia? (3) Do intracerebral nutrient steal effects influence brain tissue recovery after stroke? (4) Is the no-reflow phenomenon an important limiting factor in cerebral revascularization? (5) Does a bypass graft provide a nutritional reservoir which can protect the brain against ischemia? (6) Is there an idealized location of the graft in relation to the ischemic tissue which will make a difference in graft function and hypertrophy? (7) Will placement of the graft in the region of the infarct or in juxtaposition to it make a difference in the clinical outcome? (8) What changes in oxidative metabolism can be expected to ensue from a focal augmentation of CBF?

Oxidative Metabolism in Focal Ischemic Insufficiency

The patterns of oxidative metabolism which develop with focal ischemic infarction were studied in 27 experimental cats in an effort to answer the first four questions. Thirteen adult foxhounds were then used to assess the protective effect of a superficial-temporal–middle-cerebral-artery (STA–MCA) bypass graft on cortical nutritional balance. The rates of blood flow and the oxygen-availability levels were measured by conventional polarographic techniques. The rate of oxygen extraction (OE) of small volumes of brain tissue was assessed by a simple modification of standard polarographic principles.(9) The cortical redox state, which reflects the balance between nutrient supply and demand, was measured on the cortical surface by recording the level of NADH in relation to the terminal anoxic levels.(5) Using these techniques, a functional "cerebrovascular unit" was analyzed, since capillary blood flow, oxygen availability, and cellular oxygen extraction could be repeatedly assessed, and the balance between nutrient supply and demand in cortical units could be determined.

Characteristics of the Evolving Ischemic Infarction

Methods

To measure the local blood flow, oxygen availability, and oxygen-extraction slope, polarographic electrodes were passed through a pial window into the cortex, using the operating microscope. This window was designed to accommodate both platinum electrodes and a fiber optic light guide.(15) These could be positioned and focused to record from ectosylvian cortex in the distribution of the MCA, or from the medially located anterior lateral gyri, in the distribution of the anterior cerebral

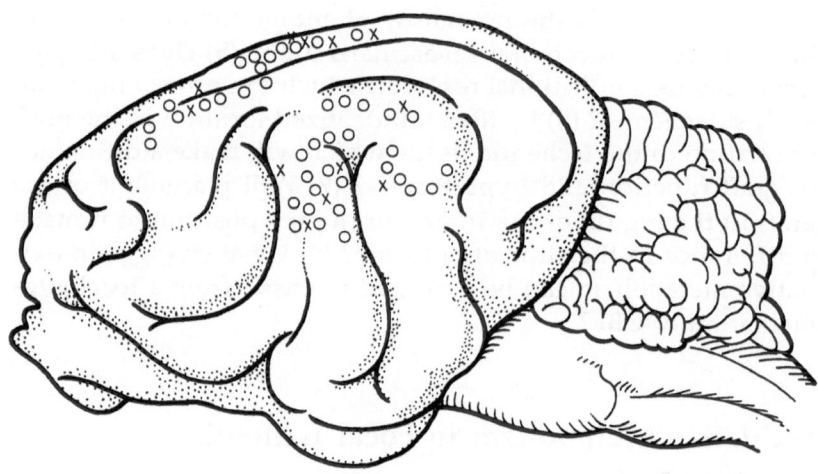

Fig. 7.4. Electrode locations in 27 experimental cat brains. O: indicates cortical placement; X: indicates subcortical placement. Electrodes placed over the convexity (ectosylvian cortex) sampled from tissue within the ischemic zone proper, whereas those placed more medially recorded from tissue peripheral to the zone of ischemia.

artery (see Fig. 7.4). The electrodes were connected by spring coil connections to copper leads on the David Kopf* stereotactic apparatus. Loose umbilical tape ligatures were placed around both common carotid arteries to facilitate transient carotid occlusion. All animals were intubated and given d-tubocurarine (0.5 mg/kg).** Respirations were controlled with a Harvard variable phase/volume respirator.*** Steady-state local (CBF) values were intermittently determined using the hydrogen-desaturation method.(7) Oxygen-availability levels were measured as described by Jamieson.(12) Appropriate arterial blood gas samples were taken and pH, Pco_2, and Po_2 were measured on a BMS-3 Mark II blood gas analyzer.° Measurements of the oxygen-extraction slope were made by transiently (10 seconds) interrupting common carotid blood flow bilaterally with the umbilical tape ligatures. This produced an immediate drop in the level of oxygen availability recorded from areas irrigated by the carotid arteries. The slope of this drop was expressed in arbitrary units as a change of voltage in a fixed time interval, and at comparable levels of oxygen availability reflected the rate of oxygen extraction by the local brain tissue. This allowed recording from within and peripheral to areas of ischemic infarction produced by transorbital occlusion of the previously exposed MCA. At the conclusion of each experiment a diathermy lesion was made through the electrodes to verify their location in relation to the area of infarction.

The level of NADH fluorescence in the cortex was measured adjacent to the polarographic electrodes. This was accomplished by using a direct-reading, time-sharing Chance reflecto-fluorometer. When the cerebral cortex is illuminated with

*David Kopf, Tujunga, Calif.
**d-tubocurarine, Abbott Laboratories, Inc., North Chicago, Ill.
***Harvard Apparatus, Mills, Mass.

a light source of a specific wave length (366 nm), the cortex will in part absorb this light and in part reflect it. In addition, it will emit fluorescent light of a higher wave length (450 nm), derived from the reduced form of pyridine nucleotide (NADH), which is excited by the 366-nm light.(5) The amount of reflectance and fluorescence returning from the cortex is influenced by scatter and absorption in the cortical parenchyma. The main absorbing substance is the circulating blood present in the field of measurement. This effect has been demonstrated previously, and a corrected fluorescence signal, free from hemodynamic artifacts, was achieved by subtracting the reflectance signal from the fluorescence signal, leaving a pure NADH fluorescence signal (corrected fluorescence). Blood pressure, blood flow, oxygen availability, reflectance, fluorescence, corrected fluorescence, and two symmetric EEG leads were recorded on a Brush 848 recorder.

Results

The Steady State

Despite attempts to position all electrodes within the cortex, 25 electrodes were placed in the right ectosylvian cortex and six electrodes were placed in the corresponding subcortical white

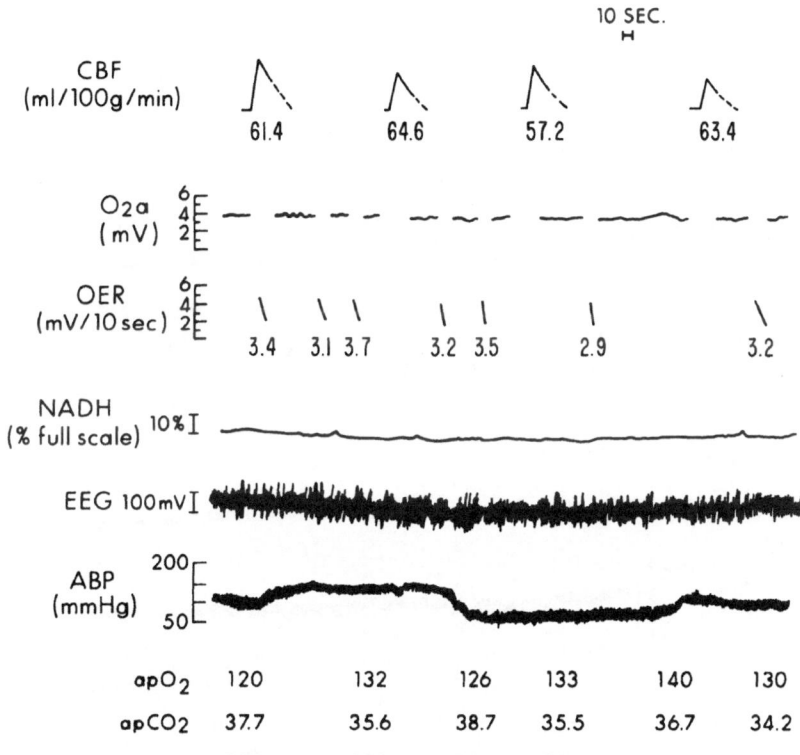

Fig. 7.5. Simultaneous measurement of CBF, O_2a, OER, NADH, EEG, and arterial blood pressure (ABP). Despite a 32% rise in ABP, there is less than a 7% change in CBF and no significant alteration of oxygen extraction or redox state.

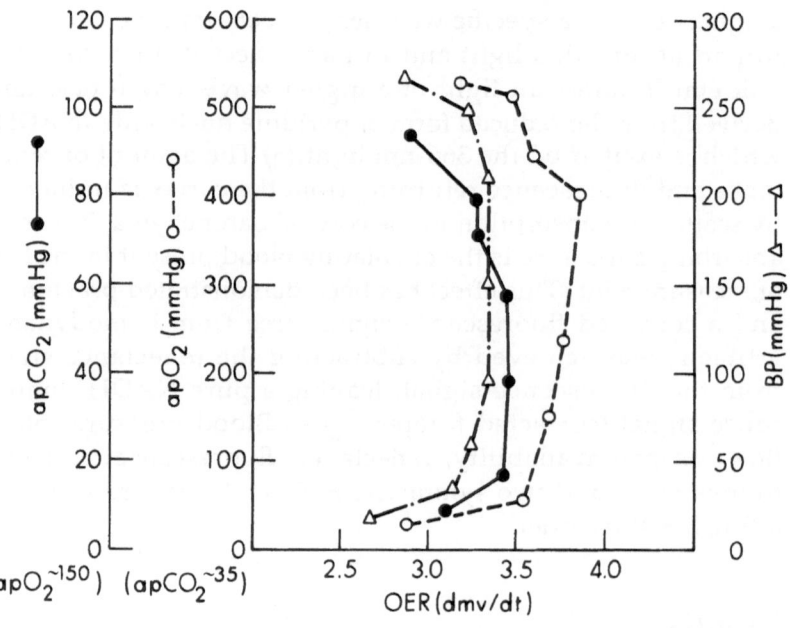

Fig. 7.6. The influence of changes of arterial Pco_2 Po_2 and blood pressure on the oxygen-extraction slopes (OER). Significant alterations of OER are seen at extremes. Observed OER change in the steady state may be related therefore to changes in the metabolic extraction rate of oxygen by the parenchyma.

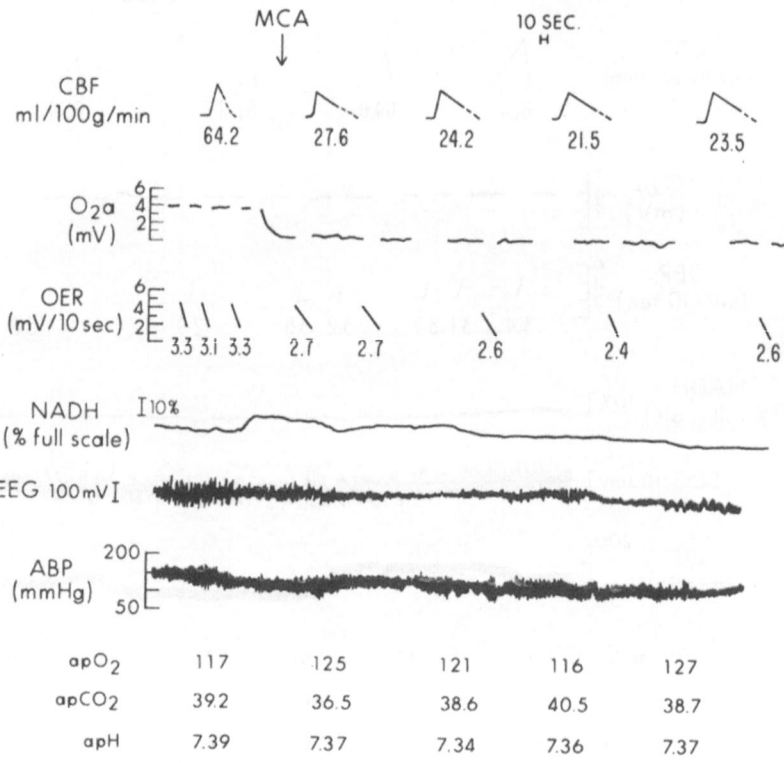

Fig. 7.7. Recording from ectosylvian electrode in relation to MCA occlusion. Rapid drop in CBF, O_2a, and oxygen-extraction rate with a redox shift indicated by a rise in NADH. Suppression of EEG amplitude and frequency after approximately 40 seconds.

Chapter 7: Oxidative Metabolism in Cerebral Ischemia

matter. Twenty-two electrodes were placed in the cortex of the right anterior lateral gyri (medial electrodes) and six electrodes were placed in the corresponding subcortical white matter (see Figure 7.4).

In the normal cat under steady-state conditions (mean blood pressure 111 ± 7 mmHg, arterial Po_2 of 97.5 ± 11 mmHg, arterial $aPco_2$ 32.0 ± 55 mmHg, and arterial pH of $7.41 \pm .07$ pH units) the mean local cortical blood flow was 67.2 ± 11.4 cm^3/100 g/minute, and the mean local subcortical blood flow was 21.6 ± 8.2 cm^3/100 g/minute. Over 96% of the hydrogen washout curves from both cortex and subcortex conformed to a single exponential, correlating (>0.9985) with a straight-line equation. Of all electrode sites, 88% showed close autoregulation of flow to Levophed (levarterenol bitartarte 2–4 mcg/minute) induced hypertension with less than 10% change in cortical and subcortical blood flow values despite a 26% increase in mean blood pressure (see Fig. 7.5). Data from electrodes showing poor autoregulation (3 ectosylvian, 4 medial) as well as the data from subcortical electrodes was not used for further analysis.

The level of oxygen availability in grey matter remained stable, with no significant change in voltage (± 0.42 mV) under basal conditions. The oxygen availability waves oscillated at a frequency of 10 to 17 cpm and at an amplitude up to 25% of the baseline voltage. Levophed-induced hypertension immediately reduced the amplitude and then the frequency of the spontaneous oxygen waves. However, the baseline levels of oxygen availability were increased to a mean of 8% and a maximum of 12% by a mean blood pressure increase of 32%.

The oxygen-extraction slopes of cortex were three to five times steeper than those of subcortex. Oxygen-extraction slopes in the ectosylvian cortex did not show a significant difference from those recorded from the medial gyri under basal conditions. The effect of hemodynamic variations on the oxygen-extraction slopes was tabulated in 14 of the 27 cats in this series. This is illustrated in Figure 7.6. There was a range of values, for arterial Po_2, Pco_2, and mean blood pressure, over which the oxygen-extraction slope remained relatively constant. At very high and very low values the slopes became dependent on physical-diffusion gradients.

The circular area adjacent to the electrode from which the NADH signal was recorded measured approximately 600 μ diameter. The cortical NADH fluorescence under normoxic conditions (100%) and under full anoxic conditions (0%) were the reference levels against which all other changes were compared. There were no significant changes in the level of cortical fluorescence from either the ectosylvian or the more medial gyri, despite the blood pressure changes previously described to test the presence of autoregulation.

Early Hemodynamic and Metabolic Response to Focal Ischemia

Within 3 to 5 seconds after closing the clip on the MCA artery a mean drop of $44 \pm 8\%$ of the steady-state oxygen availability level was seen (see Fig. 7.7) in ectosylvian electrodes. A less obvious decrease in O_2a ($12 \pm 4\%$) was seen in the medial zone where the changes in O_2a were slower in onset, less in amplitude, and usually transient. In 4 of the 20 medial electrodes, application of the MCA clip was followed by a transient (11–50-minute) period of compensatory hyperemia (10–30% increase in O_2a) (see Fig. 7.8).

Steady-state measurements of local CBF with hydrogen showed a good correlation with the oxygen-availability data. After MCA occlusion, mean local cortical blood flow of all electrodes in the ectosylvian gyrus was 34.6 cm³/100 g/minute. This was significantly lower than control values ($P<0.001$). Four medial electrodes showed an increased flow, with a mean value of 71.5 cm³/100 g/minute. By 1 hour after MCA occlusion, the mean flow of the four medial electrodes decreased to 64.7 cm³/100 g/minute. The local CBF in the remaining 16 electrodes in the medial region was 66.8 cm³/100 g/minute after MCA occlusion, which was not significantly different than control values.

The mean rates of oxygen extraction in medial cortical tissue initially showed no overall change, but they were relatively less

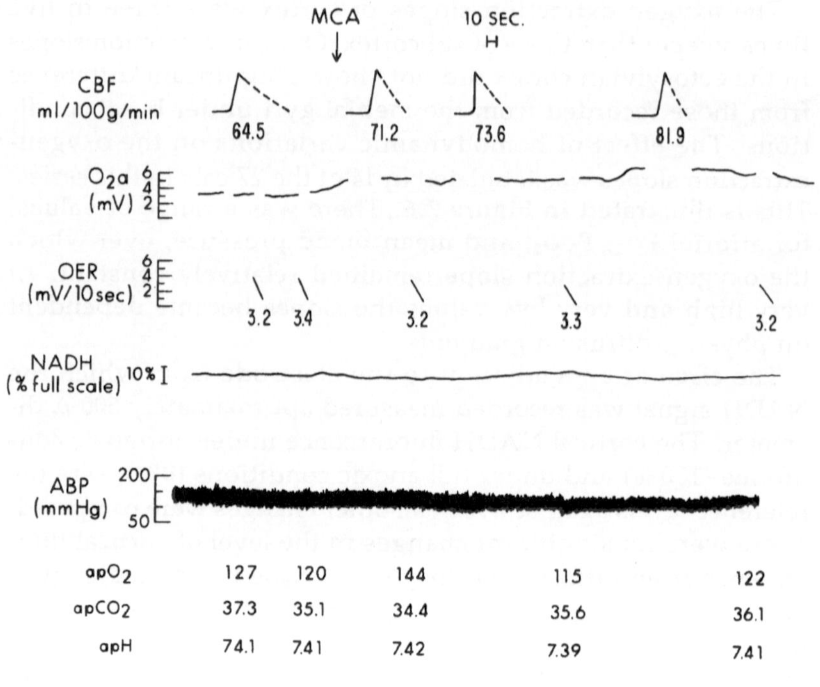

Fig. 7.8. Recording from medial zone peripheral to zone of ischemia in relation to MCA occlusion. A compensatory hyperemia is seen with no significant augmentation of oxygen-extraction rate or further oxidation of cortical NADH.

stable and changed over the course of 1 to 8 hours after MCA occlusion. Individual electrodes showed initial decreases ($n=4$), increases ($n=11$), and no change ($n=6$). In 17 electrodes the changes were transient (<2 hours), but in 4 electrodes the initial changes persisted throughout the period of serial studies (up to 18 hours after MCA occlusion). One hour after MCA occlusion the mean slope of all medial cortical electrodes was 4.27 ± 0.08 ($p<0.01$).

Within 4.5 ± 0.6 seconds after applying the clip to the MCA, a detectable increase of NADH fluorescence was seen in the ectosylvian gyrus in all 27 cats. The same change was detectable in the medial zone in 14 cats within 11.4 ± 0.5 seconds. In 4 of 14 medial recordings the NADH rise was transient, with a duration of 280 ± 42 minutes after MCA occlusion. In only 3 of 27 ectosylvian recordings was the NADH rise transient (duration 214 ± 37 minutes), while in the remaining 24 recordings the increased fluorescence persisted until termination of the experiment.

Zone of Infarction

The animals were sacrificed between 4 and 18 hours after occlusion of the right MCA (mean time to sacrifice 11.5 hours). Ischemic infarction was found in all of the brains examined, although there was a significant variation in the apparent extent of the process. These borders were not perfectly sharp, however, and the criteria for establishing them were based on a combination of gross visual observations of pallor, histologic assessment of ischemic cell change, and necrosis and palpable evidence of softening. These criteria helped to localize the electrodes either within or peripheral to the infarction zone.

Of the 25 cortical electrodes placed in the ectosylvian gyrus, 21 were clearly located within necrotic tissue. One electrode (E14) was posterior and one electrode (E20) was medial to the apparent infarction (see Figure 4).

Of the 22 medially placed electrodes, 15 were clearly in normal-appearing tissue. Three electrodes were in such proximity to the infarction that they were considered to be within the infarction zone. The zone of infarction extended far enough medially in two brains to encompass two other electrodes (M4, M17).

On this basis it was determined that 19 ectosylvian and 5 medial electrodes were within the zone of infarction, and 1 ectosylvian and 15 medial electrodes were peripheral to the zone of infarction. Since the physiologic responses from these electrodes are dependent on their relations to the infarcted zone, they will be identified as zone-of-infarction (ZI) electrodes or peripheral electrodes.

Cerebrovascular Unit in Focal Ischemia

In 19 cats it was possible to follow the later evolution (> 1 hr) of focal ischemia by simultaneous measurement of oxygen-availability and oxygen-extraction rate in the same cortical locus. These parameters, reflecting the nutrient supply and nutrient consumption, described the metabolic behavior of individual cerebrovascular units within the ischemic infarction and in the cortex peripheral to the infarction. A determination was then made on the basis of the cortical redox state (NADH) at each location as to whether the unit was ischemic or nonischemic. Within these two categories several subtypes were described by the relationship of blood flow to the oxygen-extraction slope (see Fig. 7.9).

Ischemic Cerebrovascular Units

Subtype A   Low flow, low oxygen extraction: This was the most common pattern seen within the ZI. Eleven of the 24 ZI electrodes, as well as 3 of the 16 peripheral electrodes, demonstrated low flow and low oxygen-extraction slopes. At all of these locations there was an increase of NADH fluorescence. In 7 of the 11 ZI electrodes and in all 3 of the peripheral electrodes the change in extraction rate followed a change in the O_2a by 6 to 10 minutes (see Fig. 7.10). In four ZI electrodes it preceded the O_2a change by 10, 11, 14, and 20 minutes (see Fig. 7.11).

Subtype B   Low flow, high oxygen extraction: This was seen in 3 of 24 ZI electrodes and in 5 of 16 peripheral electrodes. This subtype and subtype E (described below) were the most common patterns seen in the periphery. Subtype B is an ischemic unit, as evidenced by the significant and sustained increase in cortical NADH fluorescence.

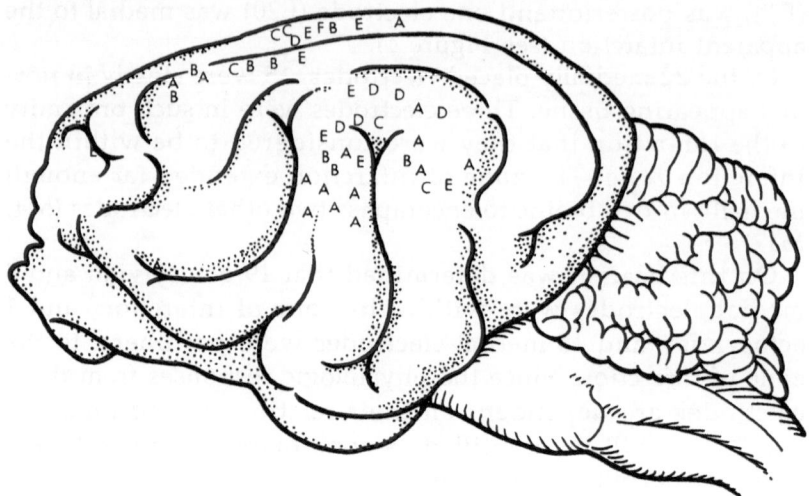

Fig. 7.9. The development of cerebrovascular units after MCA occlusion. The subtypes defined in the text were distributed in relation to the zone of infarction in the ectosylvian area and peripheral to the zone of infarction in the medial gyri.

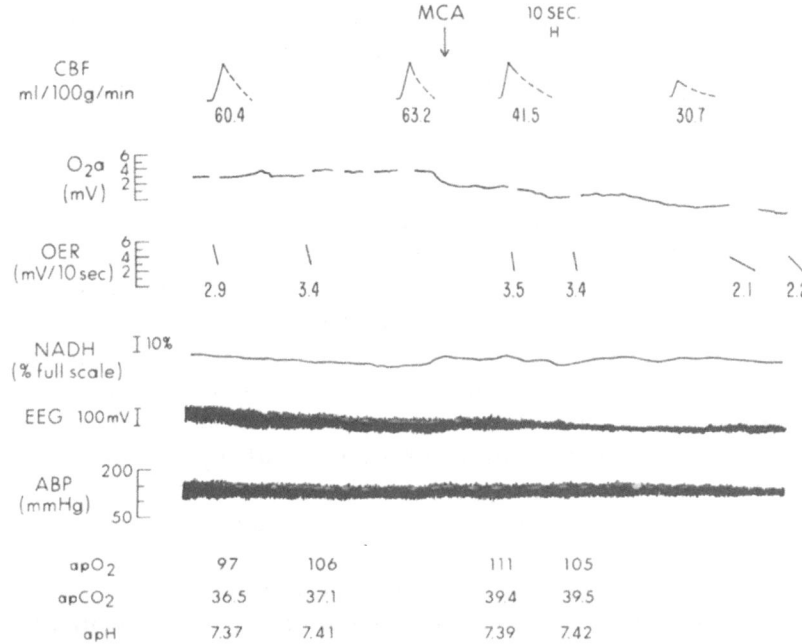

Fig. 7.10. Recording from electrode within the zone of infarction. The reduction in nutrient supply indicated by the low oxygen availability evoked an ischemic signal (NADH). A reduced oxygen-extraction rate later in the experiment was evidence of secondary injury to the cellular oxygen-extraction mechanism.

Subtype C High flow, very high oxygen extraction: Despite the relative hyperemia signified by an increased oxygen availability (170% of control), these units showed an increased cortical NADH fluorescence. The oxygen-extraction slopes were more than twice the steady-state values at 3 of 16 peripheral

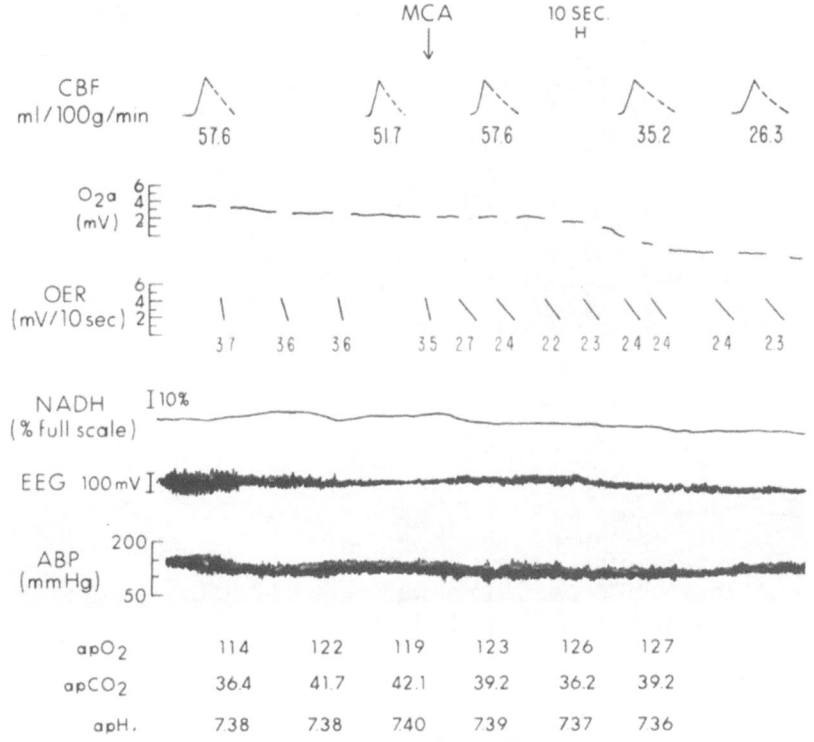

Fig. 7.11. Recording from electrode within the zone of infarction. MCA occlusion resulted in a rapid drop in oxygen-extraction rate simultaneous with a change in frequency and amplitude of the EEG. Because of the decrease in functional activity of the tissue a secondary decrease in oxygen availability was seen 11 minutes later.

electrodes. Two of the 24 ZI electrodes also showed this pattern. These were relatively unstable units; one of the peripheral units converted to a subtype D unit (described below), and one converted to a subtype E unit (described below). Both ZI units were unstable and converted to subtype D units.

Nonischemic Cerebrovascular Units

Subtype D   Low flow, low oxygen extraction: Six ZI electrodes showed low flow values, but cortical NADH fluorescence was not significantly elevated despite this apparent ischemia. The oxygen-extraction slopes at all six locations were significantly less steep than control values. There were no clear examples of this pattern peripheral to the zone of infarction. However, one unit, which had the characteristics of subtype C, showed a decrease in flow and oxygen extraction and an increased NADH fluorescence 2 to 5 hours after MCA occlusion.

Subtype E   High flow, low oxygen extraction: Four ZI and 2 peripheral electrodes showed this pattern. One additional pe-

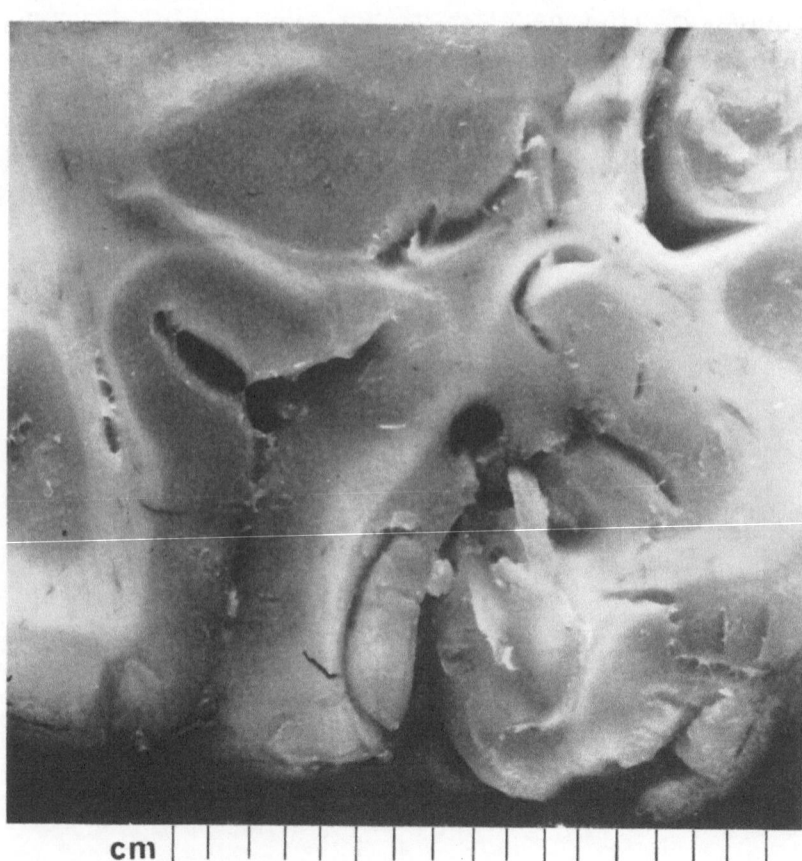

Fig. 7.12. Coronal section (spec. 107) indicating electrode location in close proximity to sulcal artery.

SPEC 107

Chapter 7: Oxidative Metabolism in Cerebral Ischemia

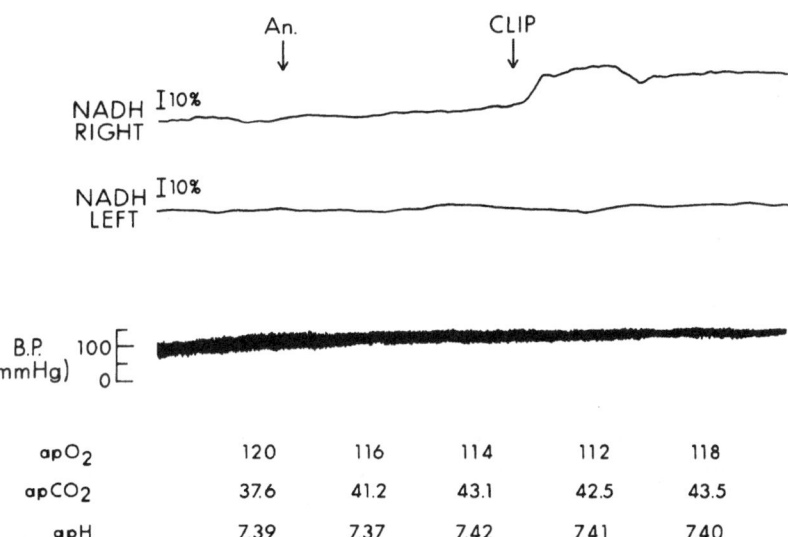

apO_2	120	116	114	112	118
$apCO_2$	37.6	41.2	43.1	42.5	43.5
apH	7.39	7.37	7.42	7.41	7.40

Fig. 7.13. Cortical redox state measured over homotopic areas of cortex. The left side protected by an STA–MCA anastomosis showed no significant rise of NADH after clipping proximal to the anastomosis. The unprotected side showed an immediate rise in NADH when a corresponding cortical artery was clipped.

ripheral site converted from type C as described. Aside from that exception, cortical NADH fluorescence did not change significantly at these locations after MCA occlusion. The oxygen-extraction rates at these electrodes were either unchanged or significantly lower than in the control state.

Subtype F Very high flow, high oxygen extraction: These units all developed steep oxygen-extraction slopes. They were accompanied by very high flow values and unchanged levels of cortical NADH fluorescence. Four units in the periphery showed this pattern; there were no such examples within the zone of infarction. One of these electrodes was in close relationship to a pial artery (see Fig. 7.12).

Protective Effect of EC–IC Anastomosis — Dog Experiments

Thirteen adult foxhounds were intubated and anesthesized with nitrous oxide/oxygen; respirations were controlled and arterial blood pressure and blood gases were monitored as described above. Bilateral craniectomies were performed and the MCA in the distal portion of the sylvian fissure was identified bilaterally. A microanastomosis between the STA and the largest visible branch of the MCA was performed on the left side. This was technically successful in 10 dogs.

A region of cortex, approximately 1 cm distal to the anastomosis and adjacent to the cortical artery, was selected for a baseline recording of the NADH fluorescence level. Small, straight Heifitz aneurysm clips were simultaneously applied to the cortical artery proximal to the anastomoses on the left and on the corresponding homotopic artery on the right side.

In 6 of the 10 dogs a significant rise of the NADH was seen on the right side within 5 seconds of applying the clip (see Fig. 7.13). In 1 dog, a significant rise of the NADH was seen on both sides, but it was transient (1.75 minutes) on the operated side and persisted for more than 5 hours on the unoperated side.

In 3 dogs there was no detectable rise of NADH on either side after clipping the cortical artery.

Discussion

The metabolic consequences of anoxia alone, or anoxia complicated by ischemia, have been elucidated by fluoremetric tissue assay techniques and kinetic enzyme analysis. These studies have led to an appreciation of the relative roles of energy failure(29) and neurotransmitter failure(4) in limiting the functional recovery from stroke.

Given an ischemic or anoxic insult of known etiology and severity in an intact animal preparation a predictable sequence of changes in glycolytic substrate concentrations, enzyme activities, and, finally, high-energy phosphate stores will ensue. Lesser degrees of ischemia will alter such sensitive electrophysiologic parameters as the EEG frequency and direct cortical response.(33) However, more prolonged ischemia is required before a level of nutritional insufficiency is attained which will produce irreversible structural alterations. The cerebral dysfunction seen clinically after a stroke may therefore be related either to irreversibly damaged neurons, to the presence of non-functional but still viable neurons, or to an admixture of both neuronal populations.

The lesions of interest to the microvascular neurosurgeon are those producing focal ischemic insufficiency. The most suitable cases for microvascular bypass surgery include symptomatic patients with an interictally normal brain. Patients with a very restricted neurologic deficit may also be candidates depending on the degree to which the area of injury is composed of ischemic rather than infarcted tissue. Within and surrounding such focal lesions, one would expect to find an admixture of tissue with varying metabolic activity which will place different demands on a bypass graft. The serial changes in oxygen metabolism of such individual subunits, however, have not been previously examined in the intact animal.

The techniques employed here for that purpose allowed an assessment of the adequacy of oxygen supply for the oxidative reactions related to energy metabolism of small volumes of tissue approximately 1 mm^3 in size. Polarographic electrode measurements of oxygen availability as an index of local CBF is well documented. A close correlation between local CBF and oxygen availability is found when oxygen-carrying capacity, arterial pH, and arterial oxygen partial pressure are normal.(12) The electrode used to measure the level of oxygen availability was also used to estimate the rate of oxygen extraction. These small tissue volumes, therefore, constitute cerebrovascular units with definable nutrient input and output functions. Presumably, a population of such units contributes to the average metabolic and hemodynamic changes recorded by more conventional assessments of regional CBF and oxygen consumption.

The model of middle cerebral occlusion consistently produced a small ischemic infarction limited to the cortical grey and subcortical white matter of the sylvian and ectosylvian gyri. In 2 animals the infarction extended into the more medial suprasylvian and anterolateral gyri. In these animals the area of softening also included the caudate nucleus, putamen, and adjacent internal capsule. However, since our main interest was in correlating the redox state of the tissue with its nutrient supply and demand, only cortical areas were studied. Although accurate placement of polarographic electrodes in cortex is difficult, a short active tip (~0.5 mm) was used and the electrodes were placed tangential to the cortex under 25× magnification provided by the operating microscope.

The artifacts encountered in fluorometric surface recording and in the estimation of oxygen-extraction rates have been treated in detail previously(15) and will not be repeated here. Suffice to say that when the methods are combined it is important to be sure that the fluorometric signal originates from the same tissue that is elaborating the signal for the oxygen electrode. Since the fluorometric signal arises from the mitochondrial NADH of the uppermost 0.5 mm of cortex, and the oxygen signal is derived from the superficial 0.5 mm^3 of tissue, it is possible to record from functionally congruous tissue volumes.

The results of these studies should be considered in the light of our present concepts of metabolic control of blood flow rates, ischemic injury to the cellular systems concerned with oxygen utilization, and the so-called "no-reflow" and "luxury" flow (luxury-perfusion) phenomenon.

Alterations in aP_{CO_2}, perivascular pH, hypoxia, transmural pressure, and perhaps neurogenic stimuli contribute to the tonic and phasic influences on arterial caliber and the rate of blood flow.(8) There is also growing evidence that rapid variations in the nutritional needs of the parenchyma act to influence the flow rate. We have previously demonstrated a close relationship of the cortical redox state to the compensatory vasodilation seen after pulsatile hypotensive stresses.(15) Bicher(3) has suggested the presence of oxygen sensors in tissue which act to vary CBF locally. Ozanne et al,(26) using oxygen polarographic microelectrodes, have shown triangular patterns of oxygen waves asynchronous with the peripheral pulse. The latter is most consistent with a capillary bed which opens and closes rhythmically in response to variations in metabolic requirements of the tissue. Increases(17) and decreases(8) in cerebral functional and presumed metabolic activity have been correlated with predictable alterations in local blood flow rates.

The close relationship of metabolic rates and blood flow rate seen in the normal brain, however, was significantly perturbed by the focal ischemic insult produced in these studies. Six characteristic unit subtypes emerged after ischemia. In two of these (subtypes B and E) flow changes and metabolic changes occurred in opposite directions. Furthermore, the time course of metabolic changes was not predictable in relation to a corresponding change in blood flow rate. Several units within the zone of ischemia showed a decrease in oxygen-extraction rate prior to a decrease in oxygen availability. Presumably, this could occur if these units were functionally suppressed by a reduced electrophysiologic input from adjacent units.(10) A decreased oxygen-extraction rate may then have acted to reduce the local oxygen-availability rate secondarily.

In the steady state there was little influence of changes in hemodynamic parameters such as CBF, oxygen availability, and arterial Pco_2, on oxygen extraction rate over a wide range (see Fig. 7.6). This has also been demonstrated for the effect of total CBF on whole-brain oxygen consumption. As flow is reduced there is more efficient utilization of oxygen delivered to tissue and an increase in the arteriovenous oxygen difference. At a certain threshold level this compensatory mechanism fails, and whole-brain oxygen consumption decreases.(14) In the ischemic units sampled by our electrodes a fall in CBF resulted first in a transient increase in oxygen extraction at most ZI electrodes. This fall in oxygen-extraction rate may have been the result of a desaturation of enzymes such as *cytochrome* oxidase in the presence of a reduced oxygen availability. Using uncalibrated polographic electrodes we have been unable to assess the threshold level below which oxygen availability itself limits the rate of oxygen extraction.

The persistent decrease in oxygen extraction seen after 1 hour of ischemia may be related to an injury to the mitochondrial apparatus itself. There is some evidence from in vitro studies that mitochondria may be relatively resistant to anoxic injury. Schutz et al(29) found that mitochondrial suspension retained their ability for oxidative phosphorylation despite 37 minutes of ischemia. Conversely there is suggestive evidence(23) that the flavin adenine nucleotide and coenzyme Q components of the elctron-transport chain within mitochondria may act as free radicals to destroy lipid membranes after an anoxic injury. In either case, when mitochondrial electron transport is slowed by anoxia, reducing equivalents accumulate at flavoprotein and pass through the shuttle system described, as well as at four sites on the TCA cycle (see Fig. 7.1) resulting in accumulation of NADH and lactate. The increased fluorescence is therefore a useful indication of ischemic anoxia. Ischemic cerebrovascular units may be localized by the increased NADH levels whenever oxygen supply is outstripped by oxygen consumption and a relative increase in anaerobic glycolysis occurs.

It is not surprising that the areas of ischemia are more widespread than the zone of infarction determined at postmortem examination. It is of interest to note, however, that the ischemia defined in such terms may evolve either from a relatively inadequate oxygen supply or a relative increased rate of oxygen utilization by the tissue. Examples of both types of changes were to be found in both areas examined, but more units within the zone of infarction showed evidence of ischemia resulting from failure to maintain normal flow rate. In the periphery there was evidence that metabolic demand was abnormally high and exceeded the ability of the injured cerebrovascular bed to meet these demands.

It is apparent that revascularization of the brain implies that the intrinsic cerebral vasculature is still patent and capable of reflow. Impaired reflow following diffuse ischemia was found by Ames et al(1) using several methods for its demonstration and has been attributed to capillary blockade from microthrombic and/or mural swelling. A persisting circulatory failure has thus been invoked to account in part for the failure of recovery from ischemia. Within the zone of focal infarction in our experiments, however, there were no regions found to be totally devoid of flow when assessed by either oxygen availability, hydrogen wash-in, or wash-out determinations. On the other hand, there were four examples of near-zero oxygen extraction in the presence of high or normal oxygen availability (type E). Within a small focal infarction some units may be nonviable as a direct result of neuronal injury apart from a failure of reperfusion. We would not expect surgical augmentation of flow to result in improved function of units such as these, but rather of units whose rates of extraction are persistently limited by rates of nutritional supply. Within the zone of infarction the nutritional requirements appear to be less than at the periphery of the lesion.

There were a large number of units in the periphery as well as a few units within the infarct with an increased rate of oxygen extraction (subtypes B, C, and F). Subtypes B and C were ischemic with very high NADH levels. The oxygen-extraction rates were apparently greater than the associated levels of oxygen availability. Subtype F units also had increased oxygen-extraction rates, but the demands of these units were satisfied by equally high rates of nutrient supply. The behavior of such cerebrovascular units may underlie the luxury-perfu-

Table 7.1 Cerebrovascular unit characteristics in focal ischemia

Ischemic Unit (NADH)	Electrode Locus	
Subtype	ZI	Periph
A. Low F[a], low OE[b]	11	3
B. Low F, high OE	3	5
C. High F, very high OE	2	3
Nonischemic Unit (or normal NADH)		
D. Low F, low OE	6	1
E. High F, low OE	4	3
F. Very high F, high OE	0	4
[c]Total Units	24	17

[a]F: flow based on oxygen-availability level

[b]OE: oxygen-extraction slope.

[c]Units appearing twice indicated by dashed line.

sion phenomenon first described by Lassen(18) to explain the hyperemia around an area of ischemia infarction. Lassen related this to vasodilatation in response to local tissue acidosis — in effect, a passive vasodilatation. The increased rate of oxygen extraction found in many of these units suggests, however, that the hyperemia may be an appropriate response to increased metabolic activity. It is also of interest that there is a wide degree of inhomogeneity of these metabolic rates in adjacent cerebrovascular units. Comparable areas of inhomogeneous glucose metabolism have, however, also been found by Ginsburg et al(11) in a focal ischemic insult produced in the cat by simultaneous occlusion of the MCA and common carotid arteries. A zone of greatly depressed (CMR) glu occurred consistently within the ischemic caudate nucleus but peripheral to that was a rim of increased (CMR) glu, suggesting enhanced anaerobic glycolysis. The increased oxygen extraction found in regions peripheral to the zone of ischemia in our studies suggests at least that some of this increased metabolism may be of the oxidative variety.

The units with increased metabolic activity, particularly the subtype F units found exclusively in the periphery, may act as a "sink" to divert microflow. This may reduce the nutritional supply of the zone of ischemia, further impeding recovery of this tissue. A prerequisite for recovery of tissue from ischemia may require that the metabolic needs of the hyperactive zones are first satisfied or suppressed. Agents such as barbiturates, which selectively depress neural activity, may exert their protective effect on ischemic injury in this manner.

Finally, the presence of an EC–IC bypass graft appeared to have a protective effect on the course of ischemc injury produced by MCA branch occlusion. The superficial temporal artery branch used in these grafts had a diameter 1½ to 2½ times that of the proximal cortical artery sacrificed after the anastomosis. A graft of this size may be useful in maintaining cellular nutrition in the face of a small artery occlusion or embolus. Occlusion of a larger artery may be more devastating; however, the STA–MCA graft may also provide a sufficient blood flow to maintain some cellular function until sufficient collaterals develop. The transient rise in NADH in the presence of patent grafts in 2 animals indicates that although the graft may not always completely protect against the development of ischemia, a partial effect may be useful until sufficient collaterals develop.

ACKNOWLEDGMENTS

This work was supported by NIH RCDA # 5 KO4 NS00198-02, NIH Contract # NO1 NS5-2305 and a Basil O'Connor Starter Research Grant from the National Foundation, March of Dimes.

REFERENCES

1. Ames A III, et al: Cerebral Ischemia. II: The no re-flow phenomenon. Am J Pathol 52:437, 1968
2. Bander A, Kiese M: Die wirkung des sauerstoffubertragenden ferments in mitochondrien aus ratteniebern bei neidrigen sauerstoffdrucken. Arch Exptl Pathol Pharmakol 224:312, 1955
3. Bicher HI, Bruley D, Knisely MH, et al: Effect of microcirculation changes on brain tissue oxygenation. J Physiol 217:689, 1971
4. Brown M, Carlson A, Ljunggren B, et al: Effect of ischemia on monoamine metabolism in the brain. Acta Physiol. Scand. 90:789, 1974
5. Chance B, Oshino N, Sugano T, et al: Basic principles of tissue oxygen determination from mitochondrial signals, in Bicher HI, Bruley DF (eds): Oxygen Transport to Tissue; Instrumentation Methods and Physiology. New York, Plenum, 1970
6. Davis JN, Carlsson A: Effect of hypoxia on tyrosine and tryptophan hydroxylation in unanaesthetized rat brain. J Neurochem 20:913, 1973
7. Fein JM, Willis J, Hamilton J, et al: Polarographic measurement of local cerebral blood flow in the conscious and anesthetized primate. Stroke 6:42, 1975
8. Fein JM: Brain energetics and circulatory control after subarachnoid hemorrhage. J Neurosurg 45:498, 1976
9. Fein JM, Eastman R, Moore CL: Oxidative metabolism in cerebral ischemia. Part 1. Measurement of oxygen extraction slopes of grey and white matter in vivo. Stroke, July–August, 1977
10. Fein JM: Oxidative metabolism in cerebral ischemia. VI. Electrophysiological correlates. Stroke (in press)
11. Ginzberg MD, Reivich M, Giandomenico A: Regional brain glucose metabolism during recovery from transient cerebral ischemia,

in Ingvar D, Lassen U (eds): Cerebral Function, Metabolism and Circulation. Copenhagen, Munksgaard, 1977, pp 6.6–6.7

12. Jamieson AD, Halsey JH: Regional CBF determination by the hydrogen clearance technique and comparison with oxygen availability in the rabbit. Stroke 4:904, 1973

13. Keaney NP, McDowall NG, et al: The time course of the cerebral circulatory response to metabolic depression, in Langfitt T (ed): Cerebral Circulation and Metabolism. New York, Springer-Verlag, 1975, pp 375–377

14. Kety S: Determinants of tissue oxygen tension. Fed Proc 16:666, 1957

15. Keuskamp A, Fein JM: Oxidative metabolism in cerebral ischemia. II. Assessment of rapid changes in local cerebral blood volume and cortical NADH redox state during abrupt and gradual reductions in cerebral perfusion pressure. Stroke (in press)

16. Krogh A: The rate of diffusion of gases through animal tissues with some remarks on the coefficient of invasion. J Physiol (London) 52:391, 1919

17. Larsen B, Shinhøj E, Soh K, et al: The pattern of cortical activity provoked by listening and speech revealed by rCBF measurements, in Ingvar D, Lassen U (eds): Cerebral Function, Metabolism and Circulation. Copenhagen, Munksgaard, 1977, pp 268–269

18. Lassen NA: The luxury-perfusion syndrome and its possible relation to acute metabolic acidosis localized within the brain. Lancet X4:1113, 1966

19. Lehninger AL, Rossi CS, Greenwalt JW: Respiration-dependent accumulation of inorganic phosphate and Ca^{++} by rat liver mitochondria. Biochem Biophys Res Commun 10:444, 1963

20. Lowry OH, Passoneau JV, Hasselberger FX, et al: Effect of ischemia on known substrates and cofactors of the glycolytic pathway in brain. J Biol Chem 239:18, 1964

21. MacDonald VD, Sundt TM Jr, Winkelman RK: Histochemical studies in the zone of ischemia following middle cerebral artery occlusion in cats. Proceedings of the American Association of Neurological Surgeons, St Louis, 1975

22. Meyer JS, Okamoto S, Shimazu K, et al: The question of uncoupling of cerebral oxidative phosphorylation in acute cerebral infarction, in Langfitt T (ed): Cerebral Circulation and Metabolism. New York, Springer-Verlag, 1975, pp 528–532

23. Mitamura JA, et al: Proceedings of the Annual Meeting of the American Association of Neurological Surgeons, Toronto, Canada, April 24–28, 1977

24. Moore CL: Gramicidin induced ion transport in brain mitochondria preparations. J Neurochem 15:883, 1968

25. Opitz E, Schneider M: Uber die sauerstoffversorgung des gehirns und den mechanismus von mangelwirkungen. Erbeg Physiol 46:126, 1950

26. Ozanne G, Vilnis V, Severinghaus J: Implications of O_2 wave shapes and synchrony for regulation of cerebral microcirculation, in Harper AM (ed): Cerebral Blood Flow and Metabolism in the Brain. New York, Churchill Livingstone, 1975, pp 9.3–9.7

27. Ruscak M, Quittam B: The metabolic response of brain slices to agents affecting the sodium pump. J Physiol 190:595, 1967

28. Schutz H, Silverstein PR, Vapalahti M, et al: Brain mitochondrial

function after ischemia and hypoxia. I. Ischemia induced by increased intracranial pressure. Arch Neurol 29:408, 1973

29. Schutz H, Silverstein PR, Vapalahti M, et al: Brain mitochondrial function after ischemia and hypoxia. II. Normotensive systemic hypoxemia. Arch Neurol 29:417, 1973

30. Siesjo Bo K, Plum F: Pathophysiology of anoxic brain damage, in Gaull GE (ed): Biology of Brain Dysfunction, vol 1. New York, Plenum, 1973, pp 319–371

31. Siesjo Bo K, Nilsson L: The influence of arterial hypoxemia upon labile phosphates and upon extracellular and extracellular lactate and pyruvate concentration in the rat brain. Scand J Lab & Clin Invest 27:83, 1971

32. Sundt TM Jr, Michenfelder JD: Focal transient cerebral ischemia in the squirrel monkey. Effect on brain adenosine triphosphate and lactate levels with electrocorticographic and pathologic correlation. Circ Res 30:703, 1972

33. Teasdale G, Rowan JD, Turner J, et al: Cerebral perfusion railure and cortical electrical activity, in Ingvar A, Lassen N (eds): Cerebral Function, Metabolism, and Circulation. Copenhagen, Munksgaard, 1977, pp 23.14–23.15

34. Thews G: Die sauerstoff diffusion im gehirn. Arch Ges Physiol, Pfluger's 271:197, 1960

35. Van Harreveld A, Ochs S: Cerebral impedance changes after circulatory arrest. Am J Physiol 187:180, 1956

36. White A, Handler P, Smith EL: Principles of Biochemistry, ed 5. New York, McGraw-Hill, 1973

References

85

8

Evidence for barbiturate protection in focal cerebral ischemia: A hypothesis for mechanism and clinical utility

G. F. Molinari, W. E. Lightfoote II, and J. M. Fein

Recent reports by several groups of investigators have documented an anatomic and clinical protective effect afforded by barbiturate drugs in a variety of animal models of both global and focal cerebral ischemia.(2,9,12,14) Additional pharmacologic and physiologic data support the fact that barbiturate anesthesia lowers cerebral blood flow and depresses cerebral metabolic rates of oxygen and glucose.(10,13) The potential application of hypometabolic therapy to man has been the subject of speculation and, indeed, some preliminary clinical investigation.(11) Before subjecting patients with cerebral lesions to the additional risks of hypotension and depressed respiration inherent in barbiturate therapy, it is imperative to establish a firm data base demonstrating efficacy as well as safety in large numbers of laboratory animals. Moreover, the goals of such radical treatment must be attainable and a tenable working hypothesis must be developed which is consistent with both the therapeutic objectives and the experimental data.

In order to supplement the data already available in the archival literature that empirically document the protective effects of barbiturate drugs in cerebral ischemia and to promulgate a hypothesis that fits these observations, the clinical, pathologic, and physiologic data generated in our laboratory have been reviewed in detail.

Experimental Data Base

During the past three years, a total of 95 healthy rhesus monkeys (Macaca mulatta), ranging in weight from 3.0 to 4.5 kg, have been subjected to segmental occlusion of the middle cerebral artery using an embolic method previously reported.(7)

Thirty-five experiments were performed under pentobarbital anesthesia (4 mg/kg), and another 60 were done using only ketamine (8 mg/kg) and local procaine at the site of the common carotid artery cutdown.

After embolism, the animals were used in a variety of experimental designs to evaluate the effects of the anesthetic agents on morphologic, physiologic, and hemorrhagic variables. Ten of the animals in which hemiplegia was induced under ketamine were given pentobarbital for 12 hours, administration of which was delayed for 30 minutes until the infarction process had begun.(9) Vasoactive agents including norepinephrine, angiotensin, and carbon dioxide by inhalation were given to another 19 animals(4); and compound platinum–silver wire probes were stereotactically placed in 10 animals before embolism.(8) In summary, of 95 middle cerebral artery occlusions, 40 had no barbiturates complicating the ischemic process, 35 occurred in animals anesthetized with pentobarbital before embolism, and 10 had barbiturates given only after hemiplegia and other neurologic signs had been documented after embolism.

All brain specimens were obtained postmortem. In the entire series only 10 animals died spontaneously, all in the acute ischemic period after embolism; brains removed from fatal embolisms were immersion-fixed in 10% formalin for 2 weeks. All others were perfusion-fixed in situ either as a terminal event or immediately after cardiac standstill using an intracarotid infusion of 10% buffered formalin. Photographs were made of each fixed intact specimen from the ventral, dorsal, and affected lateral surfaces.

Serial thick coronal sections were made at the tips of the temporal poles, optic chiasm, and mammillary bodies, and each

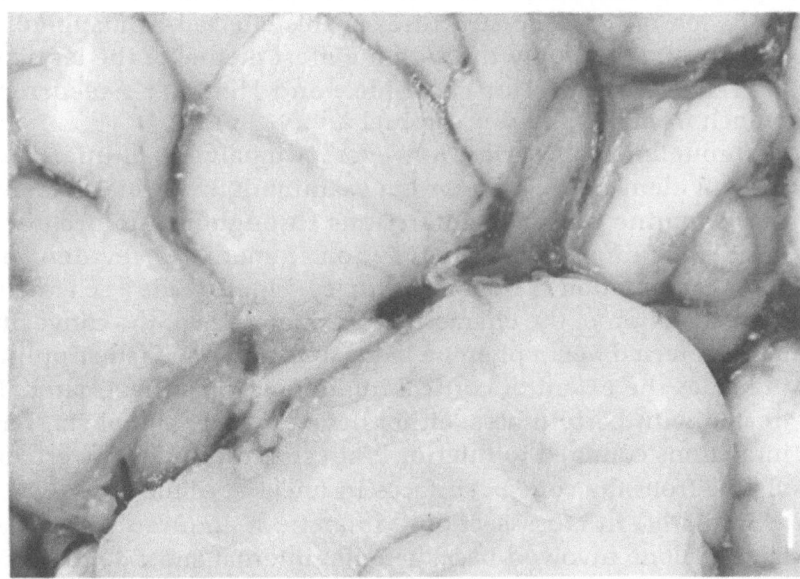

Fig. 8.1. An intravascular embolism occupying the right middle cerebral artery (MCA) of a rhesus monkey. The anterior cerebral arteries are seen to the right fusing into a common pericallosal artery just anterior to the optic chiasm. Note that the embolism is impacted distally (to the left of the photograph) at the candelabrum; the serpiginous extraparenchymal segment of a major penetrating branch is filled with embolic material; and the dead space between the proximal end of the major embolus and the occluded penetrating branch is filled with clotted blood. Throughout this large series such instances of secondary thrombosis were rare and were limited to blind pouches from which there was no outlet for arterial blood. Small segments of secondary clotting could occur either proximal or distal to the occluded surface segment, but as long as penetrating branches were patent to allow runoff for anterograde or retrograde flow, secondary intravascular clotting did not occur. Note also that the initial MCA segment arising from the circle is patent up to the point of takeoff of the occluded medial striate branch. The temporal pole has been amputated to expose the entire course of the MCA.

whole brain thick section was embedded in paraffin. Photographs were made of representative coronal sections either before or after impregnation in paraffin. Whole brain thin sections, 7 to 10 μ, were mounted and stained with hematoxylin and eosin, luxol-fast blue–PAS, and Van Gieson's stain.

Careful quantitative planimetric measurements were made in 18 specimens, ten from the postinfarction, barbiturate-treated animals and eight from the group receiving ketamine only. The analysis of this subsample is reported elsewhere.(9)

Experimental Findings

In each specimen, a continuous embolus occluded a 5 to 10 mm segment of the middle cerebral artery trunk, undercutting penetrating lenticulostriate vessels, but extending no further than the arborization of the major surface branches of the middle cerebral artery in the sylvian fissure. Short segments of secondary intravascular clotting occurred only in dead spaces between the proximal or distal end of the embolic cylinder and the first patent penetrating branch permitting outflow for circulating blood or perfusate. Figure 8.1 shows an intravascular embolus with the circle of Willis to the right. The temporal pole is amputated to demonstrate the entire intrasylvian course of the occlusion. Distally (to the left), the embolus is impacted at the candelabrum. Proximally, a small fragment fills the extra-parenchymal origin of one of the medial striate vessels. The blind pouch between the occluded penetrator and the middle cerebral occlusion is filled with clot. Yet the initial middle cerebral artery segment remains patent where the unobstructed penetrating branches, perpendicular to the plane of the photograph, permit runoff into the brain parenchyma. Therefore, perfusion of the deep structures of this affected hemisphere is still possible but only through the most medial of the lenticulostriates, the anterior choroidal, and Heubner's recurrent branch from the anterior cerebral artery.

Throughout this series, however, two patterns of infarction were evident upon postmortem examination. Animals receiving ketamine only had infarctions throughout the occluded middle cerebral artery distribution immediately evident on gross examination of the brain surface. Figure 8.2 is a schematic representation of the characteristic appearance of the convexity of the affected hemisphere; a large area of perisylvian stippling indicates the extent of cortical infarction. In contrast, animals treated with barbiturates, either before or after embolism, had infarctions confined to interior brain structures which were invisible from the convex surfaces in uncut specimens.

Similarly, in cross-sections, infarctions induced under ketamine alone involved basal ganglia; internal and external cap-

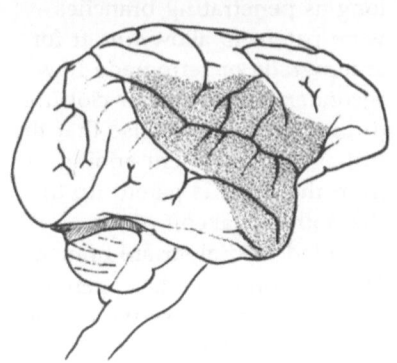

Fig. 8.2. Schematic representation of the distribution of cortical infarctions due to right middle cerebral artery occlusion using ketamine anesthesia. The stippled area conforms to the zone of pale or bland infarction involving supra- and infrasylvian gyri and the temporal tip. Middle cerebral artery occlusions sustained during barbiturate administration regularly caused lesions which were invisible from the convex surface.

Chapter 8: Evidence for Barbiturate Protection in Focal Cerebral Ischemia

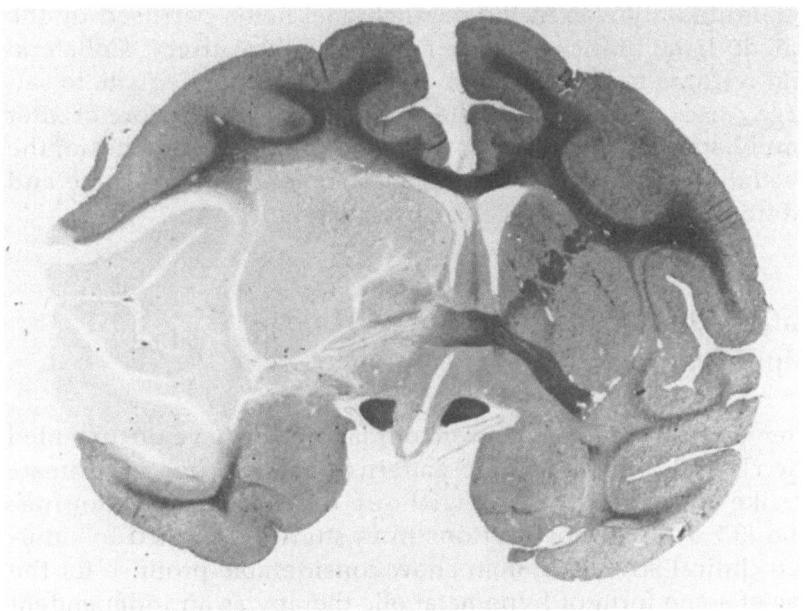

Fig. 8.3. Whole brain cross-section through the anterior commissure obtained from rhesus monkey 3 days after middle cerebral artery occlusion under ketamine. Note that in the affected hemisphere cortex is preserved only in the anterior and posterior cerebral artery distributions and in their respective watershed areas. H&E.

sules; the claustrum; extreme capsule; and the insular, opercular, and supra- and infrasylvian cortex, despite complete patency of the middle cerebral artery bed distal to the embolism (Fig. 8.3). On the other hand, barbiturate-treated animals showed lesions of basal ganglia and capsules with rare patchy extensions to insular cortex only (Fig. 8.4).

In summary, because vascular occlusions were invariably segmental, complete protection from ischemic infarction was impossible. Nonetheless, the distinctive difference between specimens treated with barbiturates in vivo and those receiving

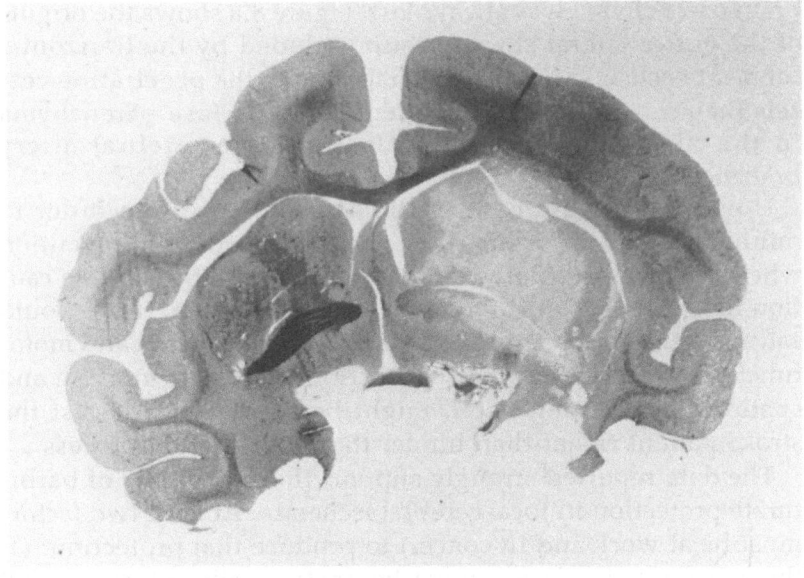

Fig. 8.4. Whole brain cross-section through the optic chiasm obtained from rhesus monkey 5 days after middle cerebral artery (MCA) occlusion under pentobarbital anesthesia. Note the restriction of infarction to the territories of the penetrating branches of the MCA, ie, the gray matter of the caudate and putamen and the white matter of the internal capsule, anterior commissure, and to a lesser extent the centrum semiovale. All of these structures are readily identified in the unaffected hemisphere to the left of the photograph.

Experimental Findings

ketamine only was in the parenchymal fields perfused by the patent distal branches of the middle cerebral artery. Collateral and retrograde circulation to those fields were adequate to salvage cortex when barbiturates were used either before or after embolism. But when ketamine alone provided anesthesia, the available collateral circulation was somehow inadequate and additional large areas of the cortex were lost.

Interpretation and Possible Clinical Significance

Previous detailed reports from our laboratory have documented the clinical and pathologic patterns observed in this primate stroke model with and without barbiturate contamination.(3,7,9) Early observations from studies designed to simulate clinical strokes in man show considerable promise for the use of some form of hypometabolic therapy as an independent or adjunctive measure in the management of cerebrovascular disease processes. Reports from other laboratories suggesting complete protection of cerebral tissue from ischemic infarction probably arise from artifacts inherent either in the species of experimental animal chosen or occlusive technique used.(6) Indeed, Smith and his group(2) noted less remarkable protection in primates than had been anticipated from their original experiment using dogs.(12)

Using an intravascular segmental occlusion, 100% of our animals had cerebral infarctions. Since multiple penetrating branches were always occluded at their origins by the embolism and since precapillary collaterals are either nonexistent or ineffectual among penetrating arteries of the brain,(1) some brain parenchyma was always lost. Figure 8.5 shows the origins of the entire lateral striate group occluded by the horizontal segment occlusion. Even collaterals among the penetrating vessels themselves would be inadequate to perfuse parenchyma in the distribution of these deep middle cerebral artery branches.

However, containment of the disease process in order to minimize sequelae is the classic goal of secondary prevention when primary preventive efforts have failed. With all due caution in extrapolation from animal models to man, if one could salvage cerebral cortex despite losses in basal ganglia and motor function, then higher cortical functions, such as language and spatiotemporal integration, might be preserved to assist the stroke patient rather than hinder the rehabilitation process.

The data reported strongly support the hypothesis of barbiturate protection in focal cerebral ischemia. At least two factors must be at work and in concert to produce that protection: (1) the collateral circulation must be anatomically intact, and (2)

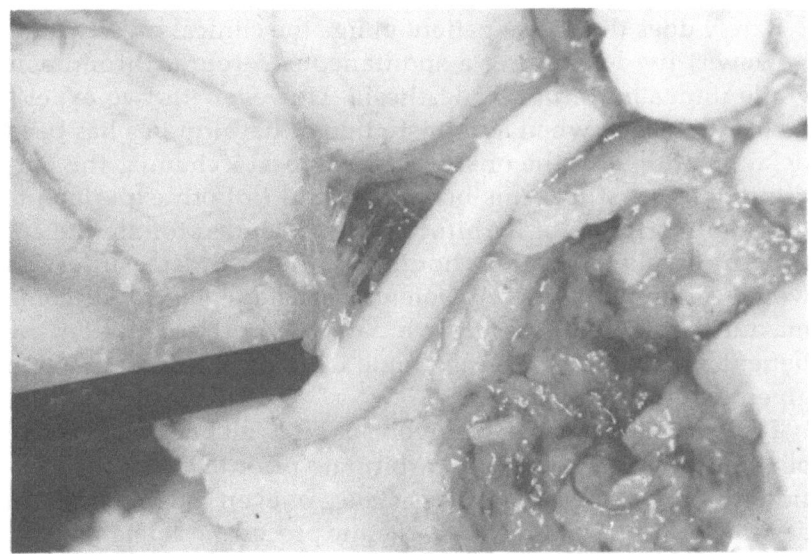

Fig. 8.5. Photograph made through operating microscope (× 6) of the occluded middle cerebral artery (MCA) of a rhesus monkey. The MCA is retracted from the brain surface to show the orbitofrontal-lateral striate artery complex. Multiple perforating branches are seen penetrating the brain substance, all arising through a single stem of the parent surface vessel. The segmental surface embolus completely occludes all of these branches to adjacent territories, making both primary and collateral circulation to the interior structures impossible. Hence, deep brain parenchyma in the distribution of such penetrators must be lost, no matter how effective or prolonged the protection afforded by pharmacologic agents.

perfusion through those collaterals must be adequate to deliver the systemically administered barbiturate agent to the zone at risk during the time interval wherein the ischemic process remains reversible. Conversely, unless the perfusion becomes adequate to sustain neuronal viability, either spontaneously through hemodynamic reflex adjustments or iatrogenically, by surgical augmentation of collateral flow, the infarction will develop nonetheless in the areas at risk as the barbiturate is eluted, excreted, or metabolized to inert by-products.

Using our experimental model, segmental occlusion does not cause secondary clotting of major vascular segments, so that the only areas totally deprived of both primary and collateral circulation are the fields perfused by penetrating vessels closed at their origins by the embolus. Only in blind pouches, from which there is no outlet or runoff, is there secondary clotting. In man, particularly in younger patients with numerous collaterals, segmental vascular occlusion is often identified angiographically by retrograde filling of distal segments with contrast medium on late arterial phase films. This retrograde perfusion, which is a slower process than anterograde flow, may be inadequate to maintain neuronal viability at presumably reduced perfusion pressures; but may be an important prognostic sign for the potential efficacy of barbiturate drugs or microvascular surgical anastomoses.

In the course of surgical intervention for primary or secondary intracranial vascular lesions, single or even multiple spring clips may be required to control bleeding. Fortunately, the anesthesiologist may select anesthetic agents prior to the event of bleeding and in anticipation of therapeutic vascular occlusions. Therefore, the protective effect of barbiturates may have considerable merit in neurosurgical operations, which by design or necessity alter normal flow patterns.

Interpretation and Possible Clinical Significance

Rarely does the stroke patient oblige the clinical investigator, however, by developing a spontaneous cerebral thrombosis while under barbiturate anesthesia. However, in two experiments,(5,9) even when administration of barbiturates has been delayed until after the onset of severe focal ischemia, the barbiturate effect still seems beneficial, and in both experiments the administration of barbiturate was extended for significant time intervals (12 and 48 hours). While such time intervals would certainly permit any potential collateral fields to become maximally efficient, in our own data we must account for the benefit provided by even a single dose of barbiturate when given before embolism.

Two mechanisms may be involved. First, all brain tissue may be uniformly perfused with barbiturate prior to vascular occlusion, thereby increasing the resistance of even the parenchyma destined for infarction to the ischemic process and delaying the onset of irreversible change. In the case of surgical occlusions using microvascular clips, the slight margin of safety provided by the increased resistance might be adequate for collaterals to become functional. Secondly, however, even a single dose of pentobarbital has a biologic half-life of approximately 4 hours. Assuming a blood–tissue diffusion coefficient of 1 for pentobarbital, the cerebral metabolic demand for oxygen and glucose, along with the products of anaerobic metabolism such as lactate, would increase gradually as the level of circulating barbiturate falls. This mechanism would translate events that ordinarily occur in an instant after vascular occlusion into a process requiring several hours to reach maximum intensity. Indeed, the mechanism of barbiturate protection, in our large experimental series of 33 animals receiving only a single anesthetic dose of pentobarbital prior to embolism, may be the retardation of the momentum of the ischemic process.

Conclusions

Hypometabolic therapy may act to retard the rate of progression of acute focal ischemia long enough to derive maximum benefit from spontaneous collateral mechanisms or to permit microsurgical intervention. Barbiturates may provide the anesthesia of choice in certain neurosurgical procedures requiring vascular ligation. Regarding the use of barbiturates after the onset of ischemia, perfusion of periinfarction zones with drugs via collateral pathways, with reduction in local metabolic activity, may tip the balance in favor of neuronal survival in marginal zones, and thereby improve the potential for high quality recovery.

Before such radical therapy may be applied to man, systems must be available to protect against the cardiovascular and respiratory complications of barbiturates in high-risk patients. As with other therapeutic modalities involving barbiturates, such as the treatment of status epilepticus, anticipation of complications is the most effective tool for their prevention. More significantly, if one is to undertake use of CNS depressant drugs in disease states, then a system must be devised for monitoring patients during their drug-induced or "therapeutic" comas to compensate for the diminished sensitivity of the neurologic examination in that setting.

REFERENCES

1. Cobb S: Cerebral circulation. XIII. The question of "end arteries" of the brain and the mechanism of infarction. Arch Neurol 25:273, 1931
2. Hoff JT, Smith AL, Hankinson HL, et al: Barbiturate protection from cerebral infarction in primates. Stroke 6:28, 1975
3. Laurent JP, Molinari GF, Moseley JI: Clinicopathological validation of a primate stroke model Surg Neurol 4:449, 1975
4. Laurent JP, Molinari GF, Oakley JC: Primate model of cerebral hematoma. J Neuropathol Exp Neurol, 1976
5. Michenfelder JD, Sundt TM: Cerebral protection by barbiturate anesthesia and intensive care for 48 hours following permanent middle cerebral artery occlusion in Java monkeys. Seventh International Symposium on Cerebral Blood Flow and Metabolism. Aviemore, Scotland, June 17–19, 1975. In Harper AM, Jennett WB, Miller JD, et al (eds): Cerebral Blood Flow and Metabolism in the Brain. Edinburgh, Churchill Livingstone, 1975, pp 12.22–12.23
6. Molinari GF, Laurent JP: A classification of experimental models of brain ischemia. Stroke 7:14, 1976
7. Molinari GF, Moseley JI, Laurent JP: Segmental middle cerebral artery occlusion in primates. An experimental method requiring minimal surgery and anesthesia. Stroke 5:334, 1974
8. Molinari GF, Oakley JC, Laurent JP: The pathophysiology of barbiturate protection in focal ischemia. Presented to Stroke Council, American Heart Association, February 27, 1976, Dallas, Texas. Stroke 7:3, 1976
9. Moseley JI, Laurent JP, Molinari GF: Barbiturate attenuation of the clinical course and pathologic lesions in a primate stroke model. Neurology (Minneap) 45:870, 1975
10. Mrsulja BB, Mrsulja BJ, Ito U, et al: Experimental cerebral ischemia in Mongolian gerbils. II. Changes in carbohydrates. Acta Neuropathol (Berl), 1975
11. Shapiro HM, Wyte SR, Loeser J: Barbiturate-augmented hypothermia for reduction of persistent intracranial hypertension. J Neurosurg 40:90, 1974
12. Smith AL, Hoff JT, Nielsen SL, et al: Barbiturate protection in acute focal cerebral ischemia. Stroke 5:1, 1974
13. Sokoloff L: The action of drugs on cerebral circulation. Pharmacol Rev 11:1, 1959
14. Yatsu F, Diamond I, Graziano C, et al: Experimental brain ischemia. Protection from irreversible damage with a rapid-acting barbiturate (methohexital). Stroke 3:726, 1972

9

Transient ischemic attacks and metabolic aspects of their relief by microneurosurgical anastomosis

G. Austin, G. Haugen, and W. Schuler

Introducton

Transient ischemic attacks (TIAs) are known to occur in 20 to 80% of persons having occlusive strokes.(6,15) As they become more frequent and more lasting, the danger of stroke increases. They may also occur in persons who have already had minor strokes. Etiologically, it is currently believed that TIAs are at least partially, based on a transient decrease in blood flow to the point at which a critical brain oxygen tension (bPo_2) is reached. At this point, brain oxygen utilization ($b\dot{P}o_2$) is decreased, with associated impaired oxidative phosphorylation. The decline in ATP formation is associated with failure of the neuronal ion pumps and depolarization. The neuronal depolarization causes abnormal nerve firing patterns manifested clinically by the symptoms of TIAs. The argument for microanastomosis rests on the further assumption that an added bypass collateral blood flow will raise the bPo_2 sufficiently to decrease the TIAs and, therefore, the likelihood of stroke. Since TIAs are frightening as well as neurologically disturbing to the individual, any improvement can be rewarding. A decreased likelihood of stroke is the major goal. The authors herein consider the various etiologies of TIAs and reasons for their relief by a bypass anastomosis which adds an additional collateral blood flow. Evidence supporting the present concept of TIAs is presented from animal and human observations.

If TIAs are due to a background decrease in bPo_2 and superimposed triggering factors that further decrease bPo_2 and $b\dot{P}o_2$, then the experimental evidence should show that bPo_2 and $b\dot{P}o_2$ are decreased by factors that simulate background mechanisms, and are further decreased by factors that simulate triggering mechanisms. Similarly, relief from TIAs should be associated with an increase in bPo_2 and $b\dot{P}o_2$

Methods

A group of 53 patients were studied as to type of TIA and the relief of TIAs by microneurosurgical anastomosis. All patients were operated on with an endotracheal anesthetic mixture of N_2O/O_2 in a ratio of 2:1. Additional drugs were used for complete muscle relaxation and immobilization. The arterial oxygen tension (aPo_2) was maintained above 90 mmHg, and the mean blood pressure was stabilized above 100 mmHg. The $aPco_2$ was maintained between 35 and 38 mmHg. In some patients intraoperative recording of relative brain oxygen tension (bPo_2), or O_2 availability at the electrode tip, was done before and after anastomosis. In a second group of 11 patients the redox level of cytochrome a and a_3 (cyt. a,a_3) was measured before and after anastomosis. Relative bPo_2 was also recorded in some patients with a 25 μ teflon-coated platinum electrode inserted into the cortex within a few millimeters of the anastomosis. The polarographic technique was used with the relative level (in nanoamps) recorded on an inkwriter. The redox level of cyt. a,a_3 was measured from the same general area of cortex using the noninvasive spectrophotometric technique of Jöbsis,[8] modified after the original instrument designed by Chance[7] for in vitro recording of isolated mitochondria. The relative redox level of cyt. a,a_3 was also recorded on an inkwriter. This technique as applied to the human cortex has been further described elsewhere.[1,4] After completion of the microanastomosis (superficial temporal artery (STA) to middle cerebral artery (MCA)), recordings were made as described. A temporary clip was then applied to the STA and the recordings repeated, thus corresponding to the states before and after anastomosis. In a few instances, some results of recording bPo_2, $b\dot{P}o_2$, and cyt. a,a_3 in cats are included.[5]

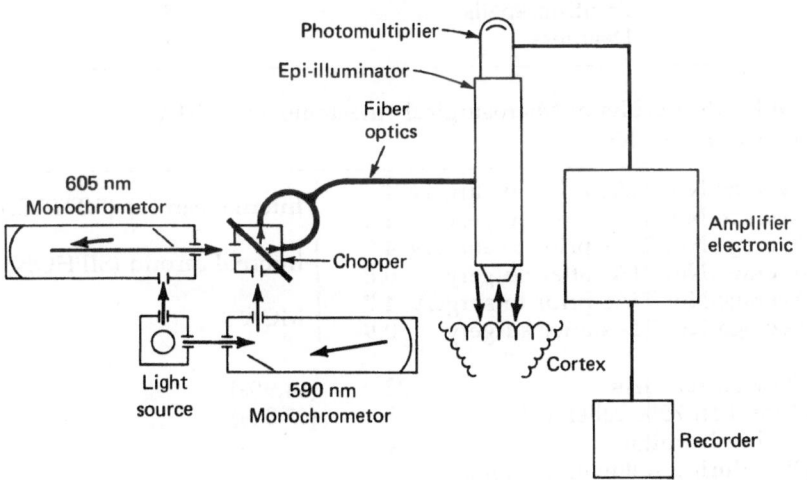

Fig. 9.1. Differential dual wavelength reflectance spectrophotometer. Absorption peaks used for recording mitochondrial cytochromes and hemoglobin by differential spectrophotometer.

Table 9.1. Absorption Peaks Used for Recording Mitochondrial Cytochromes and Hemoglobin by Differential Specrophotometer

Mitochondrial Components

	Useful Peak Absorption λ in nm
Cytochrome b	564
Cytochrome c	550
Cytochrome c_1	553
Cytochrome a	605
Cytochrome a_3	600
Flavoprotein	450

Hemoglobin Derivatives

	Useful Peak Absorption λ in nm
Red Hemoglobin Hb	555
Ox. Hemoglobin HbO_2	576–578
Isosbestic point Hb + HbO_2	584.5
Methemoglobin	578
Cyanomethemoglobin	580–590
Alkaline hematin	550–580
Heme	575

Table 9.2. Symptoms and Signs of TIAs in 53 Patients

	No.
Slurred speech	40
Confusion	32
Dizziness	34
Recent memory loss	25
Numbness-extremities	32
Paresis-extremities	27
Emotional instability	11
Blurred vision	18
Fainting spells	8
Deafness	1

Table 9.3. Results of Microsurgical Anastomosis on TIA Improvement (N=53)

Average No. TIAs prior to surgery	4	} Internal carotid (BIFURC.)
Average No. TIAs after surgery	1.1	
Average No. TIAs prior to surgery	4.7	} Internal carotid (SIPHON)
Average No. TIAs after surgery	0.8	
Average No. TIAs prior to surgery	4.7	} MCA
Average No. TIAs after surgery	0.9	
100% Relief TIAs	22	(44.9%)
More than 75% relief TIAs	33	(67.3%)
Died in hospital	4	
Died during followup at home, unrelated causes	3	

Table 9.4. Changes in Redox Level of Cyt. a, a_3 in 9 Patients[a]

Name	Date	15 to 30%	30 to 60%	Clip on-off
W.M.	29 09 75	2.7	2.1	2.6
C.B.	24 09 75	20	10	3.2
A.B.	22 03 76	10	4	10
E.C.	17 05 76	3	1	2.9
D.T.	29 04 76	6	8	5.3
A.L.	15 07 76	6	0	6.6
M.R.	19 07 76	3.3	2.5	1.3
M.L.	09 08 75	6	5	—
F.W.	09 09 76	4	1	9
Mean		6.78	3.73	5.11
SD		5.45	3.40	3.18

[a]Values in percent full scale reduction.

Table 9.5. Changes in Relative bPo_2 in 6 Patients[a]

Name	Date	15 to 30%	30 to 60%	Clip on–off
E.G.	17 05 76	5	5	23
M.R.	19 07 76	45	68	23.6
D.T.	29 04 76	30	10	130
A.L.	15 07 76	22	4.5	31.0
F.W.	09 09 76	3.3	3.9	10.0
J.W.	15 09 75	7.5	25	—
			19.40	43.52
Mean		18.80	25.10	48.93
S.D.		16.62		

[a]Values in nanoamps.

Figure 9.1 and Table 1 show the instrumentation and peak absorption wavelengths used for recording the redox state of cyt. a,a_3. The redox level of cyt. a,a_3 was measured at 605 nm compared to a reference wavelength of 590 nm. This eliminated the hemoglobin effect as previously described.(5,12,13)

Results

In this paper only the results relevant to TIAs are included. The more commonly encountered TIAs are listed in Table 2. Relief of TIAs is shown in Table 9.3. Figure 9.2 shows the typical response of cat cortex to bilateral common carotid occlusion. This indicates a prompt drop in relative blood volume, bPo_2, and the oxidized level of cyt. a,a_3, in response to a transient decrease in cerebral blood flow (CBF) occasioned by the carotid occlusion. These all occur within the first few seconds and there is a return to normal upon release of the carotids. The return occurs over a more prolonged period due to a reactive hyper-

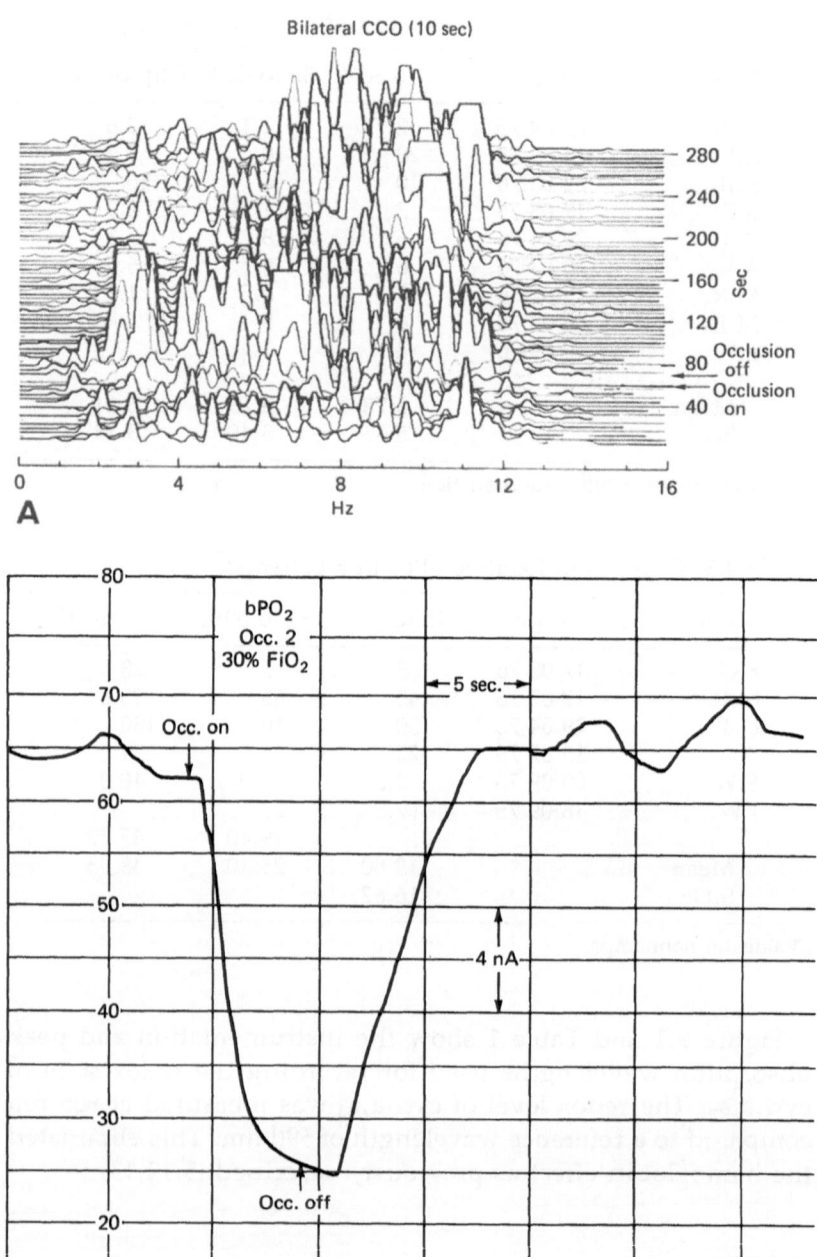

Bilateral CCO (10 sec)

A

Fig. 9.2. Frequency response expressed as compressed power spectral analysis of cat electrocorticogram in response to 10-second bilateral common carotid occlusion (CCO). Each horizontal line equals 4 seconds duration (1 epoch). Depression of bPo_2 in response to 10-second bilateral CCO. bPo_2 depressed to 36% of maximum response. Upper Trace: Reduction of cyt. a,a_3 in response to 10-second bilateral CCO. Bottom Trace: Depression of blood volume during 10-second bilateral CCO.

B

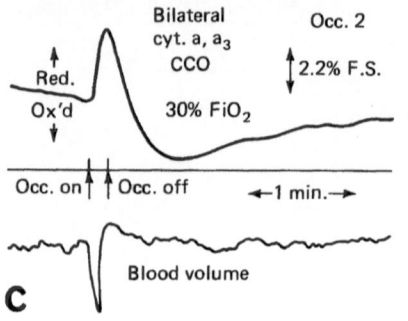

C

emia of the cortex. Figure 9.3 shows the response in relative bPo_2 (nanoamps) of the human cortex upon application and removal of the STA clip. Figure 9.4 shows a typical response of the redox level of cyt. a,a_3 to variations in the FiO_2 before and after anastomosis, ie, clip on and off. Figure 9.5 shows a similar typical response in relative bPo_2. These indicate that following anastomosis there is an increase in relative bPo_2 and in the oxidized level of cyt. a,a_3. In nine patiets the average increase in the oxidized level of cyt. a,a_3 was 5.1% ± 3.2, full scale reduction. The percent full scale reduction is a relative value and may be compared to the change in percent full scale reduction of approximately 4.4% seen with bilateral carotid occlusion in the cat (Fig. 9.2). Table 9.4 shows the redox changes of cyt. a,a_3 in nine patients in response to altered FiO_2. The response of relative bPo_2 in six patients is shown in Table 9.5.

Discussion

As mentioned in the introduction, TIAs are thought to result from a drop in bPo_2 to a critical level brought about by a decrease in blood flow. Obviously, if the bPo_2 is already lowered by some preexisting background pathology, the transient drop need not be so great. There appear to be both background and

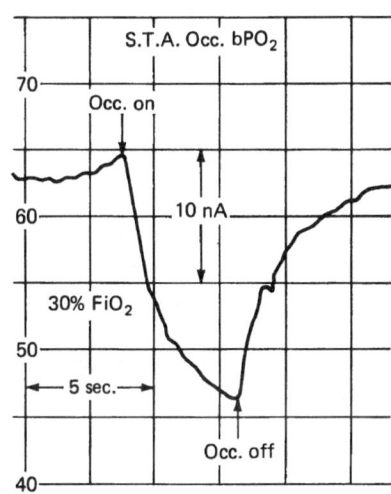

Fig. 9.3 Depression of relative bPo_2 in response to temporary clip applied to STA (condition equivalent to preanastomosis cortex). bPo_2 depressed to 70% of normal.

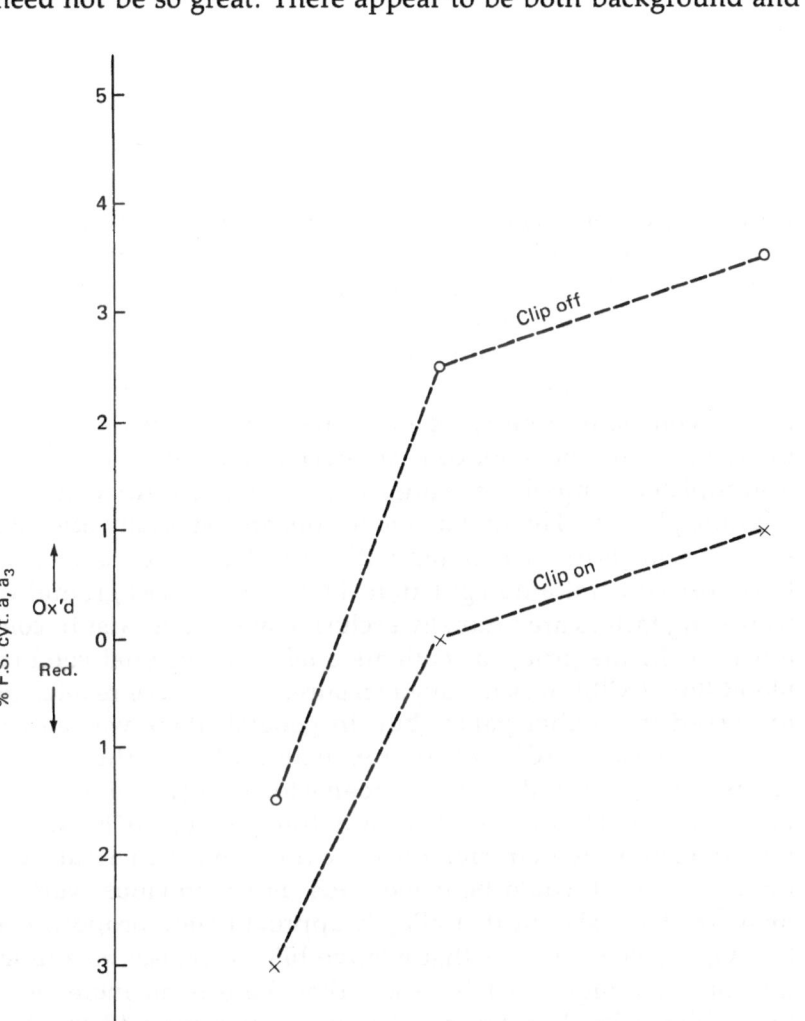

Fig. 9.4. Change in relative levels of oxidized cyt. a,a_3, comparing pre- and postanastomosis conditions. Following anastomosis (clip off) the redox level of cyt. a,a_3 at 20% is equal to preanastomosis conditions (clip on) of FiO_2 at 40%.

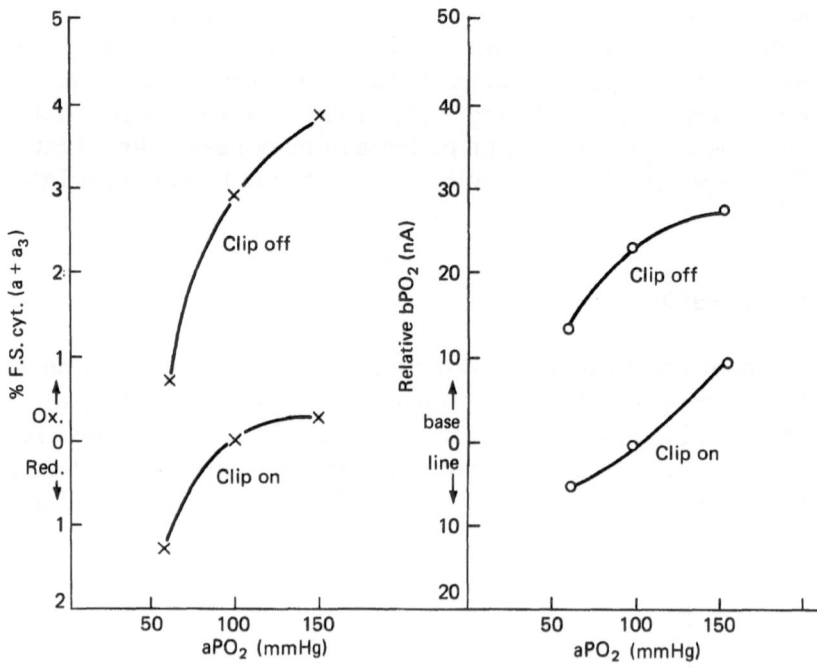

Fig. 9.5. Increase in relative bPo_2 following anastomosis (clip off) compared to preanastomosis conditions. Relative bPo_2 following anastomosis shows condition at 50 mmHg equivalent to preanastomosis bPo_2 at 50 mmHg.

triggering factors. The former includes extracranial occlusive lesions of the carotid or vertebral arteries, intracranial occlusions of branches of the circle of Willis, or cerebral small vessel disease. In addition, chronic obstructive pulmonary disease or cardiac failure may lower the aPo_2 and bPo_2. Triggering or transient factors are described as hemodynamic or embolic. The former consist of a decrease in cardiac output with a drop in blood pressure; the latter consist of activated platelet emboli or fibrinoplatelet emboli deriving from arterial or cardiac atherosclerotic plaques. Hemodynamic factors are especially effective since the majority of patients with TIAs have been shown to have lost cerebral autoregulation. None of the background or triggering factors are mutually exclusive and often exist in conjunction. In the group of patients analyzed, regional cerebral blood flow (rCBF) was usually measured.(2,3) These results are discussed in another paper; but, in general, there was an average increase in rCBF of approximately 24% in the middle cerebral territory following microanastomosis.(14) Since most patients with TIAs have a loss of autoregulation, rCBF would be proportional to perfusion pressure (PP), and even a transient mild drop in PP could be deleterious. From previous work in man, we have shown that aPo_2 is approximately proportional to FiO_2. Table 9.5 shows that relative bPo_2 increases as a function of FiO_2. Figure 9.4 indicates that there is an increase in the oxidized level of cyt. a,a_3 as FiO_2 varies from 15 to 60%. Finally, both Figures 9.4 and 9.5 show the increase in bPo_2 and oxidized cyt. a,a_3 following microanastomosis. The increase in the oxidized level of cyt. a,a_3 in response to increased FiO_2 was also shown by Rosenthal et al in the cat.(13) It is generally assumed, and there is a strong heuristic argument, that an increase in oxidation of the cytochromes in the absence of a crossover point implies an increase in mitochondrial respiration. This means an increase in electron transport and O_2 utilization as well as increased ATP formation. The only factor that could alter this situation or simulate an increased oxidized state of the cytochromes, without an increase in O_2 utilization, would be an abrupt decrease in substrate inflow from the Krebs cycle. From our results of improvement in TIAs following microanastomosis, one would logically attribute the improvements to an increase in bPo_2 and $b\dot{P}o_2$, and ATP formation. The final assumption would be that the increase in collateral blood flow yielding an increase in relative bPo_2 and $b\dot{P}o_2$, and in ATP formation, is accompanied by an increase in energy utilization. The latter is assumed to reversibly raise the neuronal membrane potential to a normal range and decrease the TIAs.

In conjunction with this, Nilsson et al(9) have suggested that ~P utilization tends to follow ATP concentrations. One other possibility remains. It has been shown that uncoupling of oxidative phosphorylation may occur with hypoxia of 10 to 60 second duration. This could also occur in hypoxic cortex of stroke-type patients and relief of this might explain the improvement in TIAs. The initial assumption of a brief transient ischemia of only seconds' duration leading to the conditions for a TIA is supported by Figure 9.3, showing a rapid drop in bPo_2 and decrease in oxidation of cyt. a, a_3 with a 10-second carotid occlusion. Although the reduction of cyt. a, a_3 implies decreased ATP formation, the latter remains unmeasured. Recent work by Siesjo et al shows that a brief 10-second period of ischemia in the rat, anesthetized with N_2O and O_2 in a ratio of 2:1, is sufficient to reduce cortical ATP and phosphocreatine, accompanied by an increase in ADP and lactate.(10,11)

From these observations of mitochondrial respiration in the cortex of cat and man, we conclude that a major part of the improvement in TIAs following microanastomosis is due to an improved collateral blood flow leading to a higher relative bPo_2. The latter is associated with a higher oxidized level of the cytochromes and an increase in energy utilization.

REFERENCES

1. Austin G, Haugen G, LaManna J, et al: Cortical oxidative metabolism following microanastomosis for brain ischemia. In Jöbsis F(ed): Proceedings of Conference on Physiology of Oxygen Metabolism. (in press).
2. Austin G, Laffin D, Hayward W: Evaluation of fast component (gray matter) by 12 minute I.V. method using analog computer

analysis. In Harper AM, et al (eds): Blood Flow and Metabolism in the Brain. Edinburgh, Churchill, 1976

3. Austin G, Laffin D, Hayward W: Physiological factors in selection of patients for superficial temporal to middle cerebral artery anastomosis. Surgery 75(6):861, 1974

4. Austin G, Schuler W, Haugen G, et al: Simulated transient ischemic attacks in cat and man. In Schmiedek P(ed): Proceedings of Third International Symposium for Microsurgical Anastomosis for Brain Ischemia. (in press)

5. Austin G, Schuler W, Haugen G, et al: Brain metabolism in the cat during brief transient ischemia. In Austin G(ed): Contemporary Aspects of Cerebral Vascular Disease. Dallas, Professional Information Library, 1976

6. Baker RN, Ramseyer JC, Schwartz WS: Prognosis in patients with transient cerebral ischemic attacks. Neurology. (Minneap) 18:1157, 1968

7. Chance B: Rapid and sensitive spectrophotometry. III. A double beam apparatus. Rev Sci. Instrum. 22:634, 1951

8. Jöbsis F, Keiser J, Rosenthal M, et al: In vivo reflectant spectrophotometry of cytochrome a, a_3 in the cerebral cortex of the cat. (in press)

9. Nilsson B, Norberg K, Nordstrom CH, et al: Rate of energy utilization in the cerebral cortex of rats. Acta Physiol Scand 93:569, 1975

10. Norberg K, Quistorff B, Siesjo BK: Effects of hypoxia of 10 to 45 seconds duration on energy metabolism in the cerebral cortex of unanesthetized and anesthetized rats. Acta Physiol Scand 95:301, 1975

11. Norberg K, Siesjo BK: Cerebral metabolism in hypoxia. II. Pattern of activation of glycolysis. Brain Res 86:31, 1975

12. Rosenthal M, LaManna JC, Jöbsis FF, et al: Effects of respiratory gases on cytochrome a in intact cerebral cortex. Is there a critical Po_2? Brain Res 108:143, 1976

13. Rosenthal M, Martel D, LaManna JC, et al: In situ studies of oxidative energy metabolism during transient ischemia in cats. Exp Neurol 50:477, 1976

14. Schmiedek P, Gratzl O, Spetzler R, et al: Selection of patients and extra-intracranial arterial bypass surgery measurements. J Neurosurg 44:303, 1976

15. Whisnat JP, Matsumoto N, Elveback LR: The prognosis and treatment of transient ischemic attacks in a community. Rochester, Minnesota, 1955–1969. Neurology, (Minneap) 22:441, 1972

III

CLINICAL EVALUATION AND DIAGNOSIS

II

CLINICAL EVALUATION AND DIAGNOSIS

10

Management of risk factors and other diseases in candidates for microneurosurgical anastomosis in cerebral ischemia

James E. Cassidy

Transient ischemic attack and, ultimately, completed brain infarction are associated with risk factors (Table 10.1) that occur singly or in combination in the majority of cases.(3) It is the purpose of this paper to examine such risk factors and to propose a set of categories into which patients bearing those risks ought to be grouped. This may help the clinician in selection of patients for surgery and also may provide a classification which would be incorporated into a randomized study of the efficacy of microneurosurgical anastomosis for cerebral ischemia. Atherosclerosis is the most ubiquitous of these risk factors and involves intracranial as well as extracranial arteries(2). It is present in 90% of patients with occluding cerebrovascular disease, and is associated with a series of collateral risk factors (Table 10.2) which should be considered as well. Cerebral embolism accounts for 8% of completed brain infarctions.

Vascular spasm occurs during the hour preceding migraine attacks. The aura period may be associated with transitory neurologic deficits and, rarely, persistent ones.(6) Hypertension, in addition to accelerating the atherosclerotic process, has been proven in experimental animals to induce intracranial vasospasm.(1,3) Of less concern here is the spasm which occurs related to cerebral or subarachnoid hemorrhage.

Thrombosis, in addition to its frequency in atherosclerotic disease, may occur in a small group of patients who do not have significant atherosclerotic disease but suffer from other vascular, as well as hematologic, disorders.

With these risk factors in mind, for the purposes of our study, we may group prospective candidates for microneurosurgical anastomosis into three categories:

Table 10.1. Risk Factors in Cerebral Ischemia

1. Atherosclerosis
   Intracranial
   Extracranial
2. Cerebral Embolism
   Associated with platelet aggregation
   In cardiac valvulitis
   After myocardial infarction
   In atrial fibrillation
   With endocarditis
3. Other Deficits in Cerebral Blood Flow
   Hypotension
   Cardiac arrhythmia
   Cardiac failure (pump failure)
   Circulatory obstruction (nonatherogenic)
4. Vascular spasm
   Associated with migraine
   In hypertension
   Related to cerebral and subarachnoid hemorrhage
5. Hypoxia
   In low blood oxygen saturation
   Related to low alveolar oxygen partial pressure
   In alveolar capillary block
   In heart disease
6. Thrombosis
   Associated with atherosclerosis
   In inflammatory vascular disease
      Lues
      Necrotizing vasculitis
      Giant cell arteritis
   In connective tissue disease
   Associated with blood dyscrasias
      Polycythemia vera
      Secondary polycythemia
      Anemia
7. Cigarette smoking

Table 10.2. Risk Factors Responsible for Acceleration of Atherosclerosis

1. Hypertension
2. Altered lipid metabolism
3. Hypercholesterolemia
4. Familial hyperlipoproteinemia
5. Syndromes sharing hyperlipoproteinemic patterns with familial hyperlipoproteinemia
   Diabetes
   Hypothyroidism
   Nephrotic syndrome
   Obesity
   Pancreatitis
   Alcoholism

Category I: Those with risk factors which, if managed, do not contraindicate surgery nor exclude patients from the study

Category II: Those with risk factors that do not contraindicate surgery, but exclude patients from the study by virtue of questionable prognosis, high incidence of complications, or continuing acceleration of the basic risks

Category III: Those with risk factors that contraindicate surgery and exclude patients from the study

The following are proposals for dealing with the specific risk factors relative to the above categories (Table 10.3). Consideration and experience may add certain other factors to the list as well as alter the categorization proposed.

Atherosclerosis

Patients with uncomplicated atherosclerosis should be placed in category I. Complicated lesions of atherosclerosis which have been unrepaired should relegate a patient to Category II.

Cerebral ischemia and infarction occur in the presence of minimal arterial disease and may be absent in the face of frank arterial occlusion. Most parenchymal effects are associated with the so-called complicating lesions(9) affecting atherosclerotic plaques (Table 10.4). Ulceration of atheromatous plaques may cause discharge of pultaceous debris into the blood stream or escape of naked collagen which, when mixed with platelets, results in aggregation. Adenosine diphosphate (ADP) is released. Fibrin–platelet aggregations are formed in the presence of calcium ion, resulting in emboli and frank thrombosis.(7)

Cerebrovascular occlusive disease is twice as frequent in the presence of complicated extracranial atherosclerosis. Patients in whom lesions have been repaired might be considered for category I. It must be realized that new lesions may develop in susceptible individuals.

Ischemic Heart Disease

In the presence of myocardial infarction, with independent cardiac compensation and arteriographic evidence of adequate coronary circulation, patients may be allowed in category II. Patients who have had myocardial infarction and cardiac failure or ventricular aneurysm should be relegated to category III. Patients with myocardial infarction and inadequate collateral coronary circulation may be amenable to coronary bypass surgery and placed in category II. The inoperable group should be in category III. This appraisal must be subjected to constant review as further data are accumulated regarding coronary bypass surgery.

Table 10.3 Suggested Disposition of Risk Factors

	Category I		Category II		Category III
1.1	Atherosclerosis	2.1	Complicated atherosclerotic lesions		
1.1.1	Uncomplicated atherosclerosis				
1.1.2	Repaired complicated lesions				
		2.3	Post–myocardial infarction	3.3	Post–myocardial infarction
		2.3.1	Compensated with adequate collateral circulation	3.3.1	With heart failure
				3.3.2	Inadequate collateral circulation
		2.3.3	Compensated with successful coronary bypass	3.3.3	Inappropriate for coronary bypass
		2.3.4	Heart block with demand pacemaker	3.3.4	Heart block
				3.3.5	Ventricular aneurysm
				3.3.6	Atrial fibrillation
1.4	Ischemic heart disease without myocardial infarction and successful coronary bypass			3.4	Inoperable ischemic heart disease with myocardial infarction
1.5	Successfully treated curable hypertension	2.5	Hypertension	3.5	Hypertension
		2.5.1	Adrenalectomized patient	3.5.1	Difficult to control
		2.5.2	Hypertension under successful medical management	3.5.2	Associated with irreversible cardiac stigmata
		2.6	Diabetes mellitus — stable and manageable	3.6	Unmanageable diabetes mellitus
1.7	Successfully controlled hypothyroidism				
		2.8	Disorders of lipid metabolism — controlled	3.8	Refractory diseases of lipid metabolism

Patients with myocardial infarction and arrhythmia should be considered as follows. The presence of atrioventricular or multifascicular block should prompt placement in category III. In cases of heart block with a functioning demand pacemaker, upgrading to category II should occur. Patients with atrial fibrillation and heart failure should be placed in category III. Transient arrhythmias may defer microneurosurgery. They will usually be discovered by monitoring with the Holter monitor.

Patients with suspected coronary artery disease who do not have myocardial infarction should be studied with stress electrocardiography. Treadmill tests have 90% accuracy if 80 to 90% of predicted cardiac response to effort can be achieved. The procedure is safe in proper hands. Patients with abnormal stress electrocardiograms should have coronary arteriographic studies. Coronary arteriography is no longer unusual. The risk involved is less than 0.5% in this procedure. The information to be gained is extremely valuable. The operable cases may

Table 10.3 Suggested Disposition of Risk Factors (*Continued*)

Category I		Category II		Category III	
				3.9	Nephrotic syndrome
		2.10	Familial hyperlipoproteinemia		
		2.11	Obesity		
		2.12	Alcoholism		
1.13	Rheumatic heart disease inactive without significant valvular dysfunction	2.13	Rheumatic heart disease	3.13	Rheumatic heart disease
				3.13.1	Atrial Fibrillation
		2.13.2	Following successful valvular surgery	3.13.2	Mitral stenosis with pulmonary hypertension
		2.13.3	Uncomplicated mitral regurgitation		
		2.13.4	Aortic stenosis without marked hemodynamic significance	3.13.4	Hemodynamically significant aortic stenosis
		2.13.5	Aortic insufficiency		
		2.13.6	Multiple valve lesions without significant hemodynamic effects	3.13.6	Multiple valve lesions with significant hemodynamic effects
				3.15	Endocarditis
1.16	Migraine — mild to moderate	2.16	Migraine — severe		
1.17	Successfully controlled anemias	2.17	Hemolytic and hemoglobinopathic anemia	3.17	Hemolytic and hemoglobinopathic anemia — uncontrollable
		2.18	Chronic pulmonary insufficiency — mild	3.18	Chronic pulmonary insufficiency — severe
		2.19	Connective tissue disease — controlled	3.19	Connective tissue disease — uncontrollable
1.20	Uncomplicated syphillis	2.20	Syphillis with cardiovascular complications	3.20	Syphillis with CNS complications
1.21	Successfully remitted polycythemia vera	2.21	Polycythemia controlled		

successfully achieve category I or II; those which are inoperable should remain in category III.

Hypertension

First the potentially curable forms of hypertension should be considered.

Table 10.4. Complicating Lesions Affecting Atherosclerotic Plaques

1. Luminal stenosis
2. Ectasia with aneurysm
3. Ulceration
4. Hemorrhage into the plaque
5. Mural thrombosis
6. Occlusive thrombosis
7. Calcification

Adrenocortical Hypertrophy or Tumor

Cushing's syndrome may be based on adrenocortical or pituitary disease. Successfully treated patients may be placed in category I. If the treatment results in endocrine deficiency requiring hormonal supplementation, category II is appropriate. Patients with aldosteronism should be categorized similarly.

Adrenal Medullary Tumor

Pheochromocytoma, if successfully treated without total adrenalectomy, should not cause a patient to be removed from category I.

Renal Vascular Lesions

Fibromuscular hyperplasia, constricting bands, and atherosclerosis may occur in renal arteries resulting in development of hypertension. The odds are low that such lesions will be found in the age group dominating this study. However, if surgical repair leads to satisfactory reduction in hypertension, the patient may be considered for category I. If additional medical management is required, category II is recommended. If surgery fails to improve the blood pressure status, of course, the patient should be considered for category III. Controllable hypertension in the presence of cardiac stigmata which do not respond to control of blood pressure should be relegated to category III. With heart lesions which are responsive to control of the hypertension, category II may be assumed.

Renal Disease

High renin-producing parenchymal disease of the kidney should cause patients to be considered for category III. Clinical judgment in some cases may indicate placement in category II if antihypertensive therapy is successful.

Diabetes

Maturity onset, stable diabetes should be treated in category II; unstable diabetes in category III. The acceleration of the atherosclerotic process in diabetics affecting the brain and heart is seven times the usual. In addition, there are microvascular effects in the kidney with complicating hypertension and renal failure. Uniform management and improved prognosis with respect to occlusive disease are unattainable, unfortunately, in the best of hands.

Familial Hyperlipoproteinemia

Familial hyperlipoproteinemias are entities of considerable interest. However, there is no good evidence that treatment, no matter how successful, alters the prognosis. Patients with familial hyperlipoproteinemias should be placed in category II and all efforts to control the syndrome should persist.

Syndromes Sharing Hyperlipoproteinemic Patterns with Familial Hyperlipoproteinemia

Hypothyroidism Hypothyroidism is associated with lipoprotein migration electrophoretically similar to that observed in types II and IV familial hyperlipoproteinemia. Management of hypothyroidism should be instituted gradually with replacement therapy and continued until all signs of myxedema, elevated cholesterol, and any cardiac impairment are eliminated. In the presence of normal thyroid studies and vital signs, these patients may then be included in category I with the stipulation that replacement therapy must be lifelong.

Nephrotic Syndrome The Nephrotic syndrome shows a migratory pattern similar to types II and IV. Because of the uncertain prognosis in nephrotic syndrome these patients should be relegated to category III.

Obesity Lipoprotein in obesity as a syndrome tends to migrate with type V hyperlipoproteinemia. The obesity question is so highly complex that adequate discussion here is not appropriate. Management has been notoriously unsuccessful and uniform management impossible. Generally speaking, obese patients should be placed in categories I or II depending upon the seriousness of the disorder. Their outlook for continued good health is such that they could create serious adverse bias in the study.

Diseases Resulting in Altered Lipid Metabolism Other diseases resulting in altered lipid metabolism and hypercholesterolemia may be handled in category II, if controllable. Levels at which hypercholesterolemia is considered controlled in this country are probably too high. The risk of further occlusive vascular disease continues, even in the face of moderate cholesterol levels. Uncontrollable hypercholesterolemia should warrant exclusion from this study (category III).

Alcoholism

Alcoholism similarly defies discussion at this time. Certainly these patients should be in category II if they are free of liver failure, pancreatitis, or serious extracranial atherosclerotic complications.

Emboli

With respect to emboli, the previous discussion of complicated or ulcerated atheroma should apply. In addition, other entities that produce embolic phenomena must be considered.

Rheumatic Heart Disease

If rheumatic heart disease with mitral stenosis is associated with atrial enlargement, the patient should be treated in category II. If associated with atrial fibrillation, there is no evidence that cardioversion alters prognosis for cerebral embolism. Therefore, these patients should be treated in category III.

Patients with endocarditis, whether bacterial or not, should be placed in category III because of the serious risks involved. Those bacterial endocarditis patients who have been treated successfully should be evaluated for severity of valvular damage and that evaluation should dictate disposition.

Pulmonary hypertension associated with mitral stenosis is usually not totally reversible. If improvement follows valve surgery, patients should be placed in category II. Without improvement or surgery, these patients should remain in category III. Mitral insufficiency without significant hemodynamic effects, treated with prophylactic penicillin, may be admitted to category II. With significant hemodynamic changes, pulmonary hypertension, atrial fibrillation, or reduction in cardiac output, the outlook should be less optimistic.

Aortic stenosis requires a 75% reduction in the valve orifice to produce significant hemodynamic or clinical changes. If these changes are significant, the patient should be placed in category III. If valve damage has been surgically repaired with success, category II may be appropriate. Less than 50% reduction in valve orifice may allow these patients to be placed in category I. When aortic stenosis is associated, as is usual, with mitral lesions, patients should be relegated to category II or III depending upon evaluation of status.

Aortic insufficiency has its chief defect in that patients fail to develop adequate cardiac output with effort. They may be placed in category II or III depending on ability to perfuse the brain under stress.

Vasopasm

Mild or moderate migraine with good response to therapy may be treated in category I. Severe migraine should be relegated to category II. As previously observed vasospasm also occurs in uncontrolled hypertension and should be relegated to category II.

Anovulatory Agents

There will be some women in the study who are using birth control pills. Those who are should discontinue their use.(4,5,8) Once the altered physiology due to medication has disappeared, these patients may be placed in category I. An increased incidence of cerebral thrombosis and embolism as well as alteration in cerebral vasculature occurs in patients using anovulatory drugs. Increased incidence of hypertension is well documented, and there may be an increase in the incidence of migraine.

Hypoxia

Hypoxia may be secondary to anemia which is diagnosable and treatable. Those types which are treatable allow patients to be placed in category I. Those anemias such as iron deficiency anemia treated with iron, pernicious anemia treated with B_{12}, and spherocytosis treated with splenectomy are examples of such entities. The untreatable types include some of the hemoglobinopathies and certain hemolytic disorders; these should be placed in categories II or III depending upon their severity.

Chronic Pulmonary and Respiratory Syndromes

Chronic pulmonary and respiratory syndromes, few of which are reversible, should be relegated to categories II or III, depending upon the degree of deterioration in pulmonary function and the effect on the general physiology.

Arterial Disease

Thrombosis and occlusion may be due to nonatherosclerotic arterial diseases including those related to lupus erythematosus.

Lupus Erythematosus

Discussion and consideration of lupus erythematosus deserves some renewal. In 1956, 15% of patients did not survive a year, and 50% did not survive five years. At present, 90% without renal disease survive past the fifth year; 90% of those patients with significant renal involvement survive the fifth year. The former should be placed in category II; those with renal involvement should be placed in category III.

Progressive Systemic Sclerosis and Polyarteritis

Scleroderma and polyarteritis patients should be placed in category III.

Arteritis

Giant cell arteritis or temporal arteritis is a self-limited disease which has good response to steroid therapy. If treated successfully, patients may be placed in category I.

Lues

Lues without cardiac, aortic, or central nervous system complications may be considered for category I following suitable treatment. Where cardiac and aortic difficulties exist, patients adequately treated may be placed in category II. If central nervous system impairment is present, the patient should be relegated to category III.

Polycythemia

Polycythemia vera may be treated successfully and included in the study (category I). Secondary types of polycythemia must be judged depending on etiology. While they are not associated with platelet dyscrasias blood viscosity remains high, leading to uncertain prognosis. The basic etiology may exclude patients from either study or surgical intervention.

Management

Some discussion may be appropriate with respect to treatment of entities in category I that require ongoing management. As noted before, sober consideration and experience may "promote" some diseases from category II into category I. At that time uniform management will be essential if studies of effectiveness are to have validity with respect to microneurosurgical anastomosis.

Among the manageable diseases in category I is myxedema. It is suggested that hypothyroidism be managed throughout the study with levothyroxine (T-4), which provides the smoothest and most easily controlled therapy for these patients. Clinical monitoring of the euthyroid state of the patient is the most practical form of follow-up observation; but normalization of TSH is an excellent objective indicator of adequate therapy.

In those patients with rheumatic heart disease prophylaxis against recurrence and against bacterial endocarditis is essential. The usual prophylaxis against rheumatic fever is oral penicillin, 250,000 units twice a day. In patients where there is question of compliance, 1.2 million units of benzathine penicillin G should be administered intramuscularly on a monthly basis. Dental and surgical procedures in which the possibility of bacteremia exists should be treated prophylactically with additional doses of either penicillin or ampicillin. In situations where penicillin cannot be tolerated, erythromycin or vancomycin should be used. Under these circumstances the antibiotic should be started prior to the procedure and continued for 2 to 3 days postoperatively. In migraine which has demonstrated its ability to be controlled, control is usually at hand. It seems appropriate that a specific regimen for treatment of acute attacks be developed for the sake of this study, and the requirement that therapy be initiated at the outset of an attack should be stressed. Ergotamine tartrate combined with caffeine is undoubtedly the treatment of choice in the mild and moderate case. Two mg in repeated doses at 30- to 60-minute intervals, not to exceed a total of 6 mg ergotamine tartrate, comprises the treatment which experience has shown to be most effective in these cases.

An exhaustive discussion of the therapy of anemias is impossible. Suffice it to say, for the purpose of this study, that appropriate therapy should result in correction of anemia and maintenance of adequate hemoglobin and red cell count. Surveillance may be required to achieve this, but the presence of controllable anemia should not exclude patients from the study.

With respect to latent lues, patients with positive serologic tests, positive fluorescent treponemal antibody, and positive treponemal immobolizing antibody, but negative spinal fluid serology, should receive 6 million units of penicillin in a 10-day period followed by repeated serologic studies at 3-month intervals for the succeeding 2 years. In the face of rising titers retreatment should be instituted. The existence of persisting stable positive serologic tests should not exclude patients from the study, if adequate treatment has been administered. Patients who are sensitive to penicillin should receive erythromycin, 4 g a day for 14 days. It should be understood that the erythromycin regimen poses a serious problem with compliance and close observation is essential to insure adequate therapy.

In the treatment of polycythemia vera, the choice for the purposes of this study would appear to be administration of radiophosphorus. Phlebotomy, while reducing blood viscosity, does so intermittently and may actually induce increased platelet and vascular difficulties. Use of chemotherapy is fraught with danger and complications. Therefore, the smoothest, most predictable, and probably most uniform control of polycythemia would best be obtained for the purposes of this study with ^{32}P. The radioisotope should be administered by experienced workers at a center where radioisotope facilities are available to insure safe and adequate therapy.

I have reserved the discussion of cigarette smoking until last. Smokers have made magnificent efforts to survive and function in spite of the odds against them.(3,9) I believe that they deserve—all else being equal—to be treated in category I, the sole therapy being a solemn promise to quit.

REFERENCES

1. Dinesdale HB, Robertson DM: Cerebral flow in acute hypertension. Arch Neurol 31:80, 1974
2. Hass WK: Occlusive cerebrovascular disease. Med Clin North Am 56:1281, 1972
3. Kannel WB, Blaisdell FV, Gifford R, et al: Risk factors in stroke due to cerebral infarction. Stroke 2:423, 1971
4. Mason B, Oakley N, Wynn V: Studies of carbohydrate and lipid metabolism in women developing hypertension on oral contraceptives. Br Med J 3:317, 1973
5. Mastri RM, Silverstein PM, Gold L, et al: Multiple progressive intraarterial occlusions. Stroke 4:380, 1973
6. Millikan CH: The pathogenesis of transient focal cerebral ischemia. Circulation 32:438, 1965
7. Mustard JF, Packham MA: Factors influencing platelet function. Adhesions, release and aggregation. Pharmacol Rev 22:97, 1970
8. Okawara SH, Calkins RA: Cerebral arterial occlusive disease with telangiectasia associated with oral contraceptive. Arch Neurol 29:60, 1973
9. Strong JP, Eggen DA, Oalmann MC, et al: Pathology and epidemiology of atherosclerosis. Circ Res 62:262, 1973

11

Ocular Plethysmography and Suction Ophthalmodynamometry in the Diagnosis of Carotid Occlusive Disease

Andrew L. Carney

Introduction

The ocular pulse is the key to the carotid artery. The ocular pulse reflects the blood flow and blood pressure (BP) of the ophthalmic artery and thus the carotid artery. Normally, the pulse reflects the flow and pressure derived directly from the internal carotid artery; however, when the carotid artery is obstructed proximally either by disease or compression, it reflects the flow and pressure in distal collateral channels.

A recording of the ocular pulse requires distortion of the ocular bulb. Pressure causes indentation and suction causes protrusion. The recorded tracing using one technique is the mirror image of the other. The choroidal plexus rather than the retinal artery is largely responsible for the ocular pulse.(19) Diminished stroke output due to cardiac failure or cardiac arrhythmia will markedly influence the ocular pulse. In some patients, ocular perfusion may fall to 25% of original volume with a marked arrhythmia.(21)

Ocular and cerebral blood flow are reflected by the amplitude of the ocular pulse wave while ocular and cerebral blood pressure are best reflected by the systolic pressure of the ophthalmic artery.(3,14,18) The source of ocular blood flow and pressure is best determined by compression of the carotid artery. It is more difficult to time the pulse delays in a system where distances are short and collateral channels can be extensive.(14)

Bynke(6) recorded the amplitude of the ocular pulse in each eye sequentially using a pressure system. In patients with a fixed neurologic deficit and unilateral carotid stenosis, he noted a decreased amplitude on the side of stenosis in 80% of his patients. In 20%, the pulse amplitude was equal or paradoxically increased on the side of stenosis. He considered a 14%

difference in amplitude to be significant. Similar findings were reported with ophthalmodynamometry.(12,23)

Brockenbrough and Lawrence(5) used ocular plethysmography to evaluate the contribution of the collateral circulation by employing carotid and temporal artery compression and observing the effect on the ocular pulse. No quantitative criteria were utilized.

Ocular pressure has been measured by ophthalmodynamometry (ODM) for over half a century. Using this technique it has been determined that (1) the differences between each eye are more significant than the relation to systemic pressure; (2) a 15% difference in pressure between the two eyes is significant and a 20% difference is diagnostic of carotid disease unless proven otherwise; (3) diastolic determinations are not reliable since one-third of patients with total occlusion of the internal carotid artery have no significant diastolic pressure differences(13,18); and (4) the use of orbital compression to determine systolic pressures is associated with adverse cardiac reflexes.(12,13,23,24)

Irrespective of the great contribution of ophthalmodynamometry, the technique has significant disadvantages:

1. It is not suitable for patients with cataracts
2. Only one eye is studied at a time
3. Adverse cardiac reflexes make determination of ocular systolic pressure hazardous
4. Collateral cerebral flow is not evaluated
5. The direct recorded pressures do not correlate with ODM values(3)

While ophthalmodynamometry raises the intraocular pressure by applying pressure to the eye, application of suction accomplishes the same objective by "pinching" the ocular bulb. Galin and Best,(1) using the accepted ODM endpoints, applied up to 500 mmHg suction to the eyeball to raise intraocular pressures to 154 mmHg. They noted minimal cardiac and systemic reaction to the suction technique of ophthalmodynamometry. Furthermore, they established the relationship between the level of the vacuum applied to the eye and the intraocular pressure, eg, a vacuum of 300 mmHg applied to the eye raised the intraocular pressure to 110 mmHg.

In 1971, Gee introduced a system which applied a high vacuum to the eye and bled the vacuum at a constant rate. He noted the onset of arterial pulsations by plethysmographic techniques rather than retinal arterial pulsation. In 1974, he introduced a binocular system which permitted the simultaneous determination of systolic pressure in both eyes.(8) By combining carotid compression with bilateral ocular pressure determinations, he could quantitatively assess the collateral flow. At surgery, the "stump" pressure of the internal carotid artery was determined. From these measurements he constructed a table establishing the relationship between the level of vacuum and the stump pressure.(8) His table correlated quite closely with that of Galin and Best in midrange. High values were excluded because vacuum levels above 300 mmHg were not employed; and in the lower ranges, the recorded stump pressures were lower than the intrinsic intraocular pressure.

The instrumentation conceived by Gee facilitates the diagnosis and evaluation of the functional capacity of carotid stenosis. It permits recording of the ocular pulse and determination of systolic ocular pressures at rest and with carotid compression, both in the office and in the operating room. It furthermore has the potential of predicting the need for a shunt during surgery, and of evaluating surgical results postoperatively.

Case Material

Sixty-one ocular pulse studies were performed in 51 patients between February 1 and June 15, 1974. Two patients underwent temporal-cortical shunts. Eight patients underwent reconstructive procedures for carotid stenosis at the bifurcation. Three patients underwent reconstruction of the proximal and distal carotid arteries. Four of the 51 underwent vertebral artery reconstruction and one was found to have an arteriovenous malformation. Five patients (10%) exhibited significant cardiac arrhythmias, but only one required a permanent cardiac pacemaker for significant bradycardia.(16,22) Thus, 18 procedures were performed on 51 patients. The ocular pulse studies were helpful in making the diagnosis, selecting the patients for arteriography, eliminating unnecessary intraoperative shunting, and assessing the postoperative results.

The following selected cases are presented to show the usefulness of these techniques as adjuncts to both extracranial and newer intracranial neurovascular procedures. Ocular pressure data (in mmHg) for the resting state and after either right carotid compression (RCC) or left carotid compression (LCC) are given. Composite sketches of the angiographic studies are included and the significance of the findings is discussed.

Case 1, MD: Bilateral Carotid Stenosis

A 75-year-old white female presented with transient numbness of the left side of her body and face and right monocular visual disturbance. Examination revealed a right carotid bruit and positive Brockenbrough for right internal carotid obstruction.

The ocular pulse data that were obtained are shown in Table 11.1.

Findings were as follows:

1. Ocular perfusion: low normal bilaterally at rest; poor collateral perfusion with carotid compression
2. Marked delay of ocular pulse with left carotid compression
3. Systemic-ocular gradient, 65 mmHg bilaterally
4. Ocular BP in excess of 50 mmHg bilaterally with carotid compression

The following impressions were recorded:

1. Stenosis of the right internal carotid artery, r/o bilateral disease
2. Normal ocular pressures with low normal perfusion bilaterally
3. Carotid artery occlusion tolerated without shunt better on right than left

Angiography disclosed bilateral carotid stenosis that was worse on the right side (Fig. #11.1).

Comment In bilateral carotid disease, the amplitude of the pulse, the pulse delay, the ocular-systemic gradient, and the collateral flow may all be symmetric. Normal amplitude with the calibrated Gee instrument is 7 to 25 mm. Pulse delays may be intensified by carotid compression as in this case. Delays in excess of 0.02 second are considered significant.(23) The relationship of the ophthalmic to brachial blood pressure has been expressed as a ratio and the normal value is approximately 0.55. However, with hypertensive patients the ratio may approach 0.90.(12) More recently, direct studies employing cannulation of the supraorbital artery cast doubt on the validity of the ratio. The systolic gradient appears directly related to systemic pressures.(3,4) Therefore, we expressed the gradient between ophthalmic and systemic pressures with explicit systemic pressures. In general, pressure gradients in excess of 30 to 40 mm are significant.

In this patient, pulse amplitude was low, but symmetric. With right carotid compression, there was no pulse delay; but with left carotid compression pulse delay was 0.1 second, suggesting an inability of the right carotid artery to supply the left side. The systolic gradients were 65 mmHg bilaterally when systemic blood pressure was 170/90. With left carotid compression, left ocular blood pressure was not sustained as it was with right carotid compression.

Table 11.1 Case 1. Ocular Pulse and Pressure Data (pressures in mmHg)

Ocular Plethysmography	Right Eye (O.D.)	Left Eye (O.S.)	%Δ
Resting	8.0	7.7	96
RCC	1.0; no delay	7.5	13
LCC	7.0	1.0; 0.1 second delay	114
Ocular Blood Pressure			
Resting, 170/90	105	105	
RCC	68	108	
LCC	108	58	

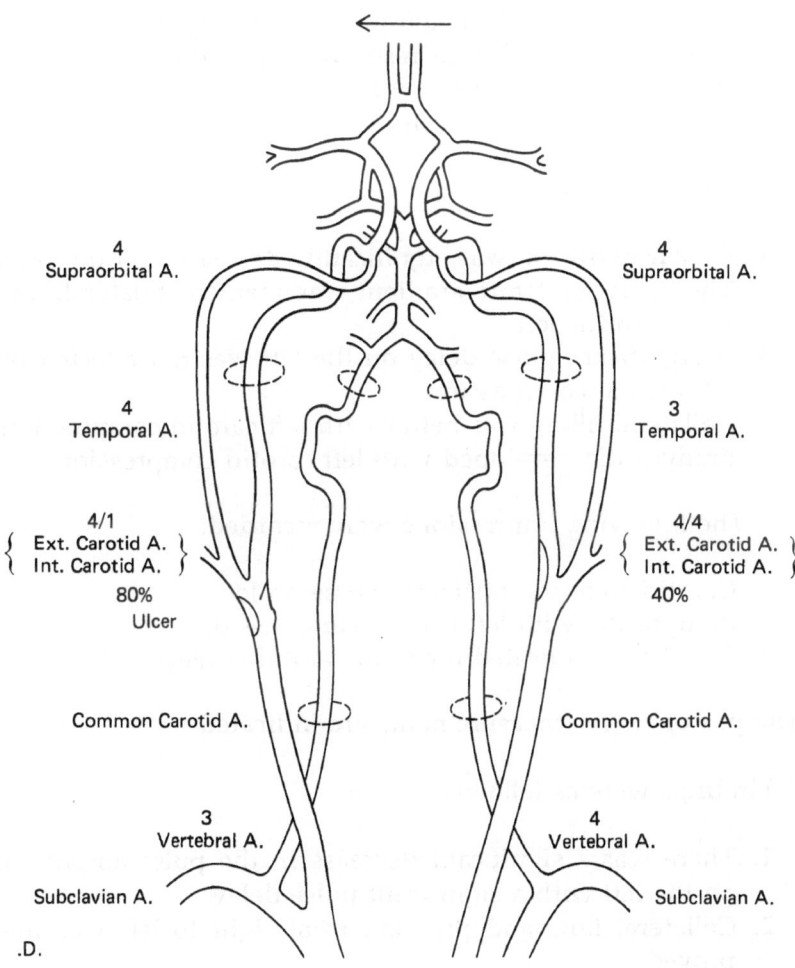

4
Supraorbital A.

4
Temporal A.

4/1
{ Ext. Carotid A. }
{ Int. Carotid A. }
80%
Ulcer

Common Carotid A.

3
Vertebral A.

Subclavian A.

.D.

4
Supraorbital A.

3
Temporal A.

4/4
{ Ext. Carotid A. }
{ Int. Carotid A. }
40%

Common Carotid A.

4
Vertebral A.

Subclavian A.

Fig. 11.1 Composite sketch of angioarchitecture in case 1.

Table 11.2. Case 2. Preoperative Ocular Pulse and Pressure Data (pressure in mmHg)

Ocular Plethysmography	O.D.	O.S.	%Δ
Resting	18.2	23[a]	79
RCC	3.2	12	27
LCC[b]	12.3	5.4	44
Ocular Blood Pressure			
Resting, 180/80	107	98	
OS Gradient	73	82	
RCC	37	72	
LCC	104	70	

[a]Delay in left ocular pulse 0.05 second; not increased with LCC.
[b]LCC produced a bradycardia, 72, to 48/minute; Δ 33%.

Case 2, MC: Carotid Stenosis with Contralateral Occlusion

A 65-year-old white male presented with right carotid bruit and transient paresis of the left upper extremity. Moderate hypertension was treated with reserpine and aldomet. Brockenbrough ± on the right. The ocular pulse data shown in Table 2 were obtained preoperatively.

Findings were as follows:

1. Ocular perfusion was significantly decreased on the right
2. The ocular-systemic gradient was marked, bilateral, and worse on the left
3. A significant pulse delay on the left was not affected by left carotid compression
4. Collateral filling was better with left carotid compression
5. Bradycardia developed with left carotid compression

The following impressions were recorded:

1. Carotid stenosis, bilateral, worse on left
2. Bradycardia with left carotid compression
3. Shunt was indicated for right carotid surgery

The postoperative measurements are indicated

Findings were as follows:

1. There was a significant decrease in the pulse amplitude on the left with a significant pulse delay
2. Collateral flow and pressure from right to left was improved

Table 11.3. Case 2. Postoperative Ocular Pulse and Pressure Data (pressure in mmHg)

Ocular Plethysmography	O.D.	O.S.	%Δ
Resting	18.0	15.3	85
RCC	1.6	4.7[a]	34
LCC[b]	13.3	10.3	77
Ocular Blood Pressure			
Resting, 180/90	110+	98	
OS Gradient	?	82	
RCC	62	78	
LCC	110+	102	

[a]Delay persists in left ocular pulse.
[b]Bradycardia with LCC 70 to 64/minute.

3. There was an improved ocular-systemic gradient on the right
4. The degree of bradycardia in response to left carotid compression decreased

The following impressions were recorded:

1. Obstruction of the left carotid artery persisted
2. There was improved right cerebral perfusion and collateral flow

Composite sketch of the angiographic data demonstrates a right carotid stenosis and a complete left carotid occlusion (Fig. 11.2).

Comment Pulse amplitude was paradoxically increased on the left side. Right carotid compression reduced pulse amplitude bilaterally. Collateral filling was best from right to left. Left carotid compression resulted in a 33% decrease in heart rate. Pulse delay on the left side was 0.05 second and was not increased by left carotid compression. The right carotid artery was the dominant vessel. The predicted stump pressure was less than 50 mmHg and the need for a shunt was evident.(2,11)

The postoperative study revealed a normalized pulse amplitude by a decrease in the left ocular amplitude. Cerebral perfusion was reduced after right carotid compression and left ocular perfusion was increased with left carotid compression. The latter was due to the decreased contribution of the left external carotid artery and increased flow from the right carotid artery. There was no change in pulse delay although pressure and flow improved. Cardiac arrhythmia in response to left carotid compression was markedly reduced.

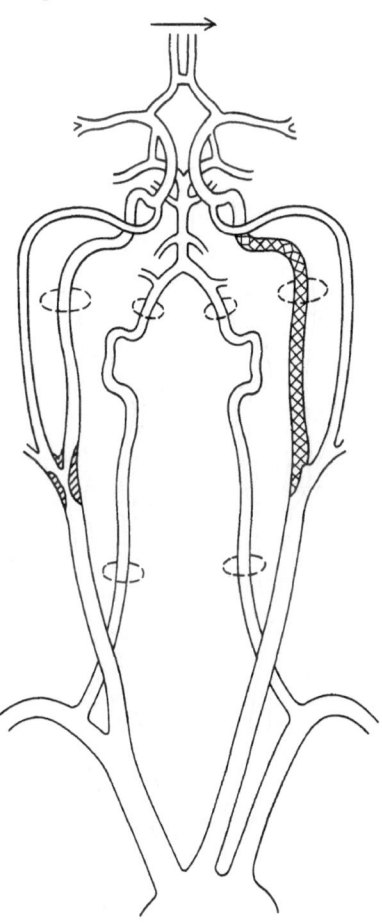

Fig. 11.2. Composite sketch of angioarchitecture in case 2.

Case Material

123

Case 3, CG: Carotid Ulceration with Embolism and Previous Contralateral Carotid Surgery

A 54-year-old white female presented in 1972 with left cerebral symptoms. Arteriography revealed bilateral carotid stenosis that was worse on the left side. At the time of surgery, ulceration of the left internal carotid stenosis with thrombosis extending to the carotid siphon was removed without incident. Two years later, she presented with recurrent emboli to the right eye. Palpation of the right carotid resulted in immediate embolization to the right eye. Right brachial arteriography revealed stenosis, with a mural thrombus and extensive ulceration of the right carotid artery. A composite sketch of the angiographic studies indicates the old left carotid endarterectomy site and the right carotid stenosis (Fig. 11.3).

The ocular blood pressure data shown in Table 11.4 were obtained before and after repair of the right carotid stenosis.

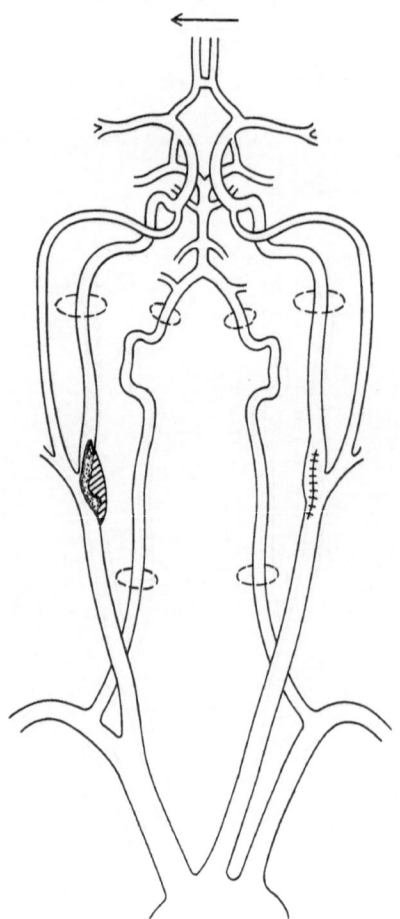

Fig. 11.3. Composite sketch of angioarchitecture in case 3.

Table 11.4. Case 3. Pre- and Postoperative Ocular Blood Pressure Data (pressure in mmHg)

Ocular Blood Pressure		O.D.	O.S.
Preoperative			
Resting, 170/90		107	110+
	gradient	63	
Pulse Amplitude		9.7	20
RCC—not done			
LCC		98	64
Postoperative			
Resting, 212/115		110+	110+

Findings were as follows:

1. The ocular-systemic gradient was greater on the right (63 mmHg)
2. There was adequate collateral flow from right to left with left carotid compression
3. Ocular blood flow on the left was two times greater than that on the right

The following impressions were recorded:

Preoperative
1. Right carotid stenosis
2. Good collateral flow from right to left was present
3. Left carotid flow was twice that of the right

4. Patent left carotid reconstruction
   Postoperative
1. Patent right carotid reconstruction

Comment The ocular pulse studies established the full patency of the left internal carotid artery and the presence of right internal carotid artery obstruction by the gradient on the right side. Left carotid compression indicated the ability of the obstructed right carotid artery to supply the left side. The safest technique to use in exposing a carotid artery containing fragile plaque is to immediately occlude the distal internal carotid artery, before any dissection of the bifurcation is performed. Arteriotomy revealed an extensive ulcer 5.0 cm. in length with an adherent fibrinaggregate type of thrombus. The patient experienced no emboli or neurologic deficit. The conduct of surgery was determined by the assessment of ophthalmic artery pressure and the status of the collateral circulation.

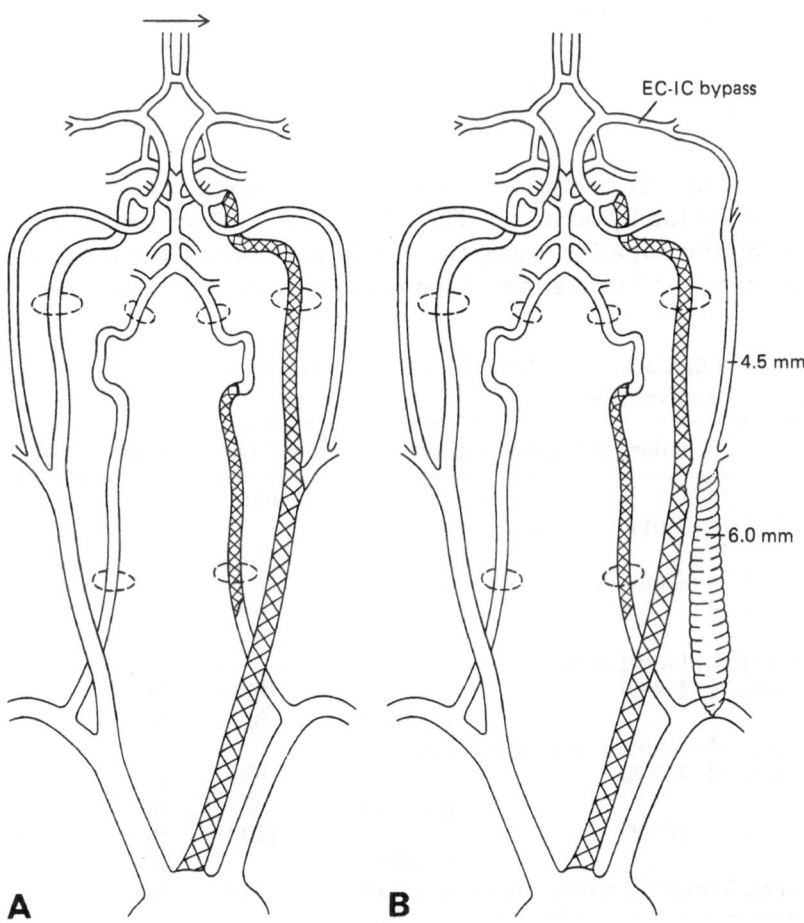

Fig. 11.4. Composite sketch of arteriograms in case 4. a. Preoperative. b. Postoperative.

Case 4, CW: Completed stroke with persistent cerebral hypotension. subclavian carotid and temporal cortical bypass

A 66-year-old white male presented in February 1974 with a right hemiparesis of gradual onset. He also suffered from defective cerebration and dysphasia. On March 4, 1974, he exhibited complete right *upper extremity* paralysis and the brain scan was consistent with cerebral ischemia or infarct. Doppler evaluation of carotid flow revealed the presence of two distinct flow patterns at the left carotid bifurcation. There were no bruits. Arteriography revealed total obstruction of the left common carotid and left vertebral arteries (Fig. 11.4a).

The left external carotid artery was reconstructed by subclavian-carotid bypass on March 15, 1974 with improvement in the ocular perfusion pressures short of acceptable levels. There was marked improvement of the right upper extremity and restoration of the brain scan to normal. On June 24, 1974, temporal-cortical shunt was performed with further improvement in cerebration, speech, and motor function of the right side. The patient has returned to normal function within his family structure. Ocular pulse and pressure data obtained from this patient are shown in Table 11.5.

Comment At operation, the internal and common carotid artery were totally occluded. The external carotid was patent, supplying the superior thyroid artery. Bypass from left subclavian artery to the bifurcation of the external carotid and superficial

Table 11.5. Case 4. Ocular Pulse and Pressure Data (pressure in mmHg)

Ocular Plethysmography		O.D.	O.S.	% Δ
3-11-74		14.6	2.3	16
3-15-74—Subclavian-carotid bypass				
4-11-74		7.7	3.0	39
6-24-74—Temporal-cortical bypass				
7-24-74		9.4	4.7	50
Ocular Blood Pressure				
3-11-74, 144/80		107	42	
	gradient	37	102	
3-15-74—Subclavian-carotid bypass				
4-11-74, 130/70		98	65	
	gradient	32	65	
7-24-74, 164/90		110+	92	
	gradient	?	72	
Left Temporal artery communication		110+	66	

temporal artery (S.T.A.) was performed with a 6-mm dacron graft.

Case 5, MR: Bilateral Carotid Disease. Use of Temporal–Middle Cerebral Shunt to Permit Contralateral Carotid Surgery

A 58-year-old white male experienced a transient paresis of the left upper extremity with dimming of vision of the right eye. Percutaneous carotid arteriography revealed a high-grade stenosis of the right internal carotid artery. At operation (2-12-74) the internal carotid was occluded and the clot was adherent to the arterial wall. Postoperatively the patient experienced retrobulbar pain in the right eye which responded to heparin and Rheomacrodex.

On March 24, 1974, a right temporal–middle cerebral bypass was performed with return of ocular pressure to normal bilaterally. Left carotid thromboendarterectomy (4-15-74) failed to enhance improvement of cerebral perfusion, but diminished

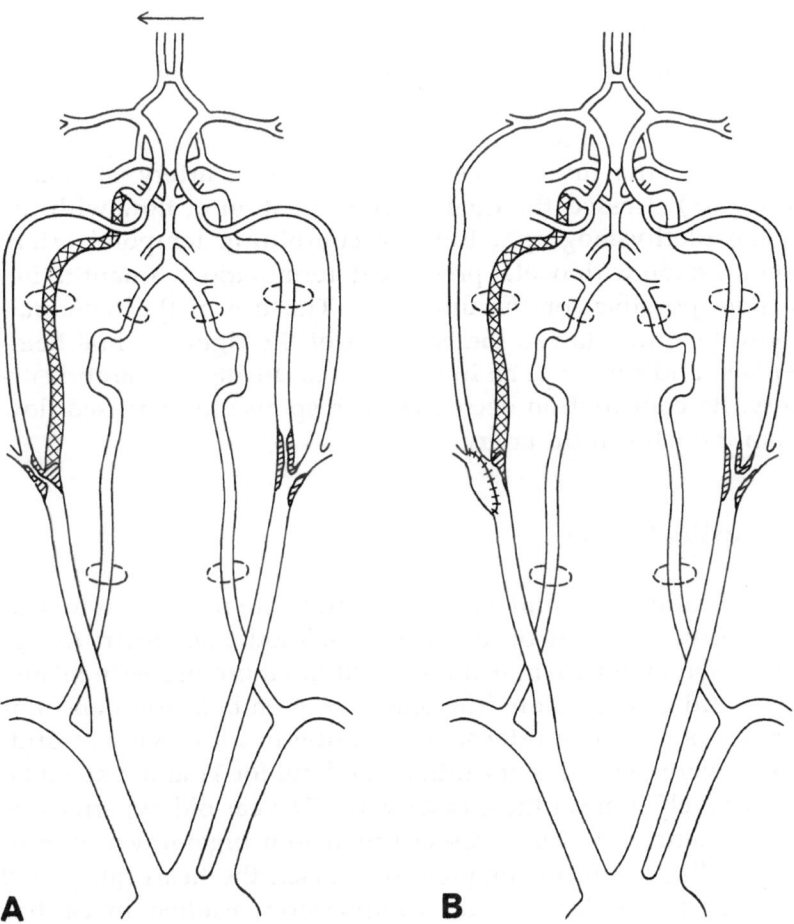

A **B**

Fig. 11.5. Composite sketch of arteriograms in case 5. a. Preoperative. b. Postoperative.

Table 11.6. Case 5. Ocular Pressure Data (pressure in mmHg)

Ocular Pressure Studies	O.D.	O.S.
2-12-74—Reconstruction of right external carotid artery		
2-28-74, 160/90	80	94
Bilateral temporal artery compression	72	88
3-14-74—Right temporal–cortical bypass		
4-11-74, 180/96	103	110
Bilateral temporal artery compression	88	110
4-15-74—Left carotid Thromboendarterectomy		
9-3-74, 176/86	102	110
Bilateral temporal artery compression	94	110

the contribution of the temporal-cortical shunt to cerebral perfusion (Figs. 11.5a, b).

In this case, the right temporal–cortical shunt served to correct cerebral hypotension, but also acted as an internal shunt during left carotid endarterectomy. Ocular pressure data obtained from this patient are shown in Table 11.6.

Comment   In this patient, carotid compression was not possible because of a short, thick neck. Bilateral temporal artery compression demonstrated the contribution of the temporal artery to ocular and cerebral perfusion. Olivarus(15) called attention to the importance of the temporal artery. Brockenbrough(5) stressed the qualitative evaluation of flow with the ocular-plethysmograph. But, by combining temporal artery compression with ocular pressure determinations, quantitation is now possible for the first time. The use of the temporal-cortical shunt relieved the ischemia of the right cerebral hemisphere and served as an internal shunt during left carotid surgery. Its contribution decreased in response to increased flow from the left carotid artery.

Complications

Complications encountered in this study are not related to ocular plethysmography or suction ophthalmodynamometry except for minor conjunctival irritation, but are more properly related to carotid compression. The one case of embolization encountered was that of an extensive ulceration in a low-lying carotid. There were two cases of cardiac standstill for 11 and 7 seconds, respectively. One of these cases was a 71-year-old hypertensive with extensive vascular disease in whom bigeminy was produced. Right carotid compression caused the heart rate to fall from 80 to 55. Left carotid compression resulted in cardiac standstill for 11 seconds. Resting ocular pressures were in excess of 110 mm/Hg bilaterally.

Discussion

Ocular plethysmography and suction ophthalmodynamometry are procedures well established in medicine. The instrumentation available now permits increased application to cerebrovascular problems.

The inherent limitations to the technique must be understood. Technical factors such as improper cup application, conjunctival edema, and prolapse occluding the cup may modify the significance of correctly derived data. The technique may be useful in defining occlusive disease of the ophthalmic artery, papilledema, intracranial occlusive lesions distal to the ophthalmic artery, and an aberrant origin of the ophthalmic artery which occurs in 3.5% of cases.(10) Moderate unilateral glaucoma does not significantly influence ocular systolic blood pressure.(9) Carotid compression may be incomplete due to calcification, slippage of the vessel beneath the fingers, or extreme muscular rigidity in the kyphotic patient. The determination of a pathologic ocular-systemic pressure gradient is predicated on a valid systemic pressure. Asymmetry of the ocular pulse wave and pressure measurements may be enhanced by position, either erect or supine.(16) Both brachial arterial disease and reflex hypotension at the time of carotid compression may produce misleading information.

Approximately 4%/(2/51) of patients develop cardiac asystole and an additional 15% develop some degree of bradycardia and/or hypotension with carotid compression. Our findings are consistent with those reported elsewhere. Electrocardiographic monitoring with facilities and medication for cardiac resuscitation is recommended whenever carotid compression is performed.(17,20)

Another aspect of carotid compression requires emphasis. Compression of one carotid artery stresses the opposite carotid and vertebral arteries by decreasing the vascular resistance and increasing the vascular bed. This permits the detection of systolic pressure gradients not apparent in states of high peripheral resistance. It also permits the assessment of collateral flow and determines the necessity for using a shunt at the time of surgery.(7)

Summary

Sixty-one ocular pulse studies have been performed in 51 patients over a 5-month period. A study of flow and pressure was accomplished with a single instrument permitting ocular plethysmography and suction ophthalmodynamometry. This noninvasive technique has been found to be safe, reliable, and without ocular complications in the evaluation of cerebrovascular lesions.

Pulse amplitude, ocular-systemic pressure gradient, and adequacy of collateral channels were determined. The complications encountered are related to carotid compression and include ocular embolism and cardiac asystole. Lesser degrees of bradycardia are more frequent.

Ocular pulse studies have proven valuable in (1) the diagnosis of significant carotid artery stenosis; (2) the selection of patients for angiography; (3) the physiologic evaluation of angiographic lesions; (4) assessing the collateral circulation; (5) determining the need for intraoperative shunting; (6) determining the success of surgery; (7) determining the adequacy of shunting; and (8) following the progression of disease and recurrence of stenosis.

REFERENCES

1. Best M, Galin, MA: Ocular pulse studies in carotid stenosis. Arch. Ophthalmol 85:730, 1971
2. Bland J, et al: Neurological complications of carotid surgery. Ann Surg 171:459, 1970
3. Borras A, et al: Ophthalmodynamometric and direct measurement of ophthalmic artery pressure. Am J Ophthalmol 67:681, 1969
4. Borras A, et al: Carotid compression test and the direct measurement of ophthalmic artery pressure in man. Am J Ophthalmol 67:688, 1969
5. Brockenbrough EC, Lawrence C, Schwenk WG: Ocular plethysmography. A new technique for the evaluation of carotid obstructive disease. Rev Surg 24:299, 1967
6. Bynke HG: Screening diagnosis of carotid occlusion by means of oculoshygmography. Neurology 16:383, 1966
7. Edwards EA: Dynamic consequences of arterial stenosis. J Cardiovasc Surg (Torino) 8:386-9, 1967
8. Gee W, et al: Ocular pneumoplethysmography in carotid artery disease. Med Instrum 8:244, 1974
9. Goldstein JE, et al: Intraocular pressure and ophthalmodynamometry. Arch Ophthalmol 74:175, 1965
10. Hayreh SS: Arteries of the orbit in the human being. Br J Surg 50:938, 1963
11. Hays RJ, Levinson SA, Wylie EJ: Intraoperative measurement of carotid back pressure as a guide to operative management for carotid endarterectomy. Surgery 72:953, 1972
12. Hollenhorst RW: Ophthalmodynamometry and intracranial vascular disease. Med Clin North Am 42:951, 1958
13. Hollenhorst RW: Carotid and vertebral basilar disease. Neuroophthalmological aspect. Trans Am Acad Ophthalmol Otolaryngol 66:166, 1962
14. Karchner MM, McRae LP: Morrison FD: Noninvasive detection

and evaluation of carotid occlusive disease. Arch Surg 106:528, 1973

15. Olivarus BF: The external carotid sign. Acta Neurol Scand 41:539, 1965
16. Reed RL, et al: Rarity of transient focal cerebral ischemia in cardiac dysrrhythmias. JAMA 223:893, 1973
17. Silverstein A, et al: Manual compression of the carotid vessels. Carotid sinus hypersensitivity and carotid artery occlusion. Ann Intern Med 52:172, 1960
18. Smith JL: Observations on ophthalmodynamometry. JAMA 170:1403, 1959
19. Suzuki I: Corneal pulsations and corneal pulse waves. Jpn Ophthalmol 6:190, 1962
20. Synek L: Evaluation of effectiveness of digital carotid compression test by EEG. Clin EEG 5:88, 1974
21. Tufo HM, Ostfeld AM, Shekelle R: Central nervous system dysfunction following the open heart surgery. JAMA 212:1333, 1970
22. Walter PF, Reid SD, Wenger NK: Transient cerebral ischemia due to arrhythmia. Ann Intern Med 72:471, 1970
23. Weigelin E, Lobstein A: Ophthalmodynamometry. Basel, Karger, 1963
24. Weiss S, Baker JP: The carotid sinus reflex in health and disease. Its role in the causation of fainting and convulsions. Medicine (Baltimore) 12:297, 1933

12

Collateral circulation of the brain

Behrooz Azar-Kia and Enrique Palacios

Arterial obstruction in the cervical or intracranial vasculature may produce a neurologic deficit, depending on the rapidity of onset of the obstruction and the anatomic nature of the collateral circulation. Gradual occlusion of any vessel is accompanied by the progressive development of compensatory circulation, ie, enlargement of preexisting collateral vessels. Sudden occlusion of a major artery is commonly associated with ischemia of the affected area.

In occlusive vascular disease the circle of Willis is the major collateral pathway. The anterior and posterior communicating arteries are the main connecting vessels between the two hemispheres and also between the carotid and basilar systems.

Besides the circle of Willis, there are a number of arteries at the base of the brain which can serve as collaterals around an occlusive lesion. The deep collateral arteries such as the lenticulostriate, thalamoperforating, posterior pericallosal, and choroidal arteries may become dilated and form anastomoses between themselves to bypass the area of occlusion. The superficial collaterals at the base of the brain consist of the ophthalmic artery and the dural branches of the cavernous segment of the internal carotid artery. The muscular branches of the vertebral arteries also serve as collateral channels by anastomoses with branches of the occipital, ascending cervical, and deep cervical arteries.

The leptomeningeal anastomosis over the convexity, between the terminal branches of the anterior, middle, and posterior cerebral arteries, is a common development with vascular occlusive disease. Over the cerebellum, however, leptomeningeal anastomosis occurs between the hemispheric and vermian branches of the posterior inferior cerebellar and superior cerebellar arteries.

132

Table 12.1. Collateral Circulation to the Brain

A. Internal Carotid to Internal Carotid
1. Superficial
   a. Anterior cerebral ⇌ Middle cerebral (Figs. 12.1 and 12.2)
   b. Middle Cerebral ⇌ Posterior cerebral
   c. Posterior cerebral ⇌ Anterior cerebral (Fig. 12.3)
2. Deep
   a. Lenticulostriate
      Middle cerebral ⇌ Anterior cerebral (Fig. 12.4)
   b. Thalamoperforating
      Posterior cerebral ⇌ Posterior cerebral (Fig. 12.5)
   c. Posterior pericallosal
      Posterior cerebral ⇌ Anterior cerebral (Fig. 12.3)
B. External Carotid to Internal Carotid
1. Ophthalmic artery (Fig. 12.10)
2. Meningeal arteries
   a. Middle meningeal (Fig. 12.11)
   b. Ethmoidal (Fig. 12.12)
   c. Accessory meningeals (Fig. 12.13)
   d. Meningohypophyseal (Fig. 12.13)
3. Arteries of the scalp
   a. Superficial temporal (Fig. 12.12)
   b. Occipital artery (Fig. 12.7)
C. Vertebrobasilar system to Internal Carotid
1. Circle of Willis
2. Persistent trigeminal (Fig. 12.6)
3. Persistent hypoglossal (Fig. 12.16)
4. Persistent otic (Fig. 12.17)
D. Vertebral to External Carotid
1. Occipital (Fig. 12.7)
2. Ascending cervical (Fig. 12.8)
E. Vertebral to Basilar
Posterior inferior cerebellar ⇌ Superior cerebellar (Fig. 12.9)

Meningoencephalic anastomoses occur by way of inconstant branches of the meningeal arteries which perforate the dura to reach the leptomeningeal arteries on the surface of the brain.

The collateral circulation in occlusive vascular disease may be very complex. Recognition of these patterns should be of considerable value as development of microneurosurgical anastomosis progresses.

A classification of the important collateral channels is shown in Table 12.1 with specific examples illustrated in Figures 12.1 to 12.15.

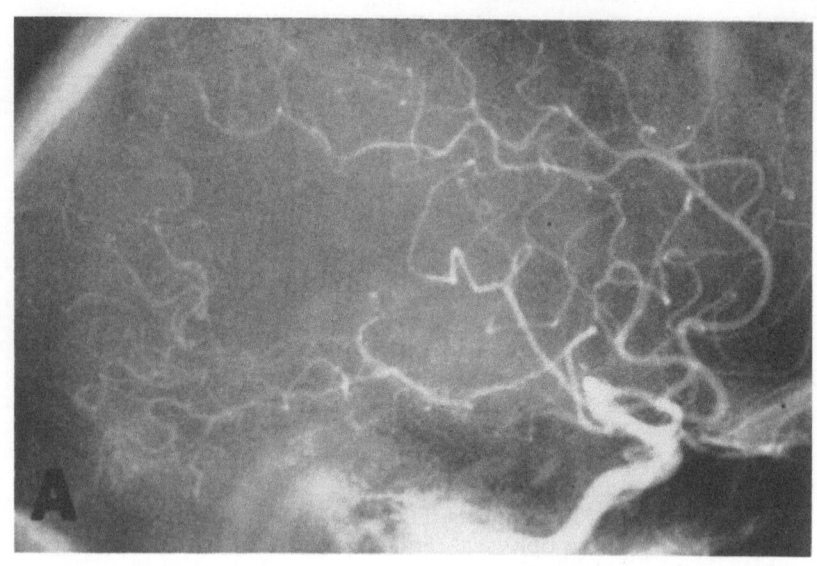

Fig. 12.1. a. Occlusion of parietal
branch of middle cerebral
artery. b. Anterior cerebral
provides retrograde filling
(▲) of parietal branches.

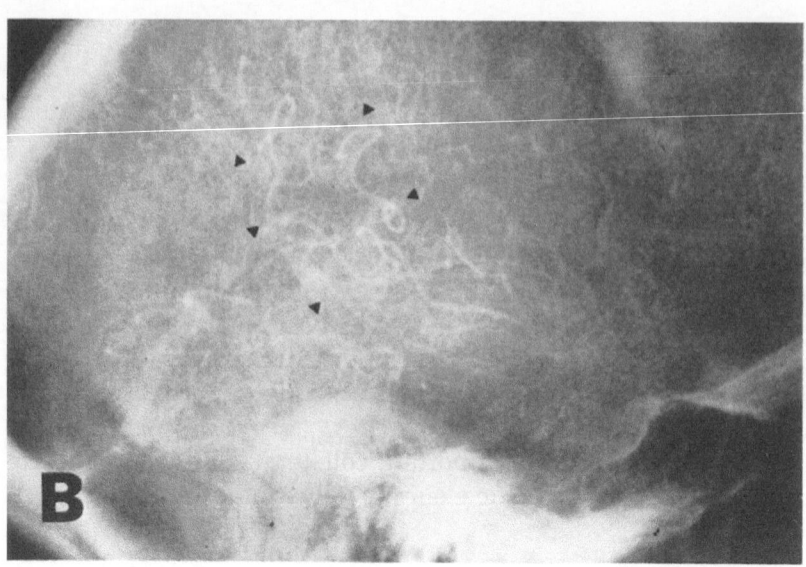

Chapter 12: Collateral Circulation of the Brain

134

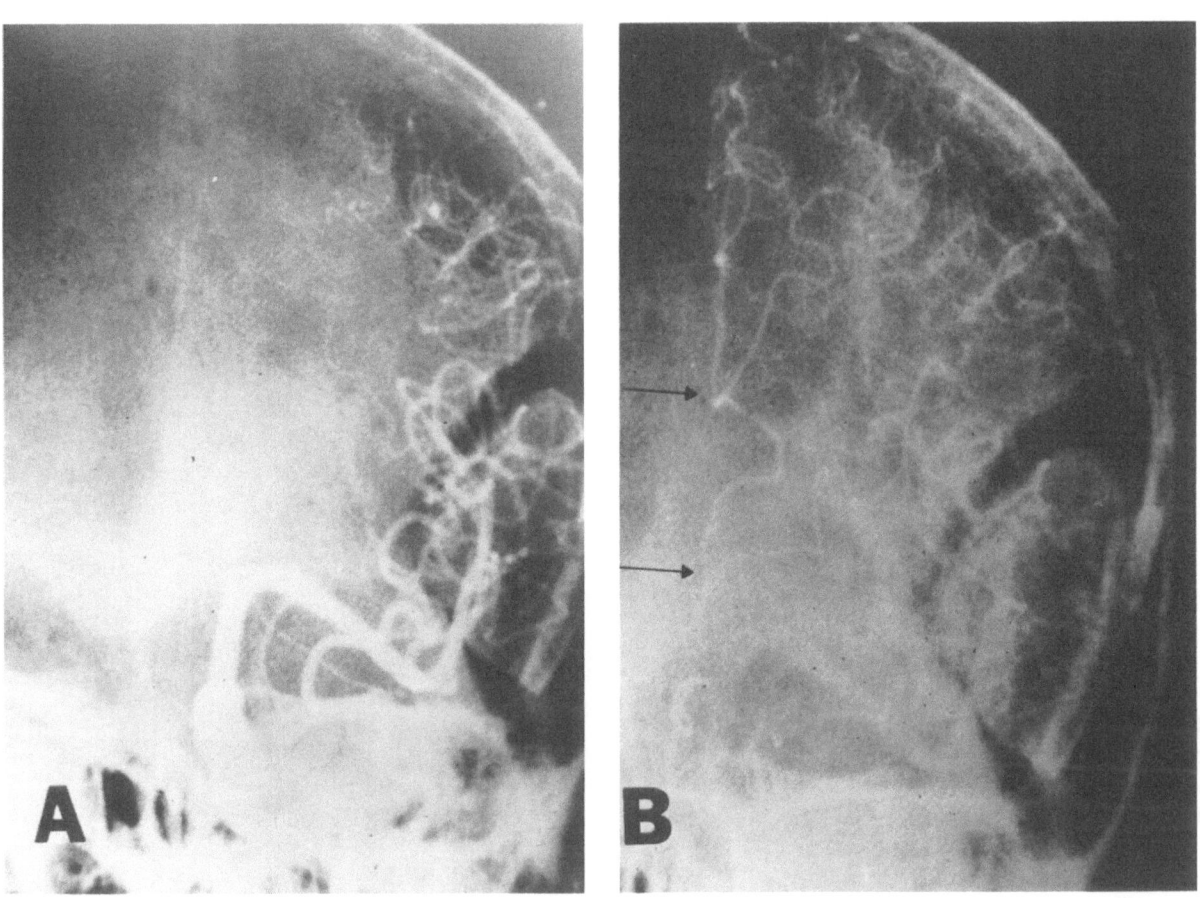

Fig. 12.2. Occlusion of anterior cerebral artery; filling through leptomeningeal arteries of middle cerebral artery (arrows).

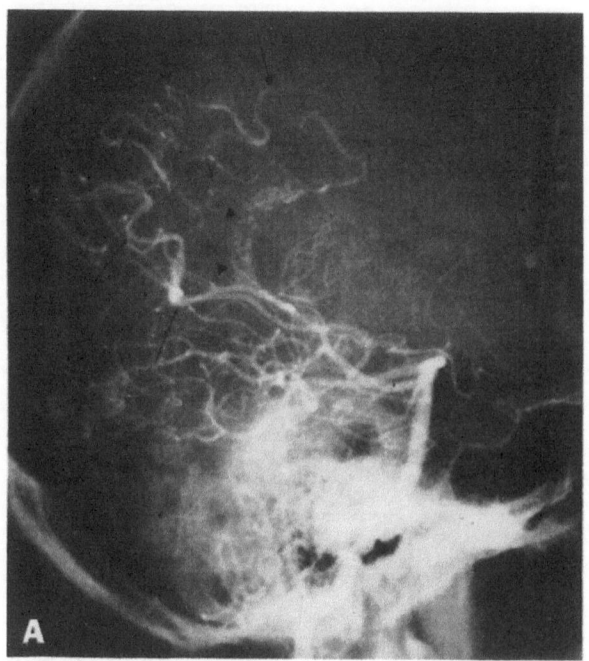
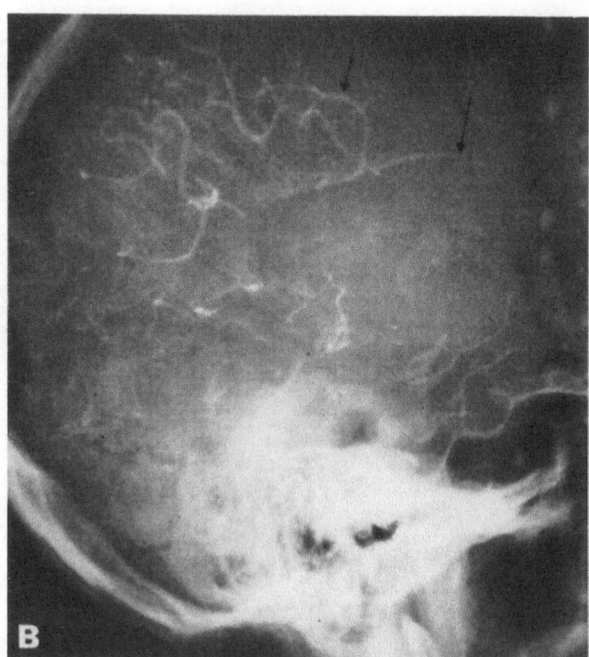

Fig. 12.3. Occluded internal carotid artery; pericallosal artery is filling through the terminal branches of posterior cerebral artery (arrows) and posterior pericallosal artery (▲).

Fig. 12.4. Stenosis of middle cerebral artery (arrows); collateral through lenticulostriate arteries (▲, moyamoya).

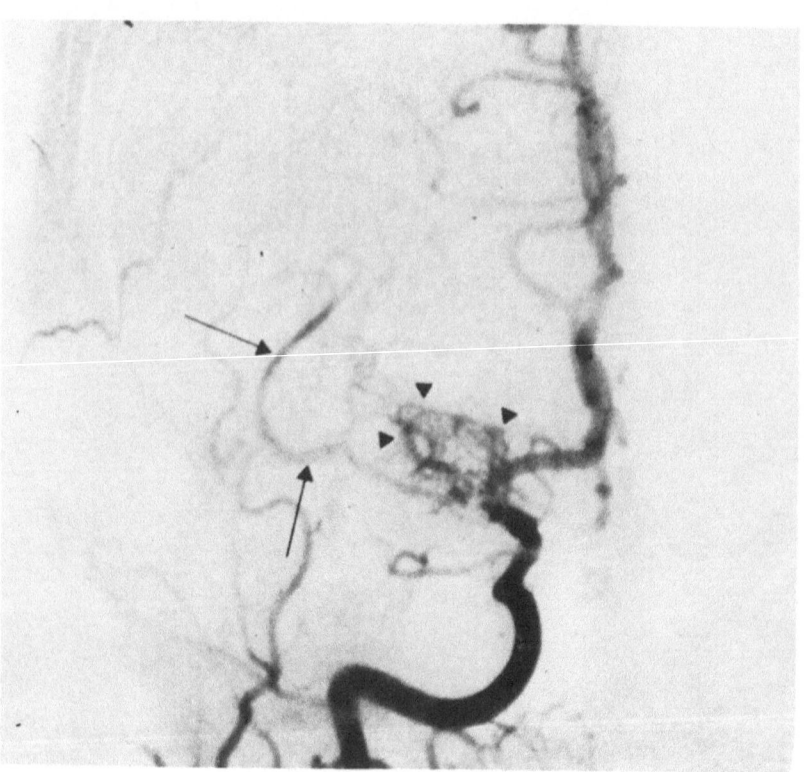

Chapter 12: Collateral Circulation of the Brain

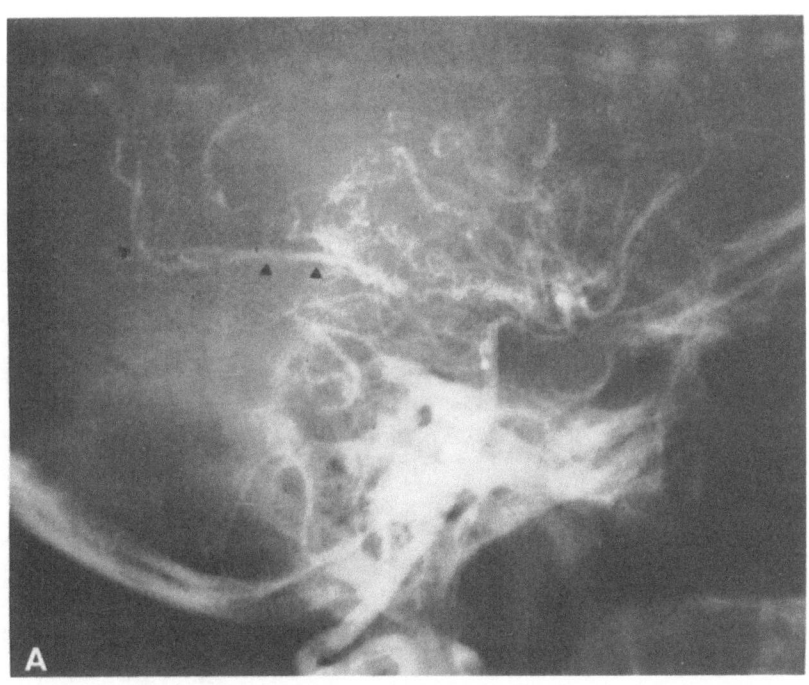

Fig. 12.5. Occlusion of posterior cerebral arteries; (▲) collateral circulation through thalamoperforating arteries (▲).

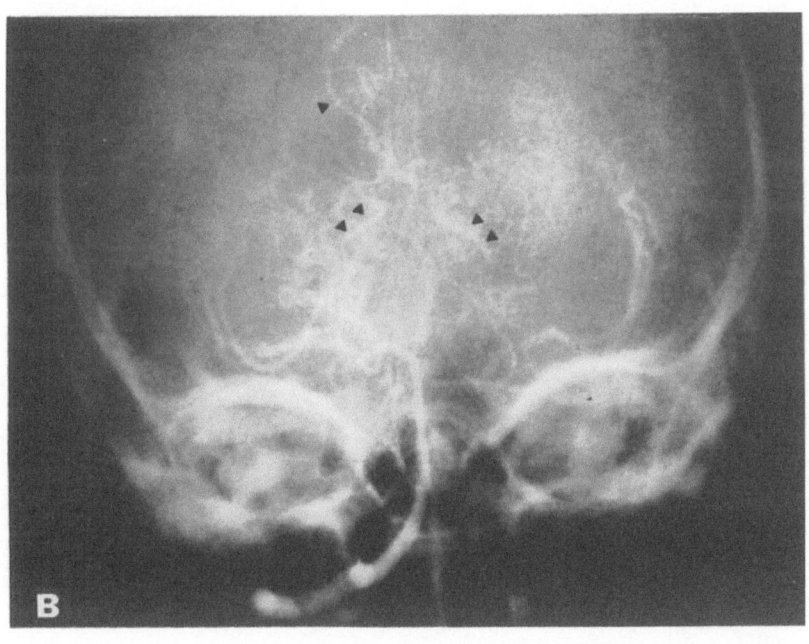

Fig. 12.6. Primitive trigeminal artery (thick arrowhead) anastomosis between carotid (thin arrowhead) and basilar artery (▲).

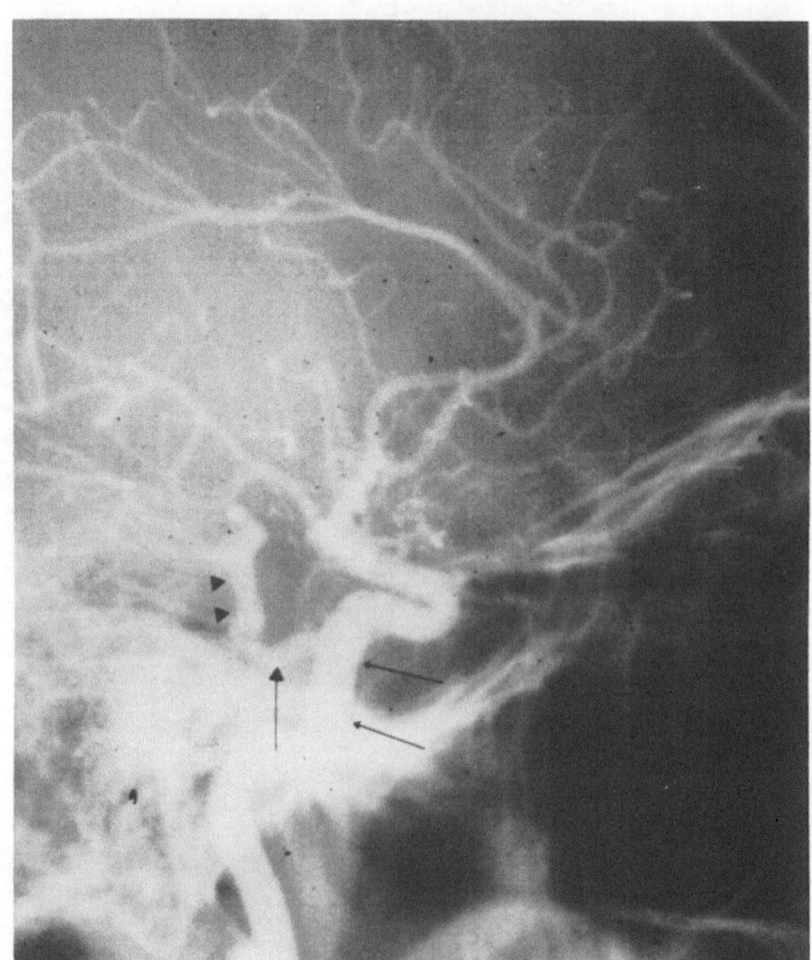

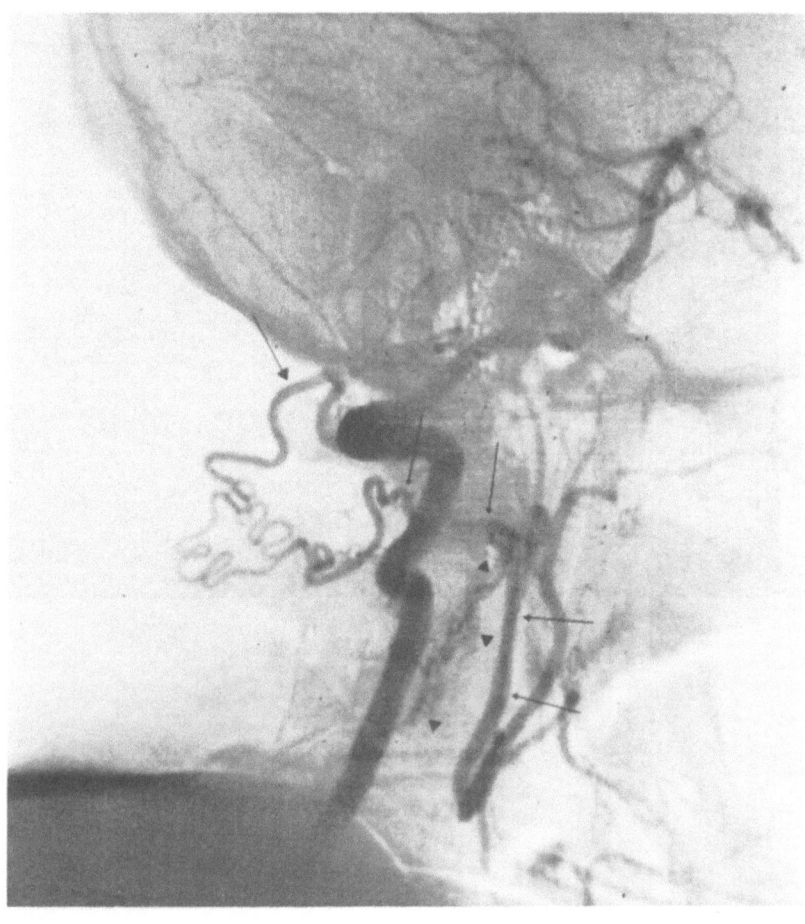

Fig. 12.7. Occlusion of common carotid artery. External carotid artery fills through the posterior occipital anastomosing with muscular branches of vertebral artery.

Fig. 12.8. Occluded vertebral (▲) and basilar arteries, which are partially filled by the ascending cervical artery (arrows) anastomosing with muscular branches of vertebral artery.

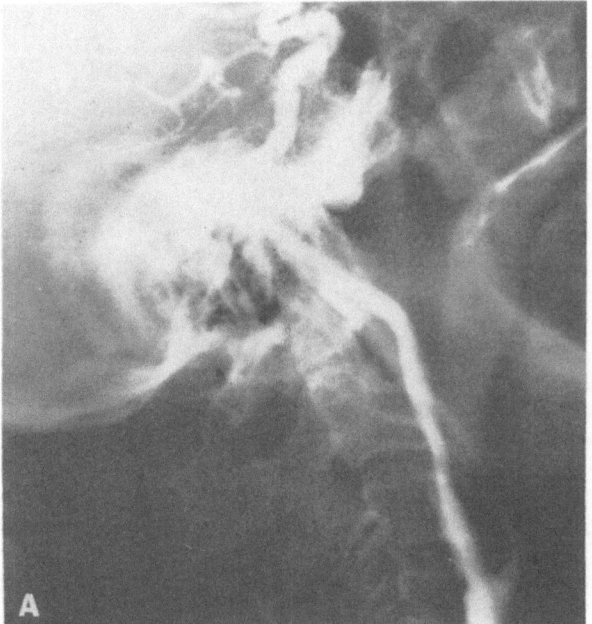

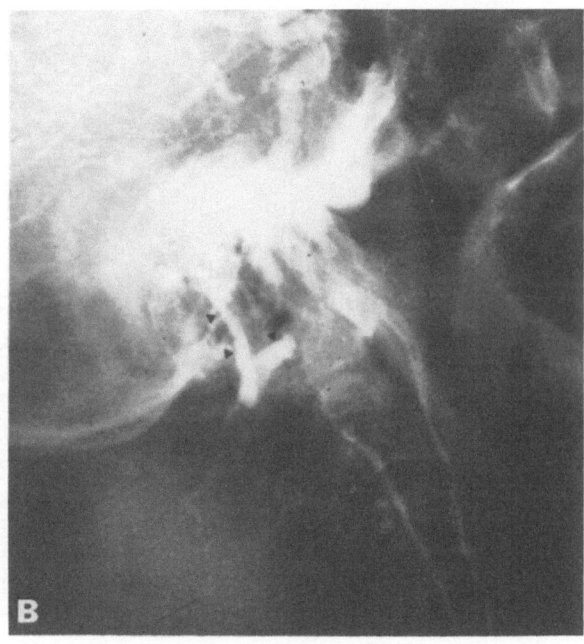

Specific Examples of Collateral Channels

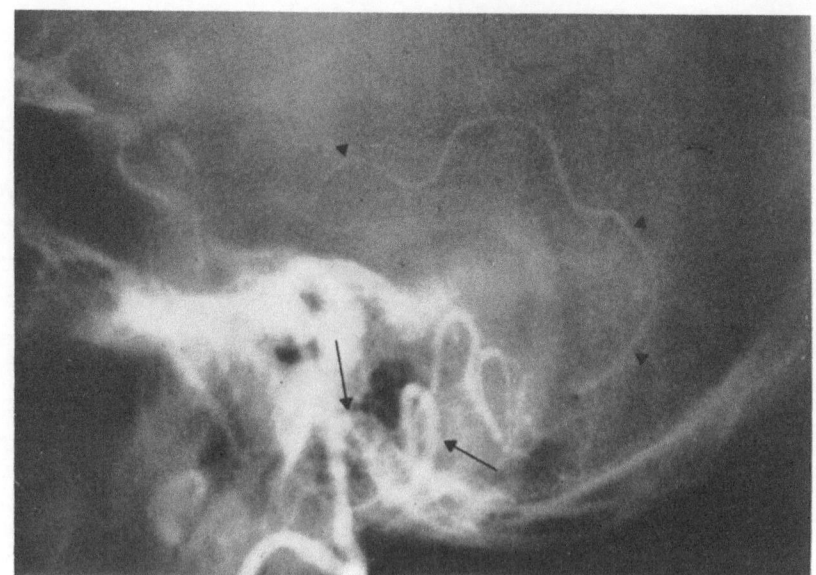

Fig. 12.9. Occlusion of the basilar artery. Collateral flow through pica (arrows) into superior cerebellar artery (▲).

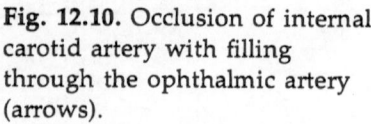

Fig. 12.10. Occlusion of internal carotid artery with filling through the ophthalmic artery (arrows).

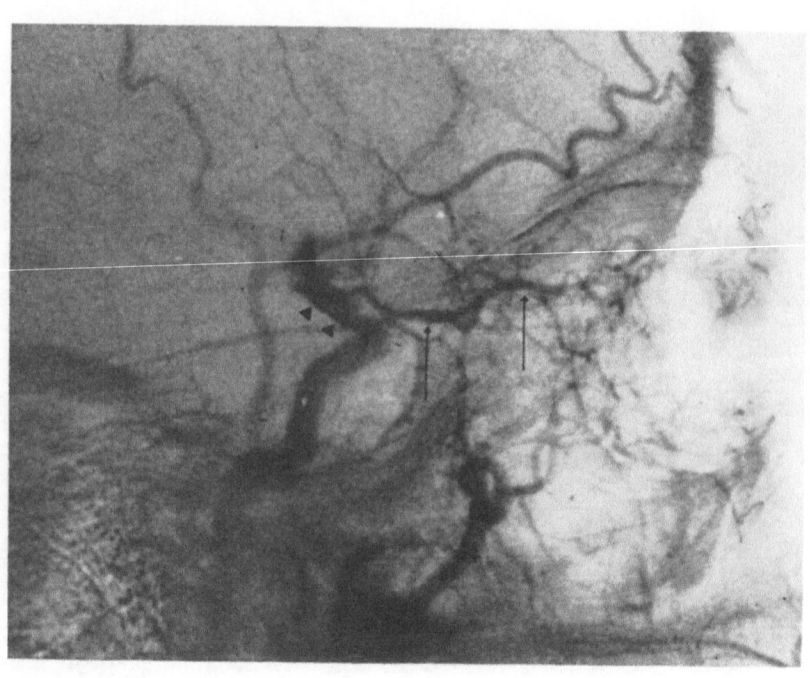

Chapter 12: Collateral Circulation of the Brain

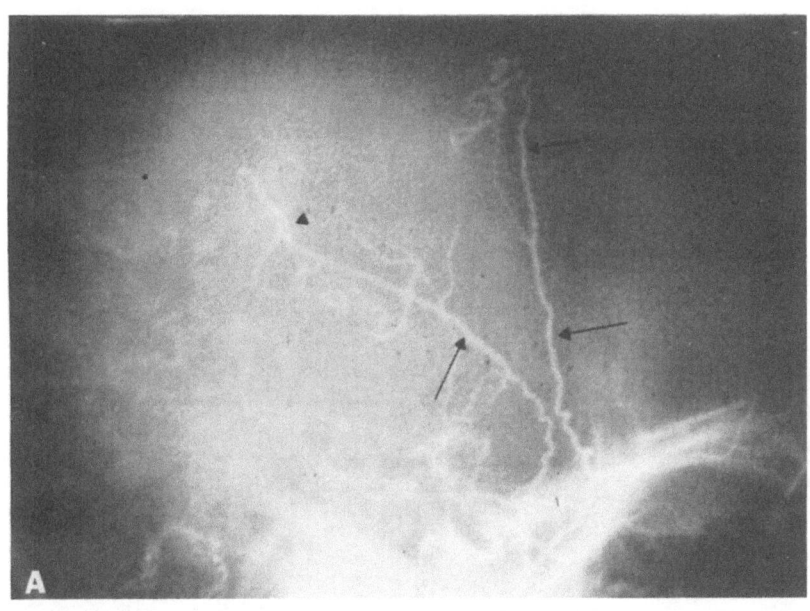

Fig. 12.11. Occlusion of internal carotid artery. Middle cerebral artery filling through leptomeningeal collaterals of middle meningeal artery.

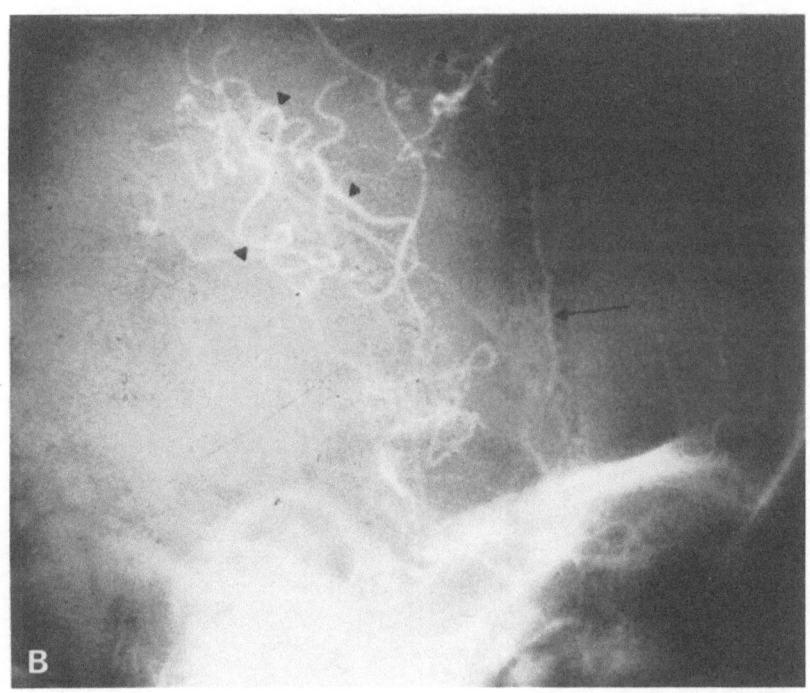

Specific Examples of Collateral Channels

141

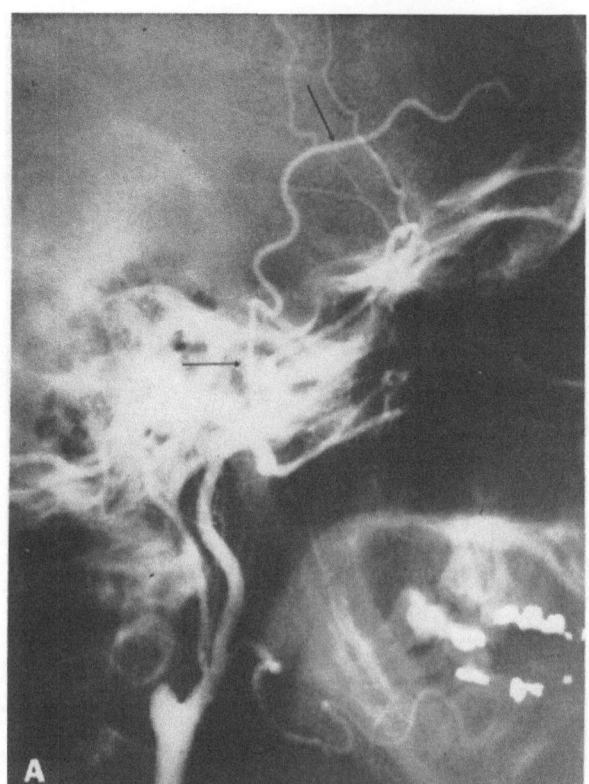
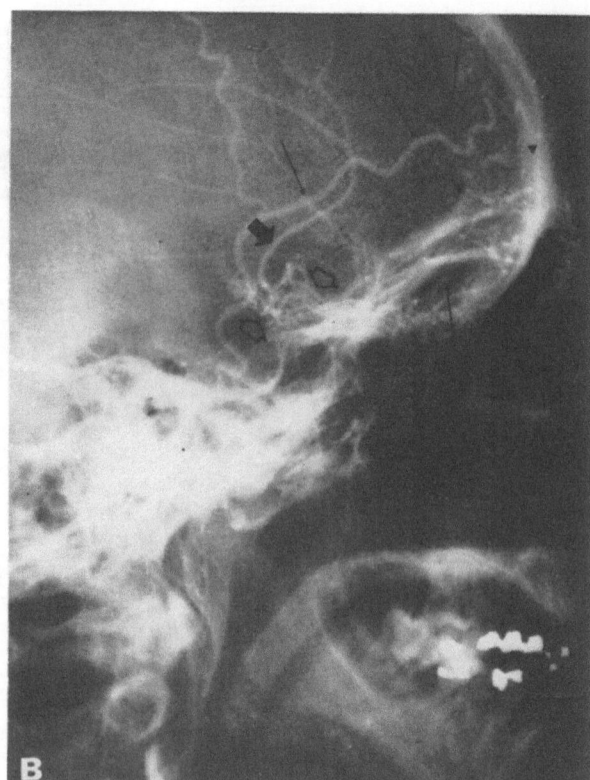

Fig. 12.12. Occluded internal carotid artery. Anterior cerebral artery (thick arrow) fills through perforating branches (▲) of superficial temporal artery (thin arrows). Note also ethmoidal collaterals (open arrows) of ophthalmic artery (crossed arrow) supplying anterior cerebral artery.

Fig. 12.13. Filiform narrowing of internal carotid artery (▲). Meningohypophyseal arteries (arrows) and meningeal branches of the external carotid artery anastomosis to bypass the narrowing of the internal carotid artery.

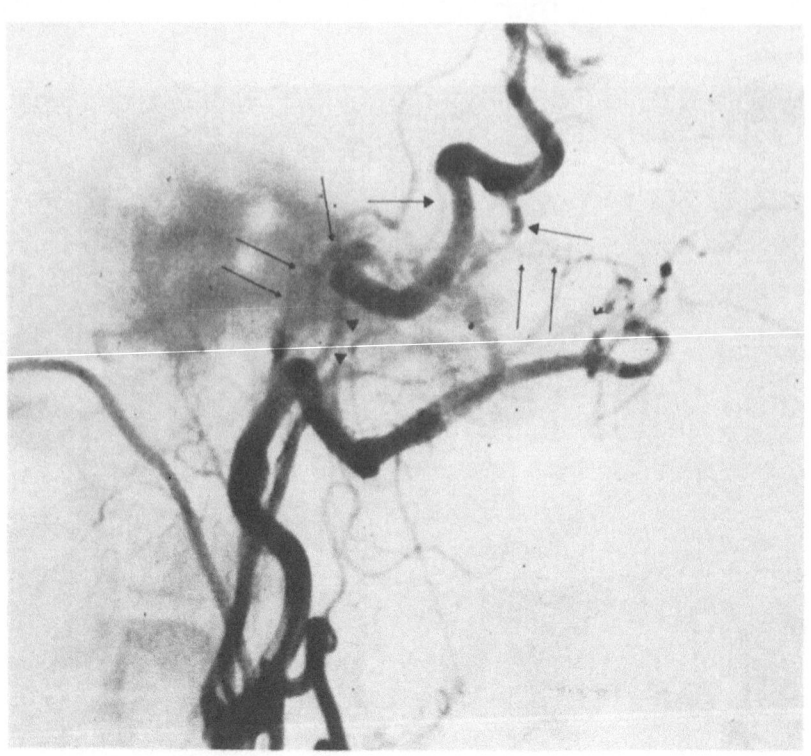

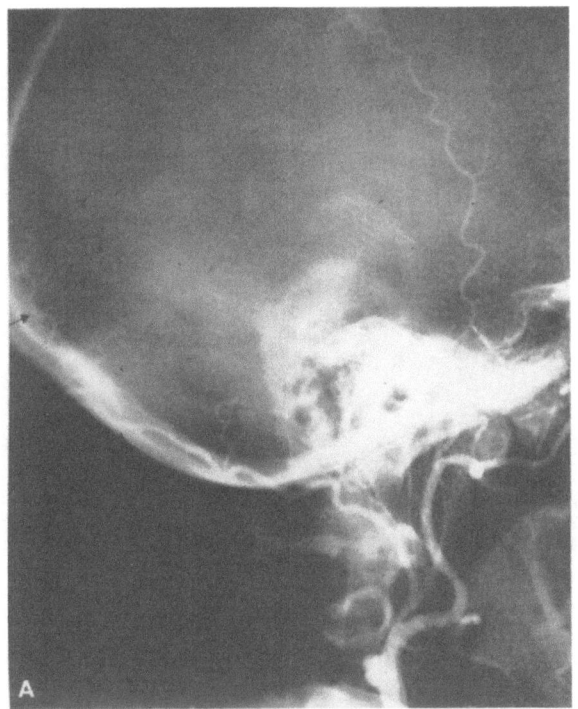
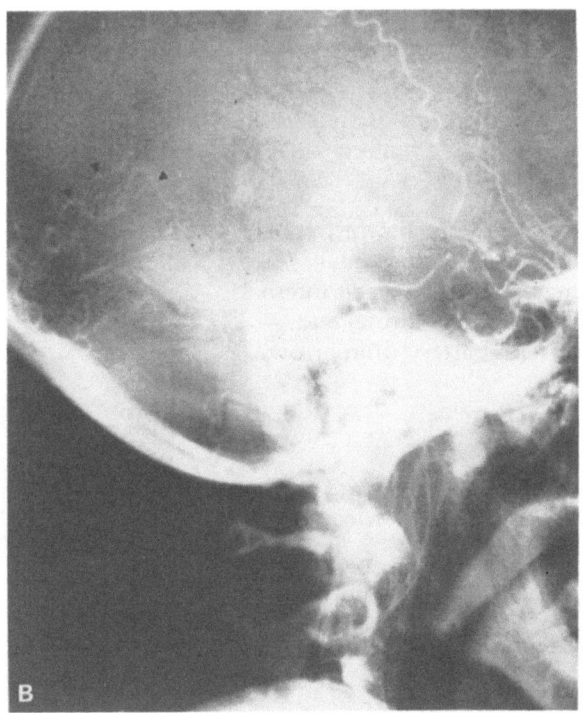

Fig. 12.14. Occlusion of internal carotid artery. Posterior branches of middle cerebral artery fill through perforating branches of occipital artery.

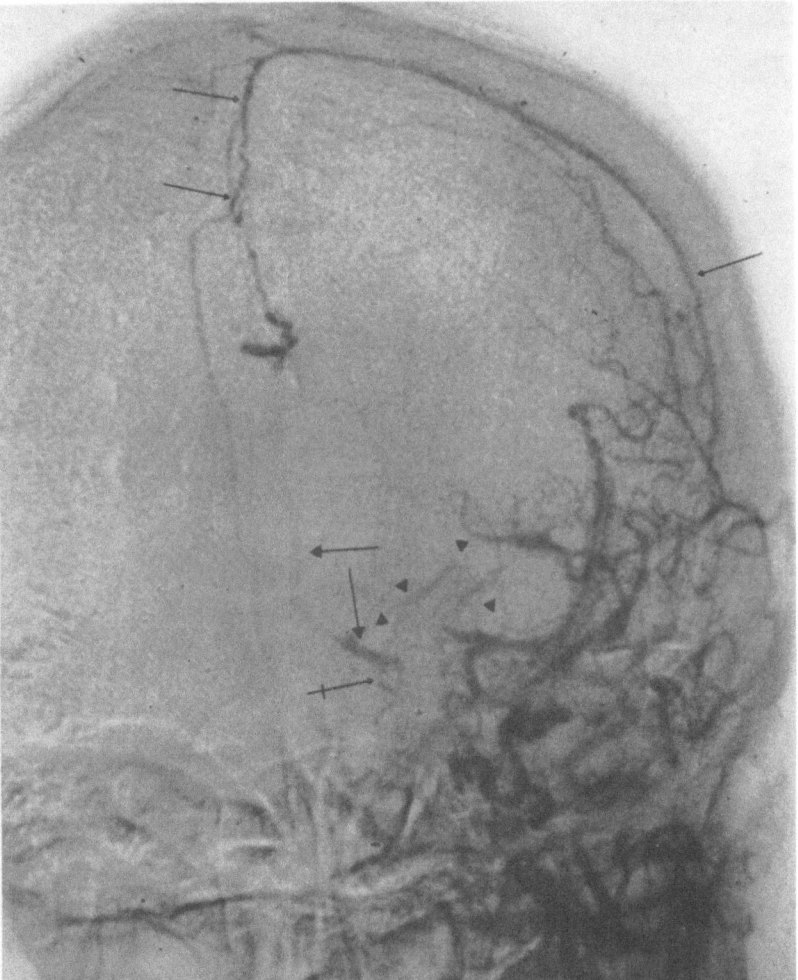

Fig. 12.15. Occlusion of the internal carotid artery. Anterior cerebral artery receives collaterals from ethmoidal (crossed arrow), middle meningeal (arrows), and lenticulostriates (▲) arteries.

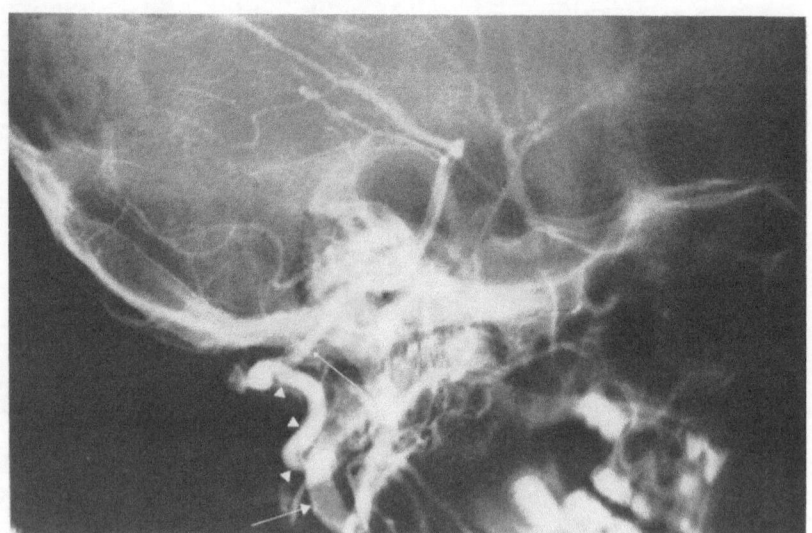

Fig. 12.16. Persistent hypoglossal artery (▲). Extracranial anastomosis between internal carotid (thick arrow) and vertebral artery (thin arrow).

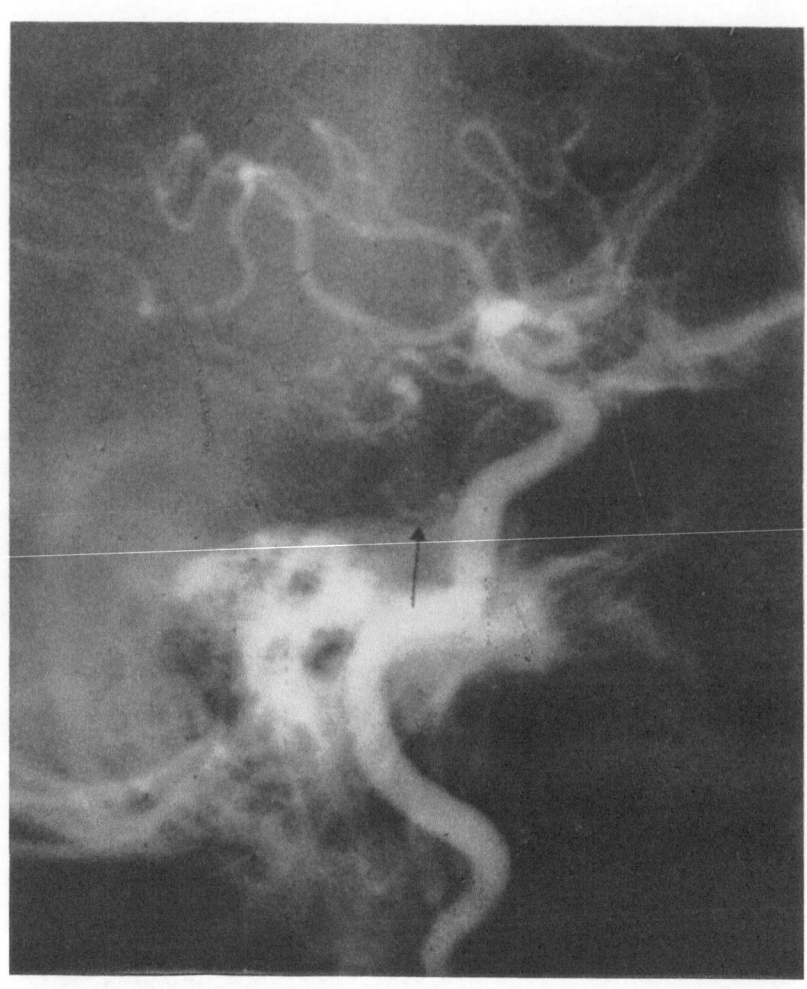

Fig. 12.17. Persistent otic artery (arrow). Anastomosis between internal carotid and basilar artery.

13

Angiographic cerebral blood flow patterns in STA-MCA anastomosis candidates

J. R. Thompson, S. A. Rouhe, G. M. Austin,
and C. R. Simmons

When severe stenosis or occlusion develops in a surgically in-accessible segment of the internal carotid artery or in the middle cerebral artery, what collateral flow possibilities exist to maintain cerebral function? How does a microneurosurgical superficial temporal artery–middle cerebral artery (STA-MCA) anastomosis contribute to preexisting collateral blood flow? Detailed descriptions of possible collateral pathways surrounding high cervical and cerebral arterial occlusions have been previously made.(1–5,7,9–11) It is our purpose to describe and illustrate the frequency of these collaterals in 26 anastomosis patients, and to give a radiologic evaluation of the contribution of these anastomoses to collateral flow.

Materials

Forty-four patients at Loma Linda University Medical Center had anastomosis of a branch of the superficial temporal artery (STA) to a branch of the ipsilateral middle cerebral artery (MCA). All patients had preoperative angiography. Twenty-six anastomoses have been studied angiographically from 9 days to 4.5 months after surgery to document patency. These 26 form the basis for this neuroradiologic study.

The completeness of preoperative angiographic visualization is shown in Table 13.1. Our policy has been to obtain complete brachiocervicocephalic angiograms in each patient.(6,8) Several patients with incomplete examinations from other hospitals did not have repeat angiography upon referral, however. One patient had only arch angiography. One patient studied at Loma Linda had bilateral proximal vertebral artery stenosis which

Table 13.1 Completeness of Angiographic Study

Angiographic Views	n
Bilateral oblique arch	1
Bilateral oblique arch, one carotid	1
Arch, two carotids	3
Two carotids, vertebral	3
Two carotids	2
Arch, two carotids, vertebral	16
Total	26

prevented vertebral catheterization. Postoperatively, each patient underwent at least a selective common carotid arteriogram on the side of STA-MCA anastomosis in the anteroposterior (AP), oblique AP, and magnification lateral projections.

Method

Observations and evaluations of cerebral collateral flow were based upon angiography. No attempt was made to compare or correlate clinical findings or nuclide cerebral blood flow (CBF) values, which will be the subject of another study. Age, preoperative occlusive lesions, preoperative collateral pathways, pre- and postoperative STA size, postoperative angiographic intervals, anastomosis function, and postoperative collateral pathways were tabulated for each patient.

For the purpose of obtaining a functional comparison of cerebral collateral pathways, a quantitative value was assigned to each according to the degree of visible opacification within cerebral vessels (Table 13.2). The term "system" and "subsystem" in Table 13.2 denote the entire territory or a portion of the anterior cerebral artery (ACA), the MCA, or the posterior cerebral artery (PCA). Of course, this method doesn't approach absolute flow values, but it does allow relative comparisons to be made. Similarly, we attempted to quantify collateral flow derived from the surgical anastomoses (Table 13.3).

Table 13.2. Angiographic Quantification of Collateral Flow

1+: Collateral vessel just visibly opacified
2+: Cortical subsystem opacification
3+: Fair cortical system opacification
4+: Excellent cortical system opacification

Table 13.3. Quantification of Anastomosis Collaterals

Flow Value	Angioanatomy	n
0	Occluded anastomosis	4
1+	Only anterograde flow in a MCA branch	2
2+	Bidirectional flow and subsystem opacification	17
3+	Full MCA system opacification	2
4+	MCA system plus adjacent system opacity	1

Cerebral Collateral Pathways

Possible routes of collateral flow to the cerebrum are listed in Table 13.4. Not all of these pathways contribute greatly to flow within the brain. It is generally understood that basal perforating arteries do not contribute significantly to peripheral flow except in those patients in whom a "moyamoya" collateral pattern has developed. The circle of Willis, the ophthalmic, and the leptomeningeal pathways are the most prominent collaterals. Scalp to dural to pial flow, although existent, is seldom demonstrated angiographically. We have found the dorsal callosal to pericallosal and posterior choroidal to anterior choroidal routes to be more important than previously indicated. These pathways are schematically represented in Figure 13.1.

The territory of the MCA is the most vulnerable to occlusive disease of all three major cerebral systems (Table 13.4). For practical purposes, from angiographic appearances leptomeningeal connections provide the only real collateral supply. In contrast, with proximal ACA or PCA occlusions, the callosal, leptomeningeal, and choroidal routes are available.

Discussion of infratentorial collateral circulation is not included here. Perhaps with the anastomosis of an occipital artery to a superior or inferior cerebellar artery for treatment of ver-

Table 13.4. Available Cerebral Arterial System Collateral Pathways

	ICA	ACA	MCA	PCA
ACA (precommunicating)	+	+		
AComA (anterior communicating artery)	+	+		
PComA (posterior communicating artery)	+			+
Dorsal callosal		+		+
Leptomeningeal		+	+	+
Choroidal	+			+
Lenticulostriate and thalamoperforate			+	+
Dural	+	+	+	+
Scalp-dural-pial		+	+	+

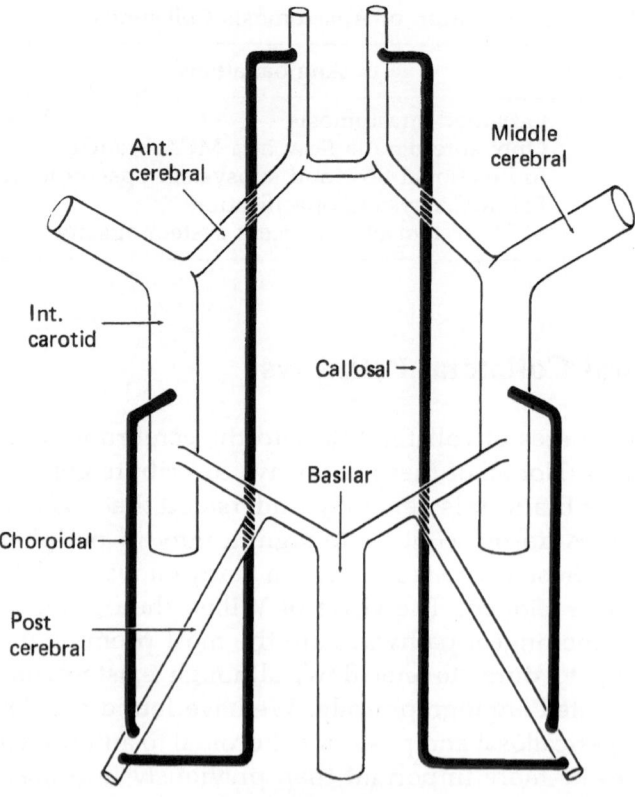

Fig. 13.1 Schematic diagram of two previously noted but overlooked posterior to anterior collateral pathways (solid black lines). Choroidal: posterior choroidal to anterior choroidal artery via choroid plexus. Callosal: dorsal callosal branch of posterior cerebral artery to pericallosal artery.

Ant. cerebral

Middle cerebral

Int. carotid

Callosal

Basilar

Choroidal

Post cerebral

Accessory cerebral collateral

tebrobasilar insufficiency, the hindbrain collateral will increase in importance.

Preanastomosis Collateral

This study group of 26 patients included 16 with internal carotid artery (ICA) occlusion (three were bilateral). Four had high carotid stenoses. Six patients had MCA stenosis or occlusion. The average age for the patients with carotid occlusions was 62. The patients with carotid stenoses and MCA lesions tended to be younger, with an average age of 46 for those with ICA stenoses and 53 for those with MCA lesions. Doubtless the average age is biased by two patients with nonatherosclerotic lesions: spontaneous dissection of the ICA in a 41-year-old man, and traumatic ICA occlusion (subsequently endarterectomized) in a 42-year-old woman. Statistically significant numbers of patients with lesions at these sites probably will show a trend closer to the average age of those with ICA occlusions.

Tabulation of collateral pathways in ten patients with complete angiography revealed a mean of 5.9 collateral sources in single ICA occlusion and 11.0 in bilateral ICA occlusion. These multiple collaterals will not be appreciated with incomplete angiographic study.

The majority of patients with ICA occlusion maintain patency of the artery at distal levels. A cavernous carotid dural branch or sometimes a pterygoid artery determines the level of reconstitution. Direction of flow in the ophthalmic artery may be retrograde or anterograde, depending upon preferential development of collaterals about the cavernous carotid. Anterograde thrombus may obliterate the ICA siphon, eliminating potential collaterals. This appears more likely to occur with embolic occlusion, however.

The many facial, pharyngeal, orbital, and scalp branches of the external carotid artery (ECA) serve as the anastomotic link to the carotid siphon. In our group this link was more commonly seen with the ophthalmic artery. Figure 13.2 demonstrates the pathways observed.

Table 13.5 shows the frequency of the more common collateral pathways seen in the study group. It also shows a quan-

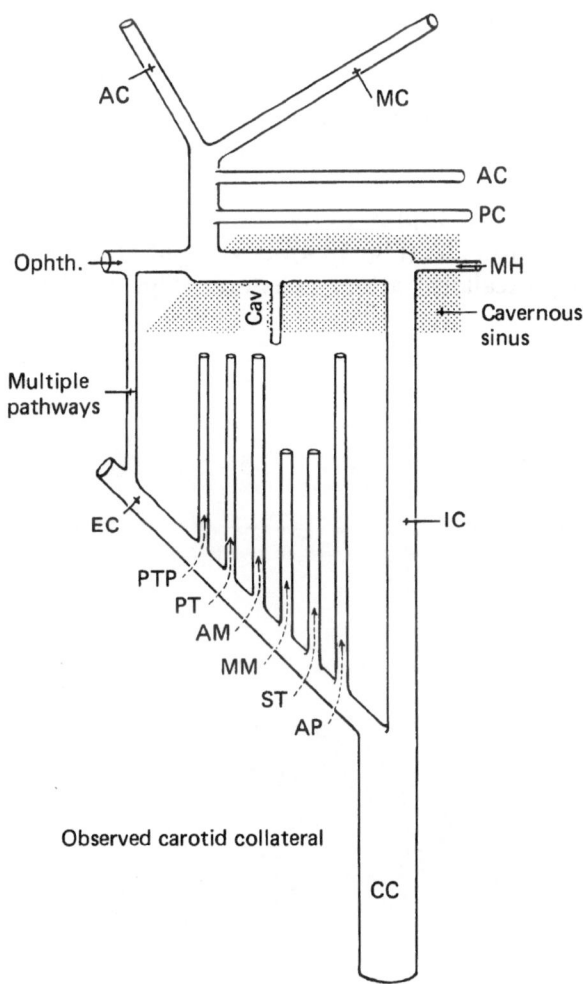

Fig. 13.2. Schematic representation of collateral pathways about the internal carotid artery (IC) observed in 26 patients. AC, anterior choroidal; PC, posterior communicating; MH, meningohypophyseal; CAV, inferior cavernous; EC, external carotid; CC, common carotid; PTP, pterygopalatine; PT, pterygoid; AM, accessory meningeal; MM, middle meningeal; ST, superficial temporal; AP, ascending pharyngeal. Nonophthalmic pathways (PTP, PT, AM, AP) all anastomose to a cavernous branch of the internal carotid artery.

Table 13.5. Common Cerebral Collateral Observed in 26 Patients

	Flow Value	n	SFV/n
Ophthalmic to ICA	23	15	1.5
PCA to MCA (leptomeningeal)	31	14	2.2
PComA to ICA	25	13	1.9
AComA to ACA	35	12	2.9
AComA to MCA	17	10	1.7
Ascending pharyngeal to ICA	10	9	1.1
PCA to ACA (leptomeningeal)	23	8	2.9
Dorsal Callosal to ACA	14	7	2.0
Internal maxillary to ICA (accessory meningeal, pterygoid, etc)	6	5	1.2

Fig. 13.3 Man, 63 years old, with occlusion of right ICA and 80% stenosis of left ICA from ulcerative plaque. (a) Opacification (4+) of right MCA from ICA via reflux through large right PComA filling from left vertebral artery injection. (b) Postoperative lateral right common carotid (CCA) arteriogram. Patent STA-MCA anastomosis (open arrow). Mainly posterior temporal artery opacification results, doubtless because of contribution to MCA from PComA. Note collateral from internal maxillary artery to inferior cavernous artery (closed arrow).

tification of these pathways in terms of the degree of opacification provided.

Although brain collateral was most frequently observed via the ophthalmic artery, the average opacification obtained (summated flow value [SFV]/n) was only 1.5+, whereas the contribution seen from the anterior communicating artery (AComA) to the contralateral ACA was 2.9+. The leptomeningeal flow from the PCA to the ACA was just as rich (2.9+), and also appeared good (2.2+) from the PCA to MCA. Flow to the MCA apparently comes more commonly from the posterior communicating artery (PComA) (Fig. 13.3) and ophthalmic arteries via the ICA. Collateral supply to the ACA is most often by way of the AComA and PCA (Fig. 13.4). Seven patients showed dorsal callosal to pericallosal artery collateral (Fig. 13.5) with an av-

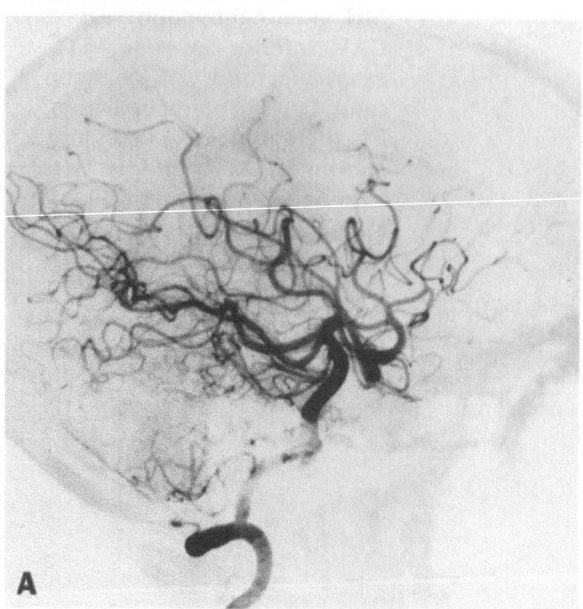

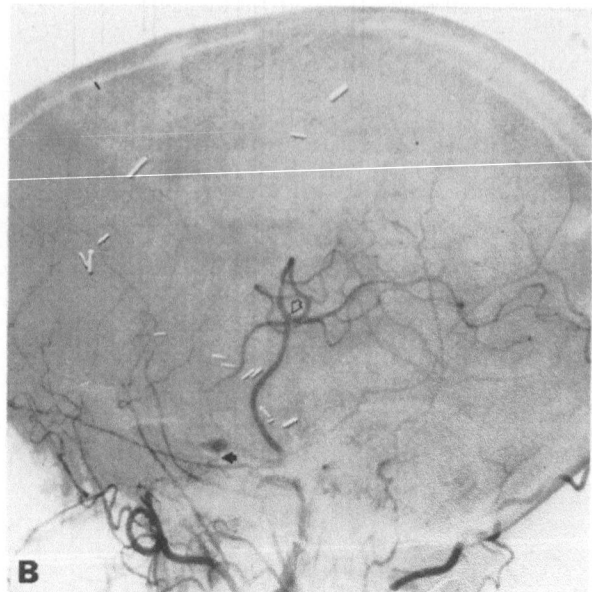

erage value of 1.7+. Posterior choroidal to anterior choroidal artery flow was seen in two patients (Fig. 13.5c). Only one dural-pial (Fig. 13.6) and no scalp-dural-pial collaterals were observed in this group. One patient with bilateral ICA occlusion showed excellent "moyamoya" collaterals (Fig. 13.7), observation of which is becoming more frequent in atherosclerotic cerebrovascular occlusive disease.

Postanastomosis Collateral

Prior to studying this group our main purpose was to determine STA patency. It is now clear that a single artery study is not adequate to determine the effect of the anastomosis on preexisting collateral circulation. A complete postoperative brachiocervicocephalic study will better help to establish the value of microneurosurgical techniques for cerebrovascular ischemia than will single artery study, and can be as easily justified to the patient.

Seven patients' examinations are suitable for evaluating effects of the STA-MCA anastomoses on collateral circulation because these examinations were more complete. Six of these seven postoperative angiograms, in comparison with preoperative studies, showed changes in flow derived from their col-

Fig. 13.4. Man, 67 years old, with right ICA occlusion. (a) Preoperative collateral flow to ACA and MCA from contralateral ICA via AComA. (b) Postanastomosis lateral right CCA arteriogram showing nearly complete right MCA opacification except for anterior frontal and anterior temporal branches. Anastomotic junction on posterior temporal branch (open arrow).

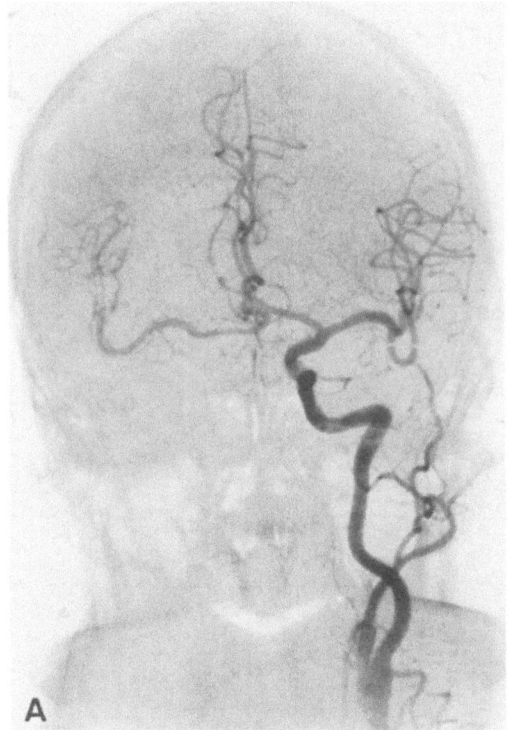 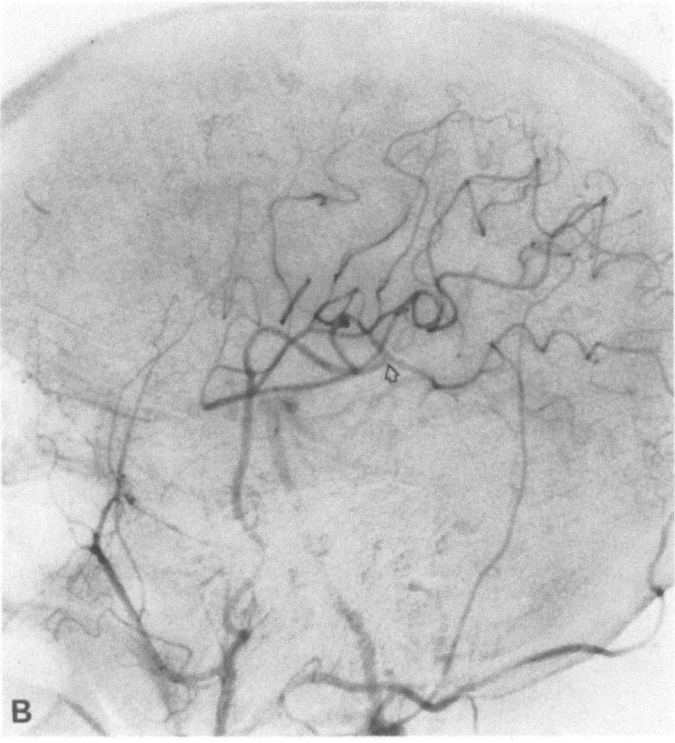

A   B

Fig. 13.5. Woman, 63 years old, with multiple occlusive lesions including occlusions of the left ICA and the left vertebral arteries. (a) Occluded right ACA fills retrogradely from MCA leptomeningeal flow (arrow). (b) Retrograde ACA opacification again shown on later sequences, lateral view (arrow). (c) Lateral right vertebral injection with retrograde *left* ACA (arrow) opacification from dorsal callosal branches (arrow 1). Faint opacification of superclinoid left ICA from retrograde flow in left anterior choroidal artery (arrow 2). (d) Left ACA opacity in AP projection of right vertebral arteriogram (arrow). (e) Functioning anastomosis to central sulcus artery (upper open arrow). Supraclinoid ICA opacification from ophthalmic (arrow 1) and inferior cavernous (arrow 2) arteries. (f) MCA branches not filled by STA later opacify from ophthalmic artery (arrow).

laterals. Examples of flow alterations from STA anastomosis were observed within the AComA, ophthalmic artery, and leptomeningeal pathways. In one patient with unilateral ICA occlusion and patent anastomosis, no such change was observed.

Superficial Temporal Artery Contribution

From Table 13.3 one can see that most angiograms (65%) demonstrated anterograde and retrograde flow at the anastomosis and less than total opacification of the MCA system. Relating the STA flow to the type and location of the occlusive lesion, no greater STA flow appears to develop with one lesion than with another. The fact that the three patients with complete MCA system opacification from the STA were in the carotid occlusion group probably does not mean that better postanastomotic flow will develop in patients with carotid occlusion. The average flow was no better for this group than for those with high carotid stenosis. Larger groups in each category are necessary for reliable conclusions to be drawn.

Another obvious parameter in evaluating STA-MCA flow is change in STA size. Seven patients' STAs could not be measured preoperatively. In the group of 19 with satisfactory pre- and postoperative STA visualization, the average preoperative diameter at the level of the sella was 1.5 mm. Postoperatively (21 days average), the average artery measured 2.0 mm. An increase of 1.3 mm² occurred which represents nearly a doubling of the calculated cross-sectional area.

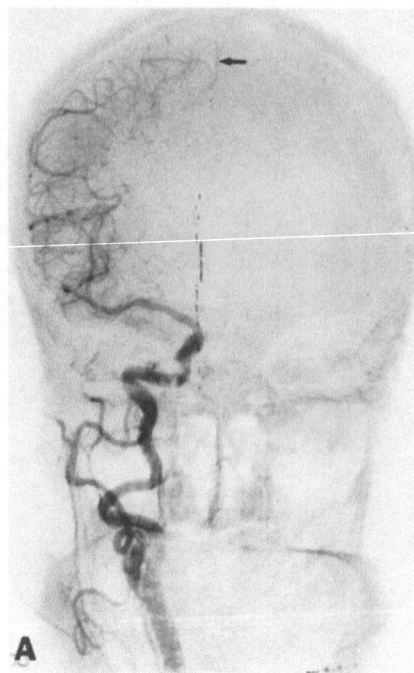
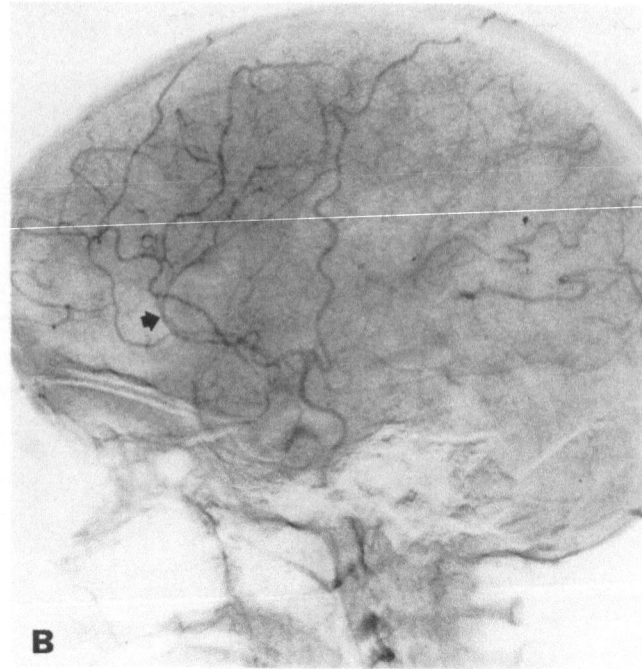

A   B

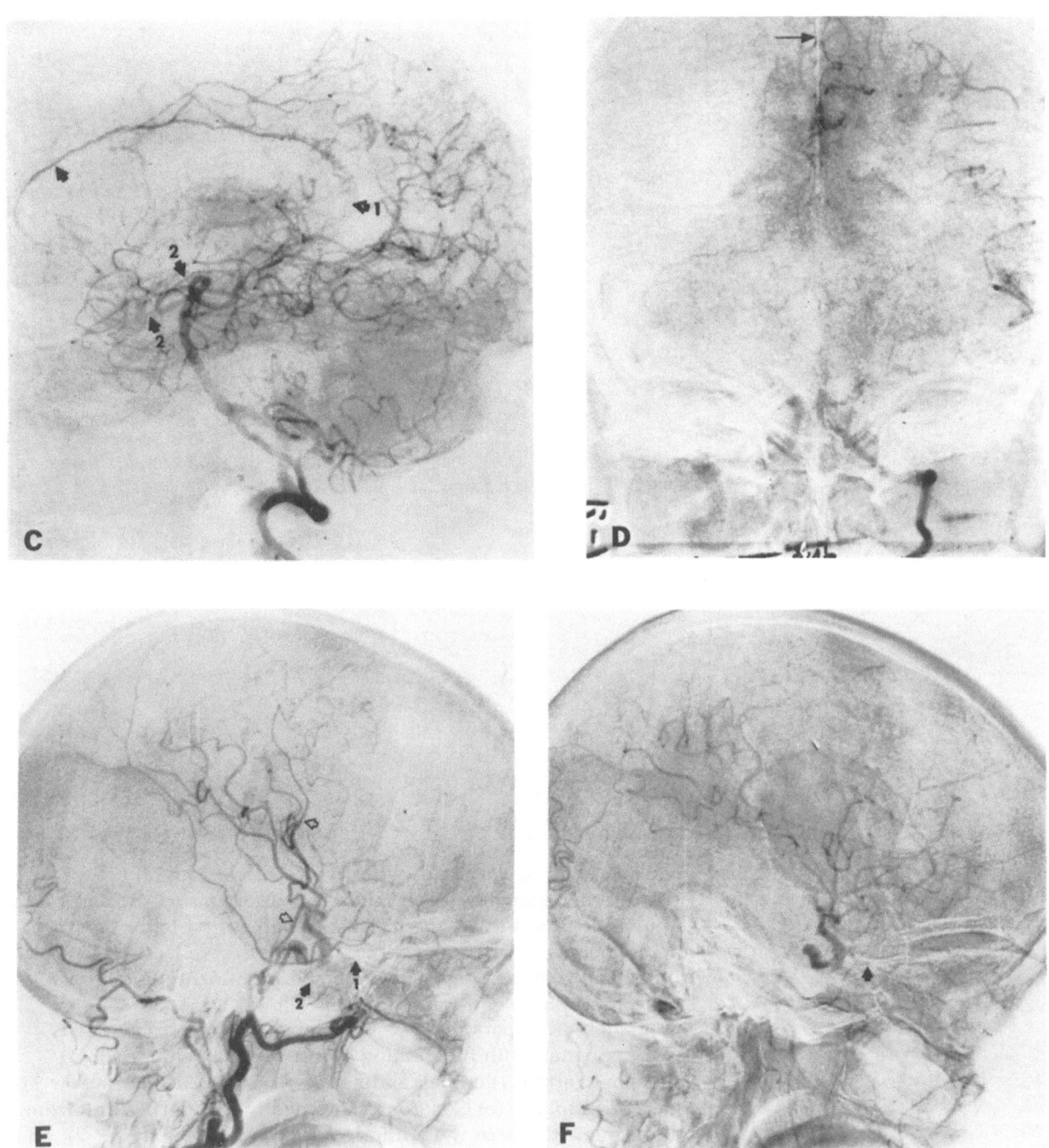

Several patients developed prominent postoperative STA enlargement (Table 13.6). The greatest was a nine-fold increase in luminal area in a patient with ICA occlusion (Fig. 13.8). The second largest increase was seven times the preoperative measurement; this patient had suffered a severe MCA stenosis which became occluded subsequent to the anastomosis.

If any conclusion can be drawn from the time interval of the

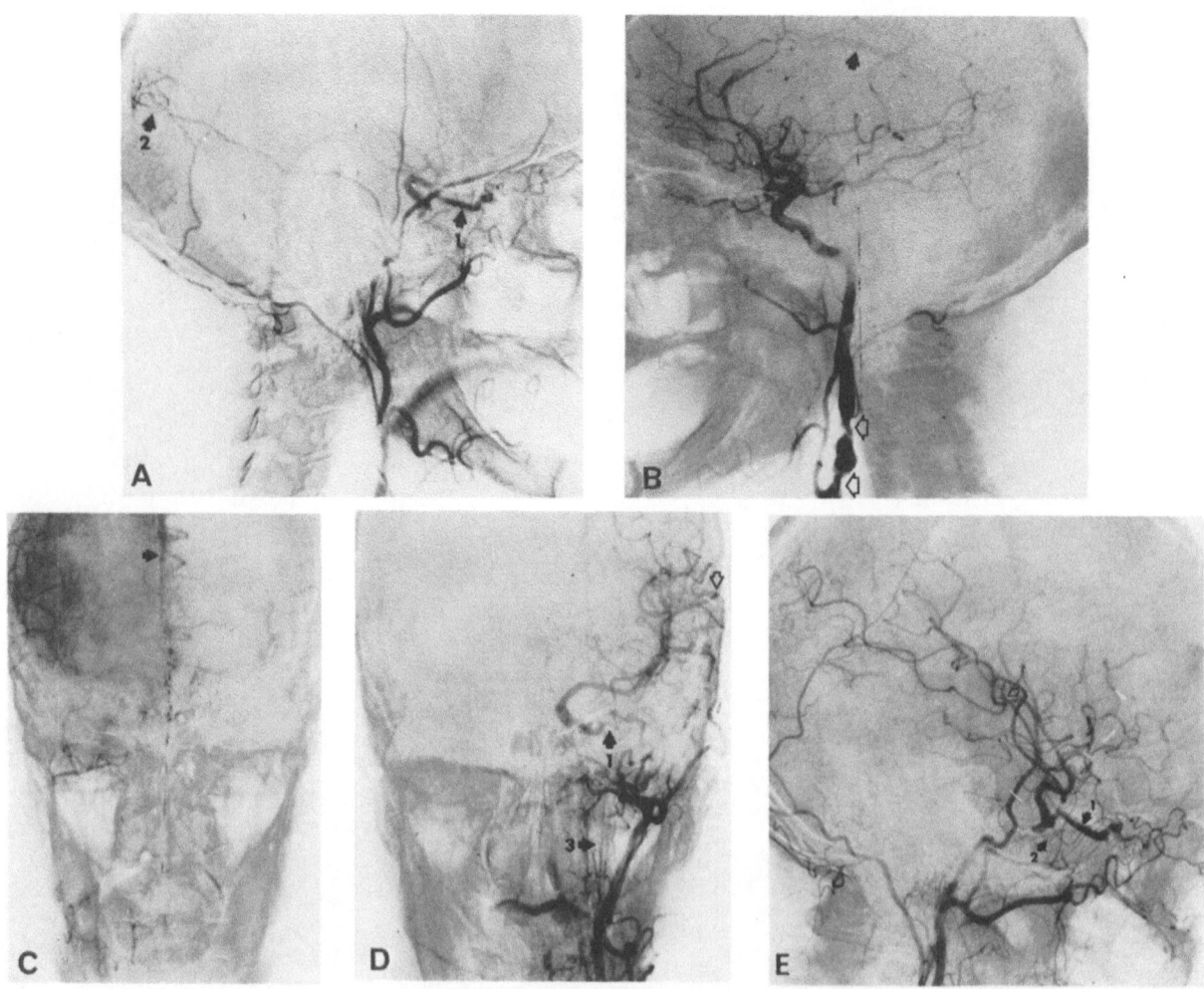

Fig. 13.6. Man, 61 years old, with left ICA occlusion. (a) Left CCA injection showing large ophthalmic artery (arrow 1). Small area of dural to cortical collateral flow via prominent posterior branch of middle meningeal artery (arrow 2). (b) Note severe tandem stenoses in proximal right ICA (open arrows) and prominent pericallosal sulcus arteries (closed arrow). (c) Opposite left ACA (arow) fills retrogradely from pericallosal connections. (d) Postoperative left CCA angiogram with functioning anastomosis (open arrow); ophthalmic (arrow 1) and ascending pharyngeal collaterals (arrow 3) to left ICA siphon. (e) Generous combined MCA opacification from ophthalmic artery (arrow 1), inferior cavernous artery (arrow 2), and STA (open arrow).

postoperative angiogram and its relation to STA size it is probably this: If an STA is going to increase in size it will probably occur early and continue for several months. This is implied by comparison of different patients with single angiograms performed at varying postoperative intervals. Serial postoperative angiograms have not been performed in individual patients. The average time interval for study in seven patients

Table 13.6. STA Enlargement in 5 Patients Showing Greatest Increase

Patient	Days Postoperative	Area Change
JB	9	3.4 ×
RC	10	7.3 ×
JS	14	2.0 ×
JB	12	6.5 ×
PN	60	9.1 ×

who showed no postoperative change was 41 days. Some of the greatest diameter changes were apparent in about 2 weeks.

Conclusions

Our conclusions, based on angiography in 26 patients, are the following:

1. Of the multiple possibilities for collateral development about ICA occlusive lesions, in the majority of patients the circle of Willis and ophthalmic artery dominate.
2. The MCA territory is the most vulnerable to ischemia because of the limited number of possible collaterals.
3. An average of 5.9 collaterals serve in unilateral ICA occlusion, but no prediction can be made of which pathways will become important in any individual.
4. Demonstration of these collaterals depends upon the pre- and postoperative performance of complete catheter femor-ocerebral angiography with radiographs coned to each area of interest, ie, arch, cervical carotid, cervical vertebral, and cephalic arteries.

Fig. 13.7. Man, 53 years old, with bilateral ICA occlusions. No ophthalmic artery filling of supraclinoid ICA was present on either side. (a). Lateral right CCA injection showing ethmoidal to olfactory to anterior cerebral artery flow (arrows). (b) Left vertebral angiogram revealing four distinct functioning collateral supplies to ICA territory: PComA (arrow 1), dorsal callosal (arrow 2), leptomeningeal to ACA and MCA (behind arrow 2), and moyamoya pattern, ie, lenticulostriate and thalamic-perforating artery accentuation.

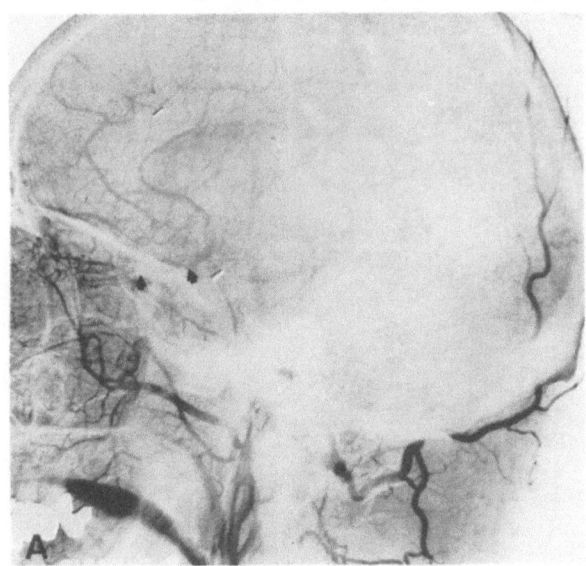 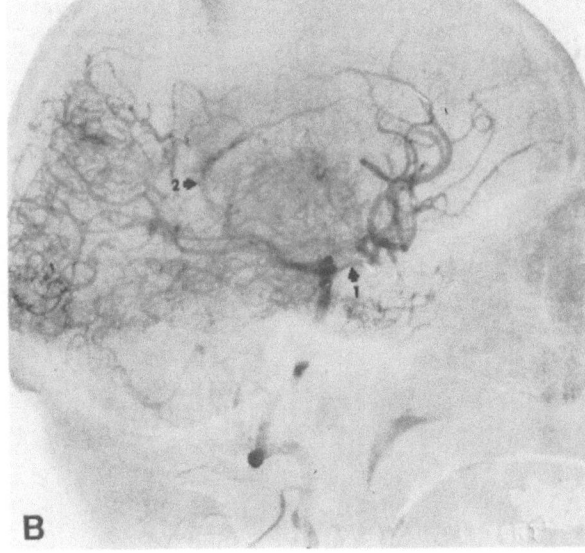

Fig. 13.8. Man, 68 years old, with bilateral ICA occlusions. (a) Note severe stenosis of left subclavian artery (curved arrow) proximal to left vertebral origin. Vein graft (open arrow) was inserted between LCC (arrow head) and subclavian artery to sustain left vertebral flow. (b) All cerebral systems opacify from right vertebral injection. (c) Postanastomosis frontal oblique angiogram demonstrates prominently enlarged STA with good MCA flow via angular artery. Oblique view helps to visualize anastomotic junction (open arrow). (d) MCA system opacification from STA (open arrow) and ophthalmic artery (closed arrow). Note faint leptomeningeal opacification of right ACA (curved arrow) and nonopacified temporal arteries (below black dots) which fill from PCA by pial connections.

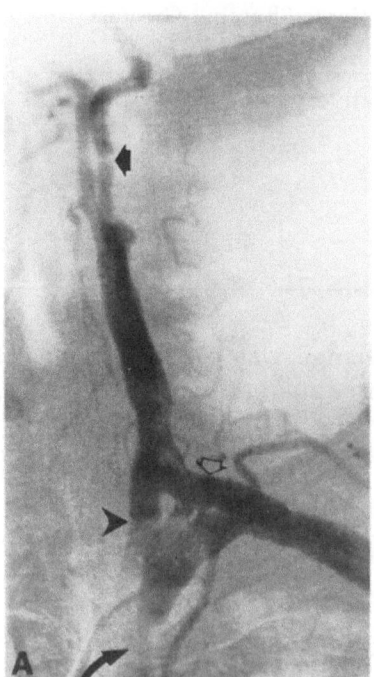

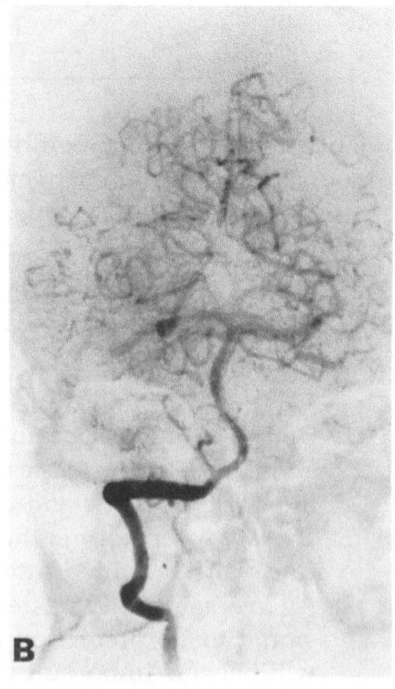

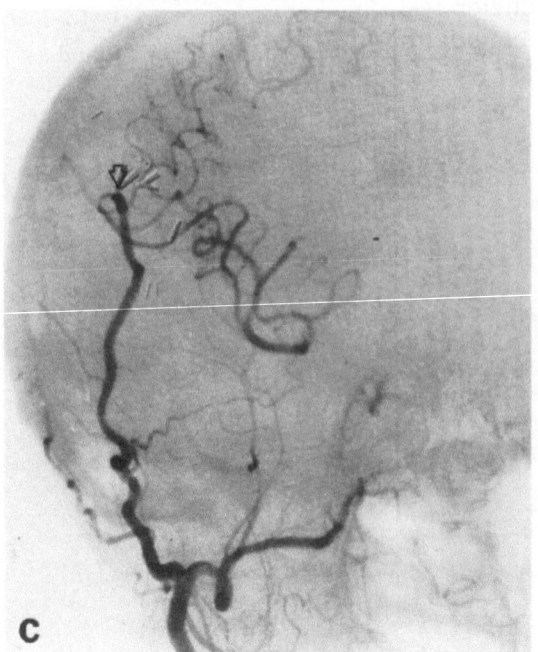

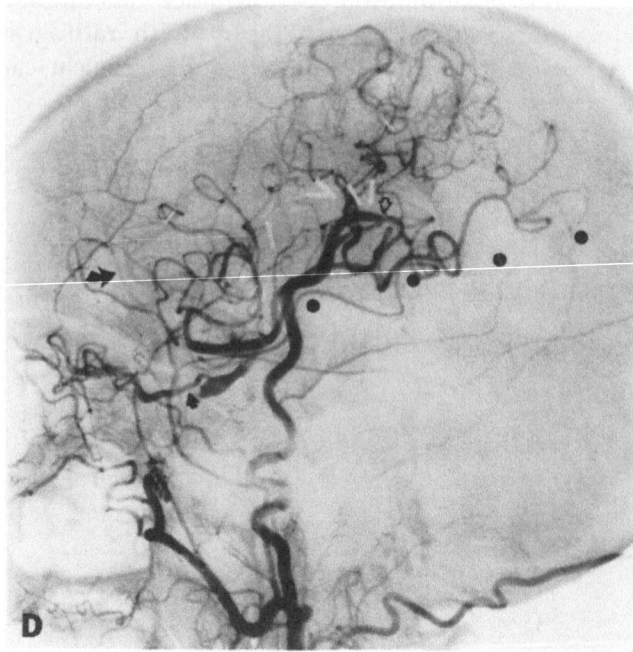

Chapter 13: Angiographic Cerebral Blood Flow Patterns

5. Average STA cross-sectional area doubled after anastomosis. One patient's STA increased nine times in luminal area.

6. The implication from comparison of different patients with angiograms at varying postanastomotic intervals is that size increases probably occur within a week or two.

7. A larger series with complete pre- and postoperative angiograms will be needed to relate postanastomotic STA size and flow to the location and nature of the primary lesion, and to more completely determine the effects of the functioning anastomosis on existing collateral circulation.

ACKNOWLEDGMENT

The authors wish to express gratitude to Ms. Brenda Holden for assistance in the preparation of this manuscript.

REFERENCES

1. Fasano V, Braggi G, Portalupi A: Investigation of some aspects of hemodynamics by models simulating cerebral blood flow. In Taveras JM, Fischgold H, Dilenge D, (eds): Recent Advances in the Study of Cerebral Circulation. Springfield, Ill., Thomas, 1970

2. Fields WS, Bruetman ME, Weibel J: Collateral circulation of the brain. In Monographs in the Surgical Sciences, Williams & Wilkins, Vol. 2. 1965, 183–259

3. Mount LA, Taveras JM: Arteriographic demonstration of the collateral circulation of the cerebral hemispheres. Arch Neurol Psychiat 78:235, 1957

4. Parkinson D: Collateral circulation of cavernous carotid artery. Anatomy. Can J Surg 7:251, 1964

5. Rosegay H, Welch K: Peripheral collateral circulation between cerebral arteries. J Neurosurg 11:363, 1954

6. Simmons CR, Tsao E, Smith LL, et al: Angiographic evaluation in extracranial vascular occlusive disease. Arch Surg, 107:785, 1973

7. Stehbens WE: Pathology of Cerebral Blood Vessels. St. Louis, Mosby, 1972

8. Thompson JR, Simmons CR, Tsao EB: Angiographic evaluation of brain ischemia and the superficial temporal artery–middle cerebral artery anastomosis candidate. Presented at the First International Symposium on Microneurosurgical Anastomoses for Cerebral Ischemia, Loma Linda, California, June 14, 1973

9. Wallace S, Goldberg HI, Leeds NE, et al: The cavernous branches of the internal carotid artery. Am J Roentgenol 101:34, 1967

10. Weibel J, Fields WS: Atlas of arteriography. In Occlusive Cerebrovascular Disease. Philadelphia, Saunders, 1969

11. Wylie J, Ehrenfeld WK: Extracranial Occlusive Cerebrovascular Disease. Diagnosis and Management. Philadelphia, Saunders, 1970

IV

SURGICAL TECHNIQUES

14

Contemporary techniques
of cerebral revascularization

Jack M. Fein

Introduction

Before the application of the surgical microscope to neurosurgery, sporadic attempts were made to remove occlusive lesions of the intracranial arteries using conventional operative techniques. This was first accomplished in 1955 by Welch, who reported the surgical removal of obstructions from the middle cerebral artery in two cases.(16) One patient had an embolectomy for an occlusion distal to the posterior temporal branch and the other patient had an occlusion proximal to the lenticulostriate branches. In 1959 Scheibert(12) reported an experience of four cases and in 1960 Piazza and Gaist reported the removal of a shotgun pellet that embolized to the middle cerebral artery(10). Subsequent reports by Shillito,(13) Driesen,(4) Chou,(2) and Woringer(17) also described technical success in repairing intracranial arterial occlusive lesions without the benefits of the surgical microscope.

Survival of brain tissue, however, is not necessarily dependent solely on the size or site of an arterial occlusion. Both clinical(9,11) and experimental evidence(14,15) indicate that the outcome of arterial occlusive or embolic insults is primarily related to the adequacy of the collateral circulation. It seemed particularly appropriate in cases of atherosclerotic occlusion to augment cerebral blood flow with extracranial sources of collateral vessels rather than to persist in attempts to remove occlusive or stenotic lesions from the deeper arteries of the brain. In fact, one of the earliest attempts to accomplish this was made by Henschen in 1944.(6) He attached a pedicle of temporalis muscle to the surface of the brain in an attempt to furnish a source of collateral circulation from the temporalis vasculature. The patient had bilateral carotid stenosis. Although he improved after surgery, no postoperative cerebral angiogram was reported. Another modification of this same concept was described by Khodaddad.(8) He implanted a scalp artery directly into the brain parenchyma after sealing the distal lumen with clot, in an effort to stimulate neovascular budding.

Extracranial–Intracranial Bypass Surgery

Anastomosis of extracranial to intracranial (EC-IC) arteries is currently the most practical technique for immediately augmenting collateral blood flow. This requires precise manipulation of arteries approximately 1 mm in diameter, and developments in this field were primarily limited by the surgeon's visual acuity and the available instrumentation. In 1960 Jacobson et al(7) demonstrated the value of the surgical microscope in the microvascular repair of 1 mm arteries. This required the development of special instrumentation for microsurgery, as well as ultrafine suture materials and needles.

The First Conference on Microvascular Surgery was held in Burlington, Vermont, in October, 1966. At that time Yazargil described the technique for creating a superficial temporal–middle cerebral anastomosis in the dog.(3) One year later Yazargil and Donaghy performed the first and second anastomoses in patients.

Unlike most other neurosurgical procedures, which one can learn in the operating room, the skills of microvascular surgery and the facility which is required to attain a high patency rate cannot be developed in the operating room alone. A series of laboratory exercises have been established which will allow one to become familiar with techniques of arteriotomy, arteriotomy repair, end-to-end and end-to-side anastomoses in vessels varying from 1 to 3 mm in diameter.(18) Furthermore, these skills should also include a familiarity with the surgical microscope and the ability to troubleshoot problems as they may arise in the operating room.

Operating Room

The design of the operating room in which such procedures are carried out should provide adequate space and a minimum of traffic flow to reduce bacterial contamination. The nurse should have ready access to microinstruments on an overhead Mayfield table. A right-handed surgeon who has an assistant at his right must still be within comfortable reach of the nurse who will pass instruments and may also guide the surgeon's hand back toward the operative field.

The Zeiss operating microscope fitted with a 200-mm objective provides approximately 8 inches of focal length between the surgical field and the objective lens. This is the surgeon's working space. In the vertical position the motor drive functions as a fine focus; otherwise focus is obtained by a coarser knob control. Various magnifications are possible and are related to: the focal length of the tube (F_t), the focal length of the objective lens (F_o), the factor indicated on the magnification changer control knob (W) and the magnification of the eyepieces (V_{ok}). The actual magnification may be calculated from the equation:

$$V = F_t/F_o \cdot W/16/V_{ok}$$

When using eyepieces of less than 20× or objective lenses with focal lengths greater than 200 mm the microscopic magnification is always less than the factor indicated on the magnification changer. Since the focal length of the tube remains constant, the effective focal length of the objective decreases with increasing magnification. This focal length can become a critical factor between 25 and 40 times magnification. When 1-mm arteries are visualized at these magnifications, it may be necessary to use the vertical motor drive control to focus on different parts of the anastomosis.

The diameter of the field of vision (d) is also inversely related to the magnification by the equation $d = 200/V$. With the commonly used 200–400 mm objective lenses and 10–20× eyepieces, the range of the diameter of the field of vision is 5–133 mm. It may be necessary to use the wider field when preparing to tie sutures. Between sutures, both the depth and the diameter of field may need to be changed.

The microinstruments should be short enough so that one can work comfortably within a relatively superficial craniotomy field. One of the new bicycle chairs may make it more comfortable for the surgeon during the lengthy procedure. Pin fixation of the patient's head provides a stable operative field and obviates the development of pressure sores, which may result from the various "doughnut" rests used to hold the patient's head.

Videorecording

Television monitoring through the microscope allows nurses, aides, and students to participate in the procedure. By looking at the monitor, the scrub nurse can anticipate what intruments will be required next, and this allows for smoother flow of one part of the procedure into the next. The anatomy is magnified for better illustration and instruction of students and visitors. The video tape can be used to store all or part of the procedure as a permanent record. This can then be reviewed later for analysis of errors in technique.

We have utilized the Magnavox Chromavue 400[1] color television camera, mounted on the left side of the Zeiss beamsplitter using a photo adapter. This allows f stop settings between $f/44$ and $f/8$. A condenser type microphone is mounted in the lens end of the Magnavox camera for recording a narrative description of the operation. Both audio and video channels are fed into a processor unit which contains the power supply, sync generator, and most of the signal processing circuits. The composite audio and video signals are then connected to a Sony U-matic video-cassette recorder.[2] The video recorder output signals are connected to a Sony Trinitron CVM-1720[2] color monitor via 75 Ω coaxial cable. When considering the use of mul-

[1]Magnavox Co.

[2]Sony Corp., Woodside, N.Y.

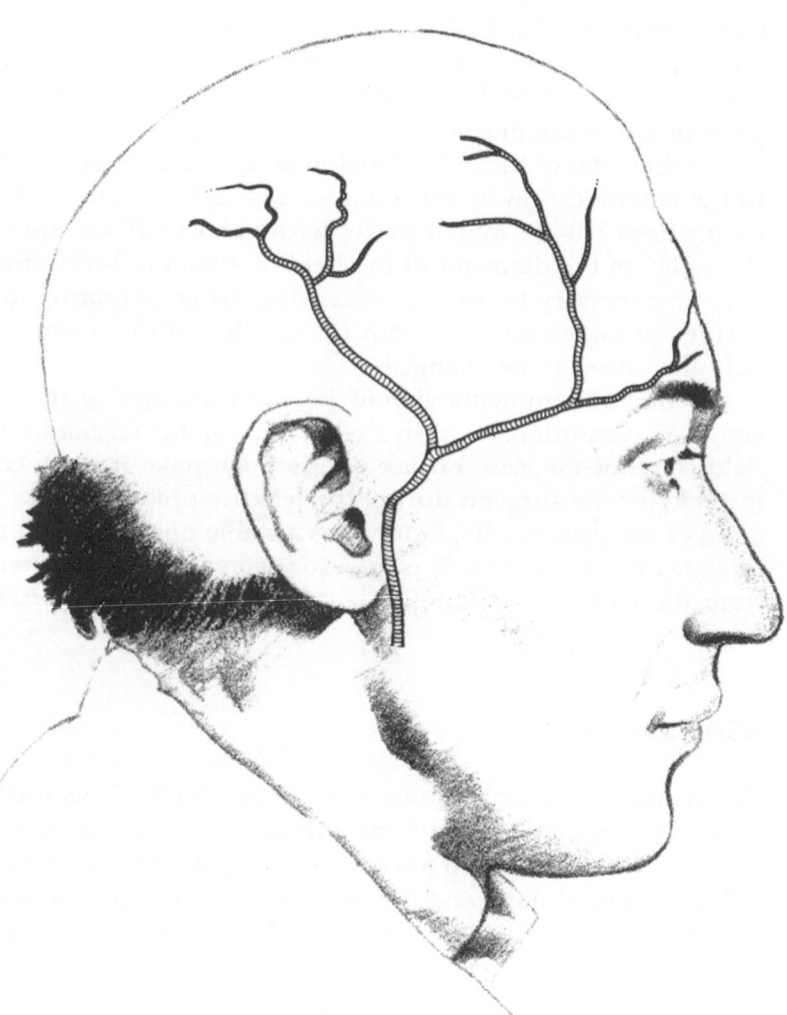

Fig. 14.1 The superficial temporal artery divides into a parietal branch and a frontal branch. These can be recognized by their sinuous course and branch approximately 1 cm anterior and superior to the external auditory meatus.

tiple monitors, it is important to remember that if the connecting cable is longer than 165 feet, there is usually some degradation of the picture quality. However, this can be mitigated with a line amplifier if longer cable runs are desired (e.g., to a conference room). To obtain both 35-mm slide photography and video recording we have used a recently developed optical switch(1) instead of the photo adapter on the microscope. This allows one to direct the image coming from one part of the beamsplitter to either the 35-mm or television camera so that both types of photodocumentation can be achieved.

Anesthesia and Perioperative Treatment

Anesthetic and ancillary aids for the EC-IC bypass have been simplified. The major requirement is the selection of a general anesthetic which will maintain cerebral perfusion pressure and which does not place increased demands on cerebral metabolism. We have employed 1% Halothane with controlled respirations for this purpose. Arterial catheters are placed percutaneously in either the radial or dorsalis pedis artery to sample and monitor the blood gas values as well as the blood pressure. A high normal arterial pCO_2 (between 38 and 44 mmHg) and a high normal blood pressure is maintained throughout the procedure. The flow rate becomes especially critical after a fresh anastomosis is completed. Intraoperative heparinization is not utilized. However, Rheomacrodex (low molecular weight Dextran) is infused through a separate catheter after the new graft is completed, and a slow drip (50 cc/hr) is maintained for 24 hr postoperatively.

Flap Design

The design of the craniotomy incision depends on the scalp artery which is selected as well as on the branch of the middle cerebral artery to be used as a recipient vessel. The superficial temporal artery divides into a frontal and parietal branch approximately 1 cm anterior and superior to the external auditory meatus (see Fig. 14.1). Each branch can usually be palpated separately and its pulsations are often visible when the scalp is shaved. The branches are identified definitively on the angiogram. They should not be confused with meningeal arteries, which are usually narrower and run a straighter course in the meningeal grooves on the inner table of the calvarium.

The appropriate scalp artery is chosen and the skin is prepared, marked and draped. Some surgeons prefer to make an incision parallel to the branch of the superficial temporal artery and dissect the artery from the subcutaneous tissues. If a formal

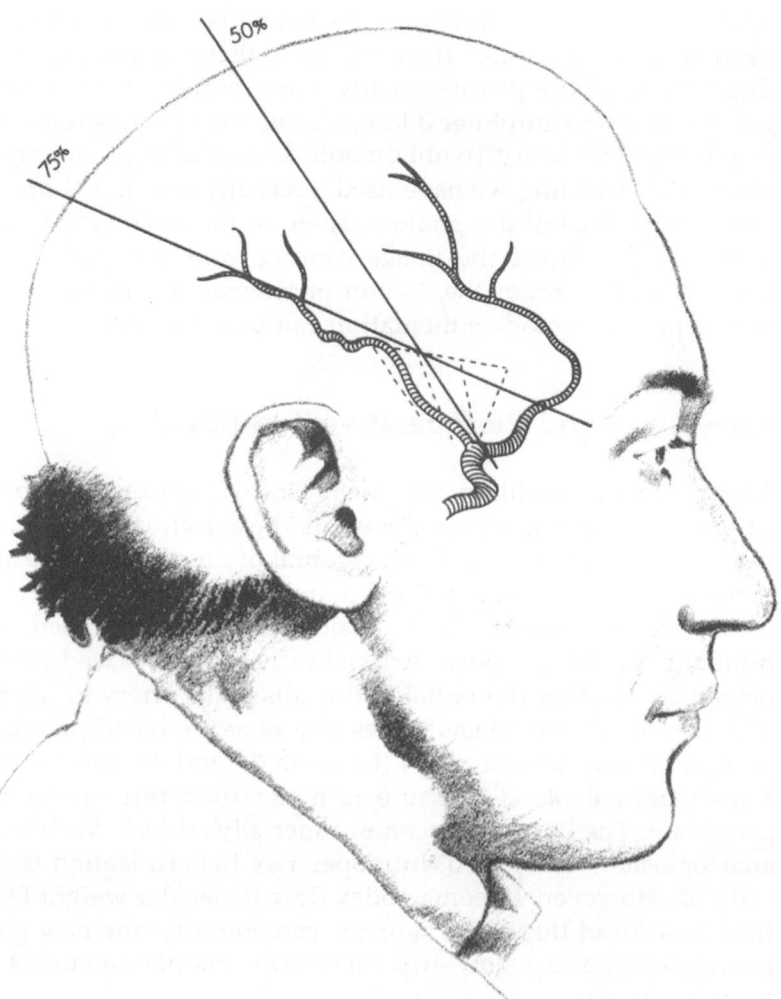

Fig. 14.2 It is helpful to design the flap in relation to the Sylvian fissure and central sulcus. For this purpose the Sylvian fissure can be superimposed on a line drawn from the external angular process of the frontal bone to a point located 75% of the circumferential distance from the nasion to the inion.

flap is used, hemostats rather than clips should be used on the flap edges.

After the superficial temporal artery is identified in the galea, a separate T-shaped incision in the temporalis muscle is made. Flaps of muscle are undermined and held apart by fish hooks. The muscle incision should be designed so that a cuff of fascia is preserved at the temporalis insertion which will allow this layer to be closed separately.

Craniotomy Design

A 3.5-cm trephine opening will provide the necessary exposure and protection of the anastomosis when the flap is replaced. In those cases where an infrasylvian exposure is appropriate, a craniectomy may be sufficient. In either case the bony opening should be positioned in relation to the Sylvian fissure which is located on a line between the external angular process of the frontal bone and a point along the sagittal midline located 75% of the circumferential distance from the nasion to the inion. The central sulcus may be superimposed on a line drawn from a point 2 cm posterior to the midpoint of the nasion–inion circumference and the middle of the zygomatic arch (see Fig. 13.2).

For the occasional suprasylvian exposure the trephine is placed so that the Sylvian fissure lies in the caudal one-third of the opening. For the infrasylvian exposure, the Sylvian fissure should lie in the cephalad one-third of the trephine opening.

If the bypass graft is done in preparation for a procedure at the base of the brain (e.g., trapping of the internal carotid or middle cerebral arteries), a posteriorly placed branch such as the angular artery is chosen. In this position the anastomosis will not be displaced by the frontotemporal retraction required for exposure of the supraclinoid internal carotid artery at the base.

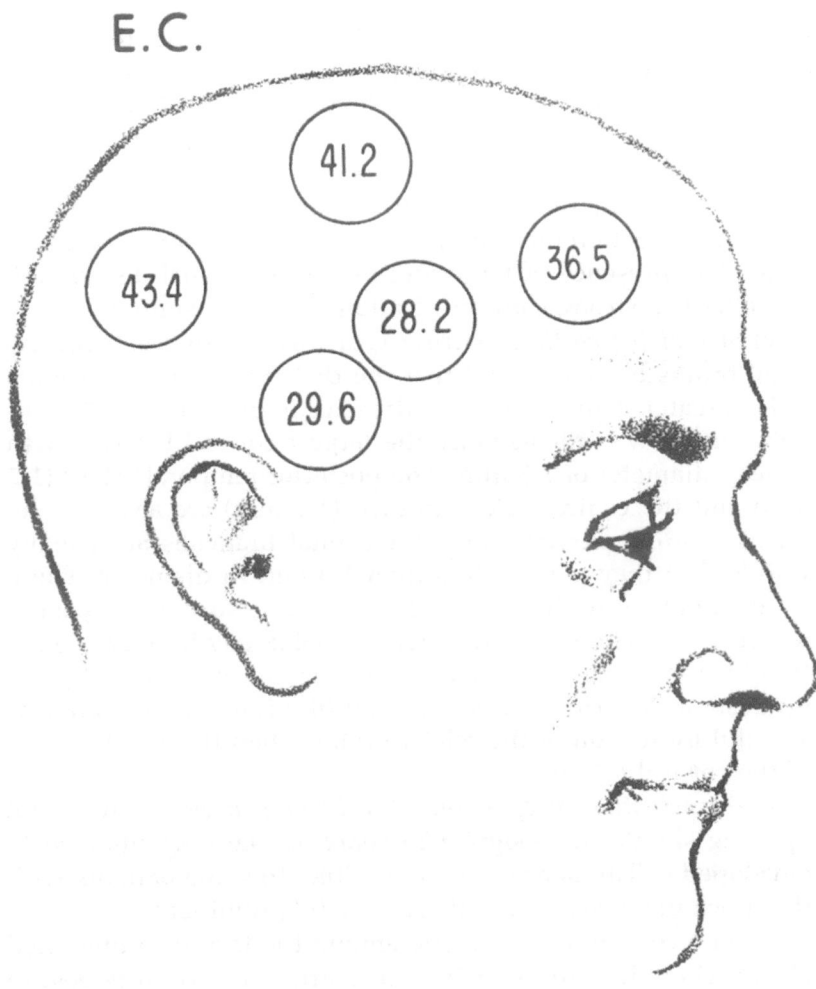

E.C.

Fig. 14.4. Regional cerebral blood flow study in a 43-year-old patient with a right middle cerebral artery occlusion. The focal ischemia is an objective functional parameter which confirms the location of the cerebral regions at greatest risk.

After the bone flap is removed the Hall air drill is used to make small angled holes around the periphery of the cranial defect and at three equidistant points on the flap. Twenty-eight gauge wire is passed through the three corresponding holes on the edge of the defect and the dura is apposed to the inner table at each hole with 4-0 silk. The dura is then opened in stellate fashion aligning one of these limbs with the intended course of the superficial temporal artery.

The cortical artery which is selected for anastomosis should be chosen carefully. This decision may be influenced by the following information:

(a) *The clinical syndrome*: In most cases this is only useful in differentiating a more anterior from a more posterior syndrome. An anterior ischemic syndrome may include adversive eye movements, but usually consists of paresis and on the dominant side, a nonfluent language disorder. A posterior syndrome includes a fluent language disorder and a hemianopic defect.

(b) *Preoperative laboratory studies*: Some patients suffering from transient ischemic attacks will have interictal evidence of impaired hemodynamics. Despite the relatively poor resolution of the dynamic brain scan such studies may help to confirm the location of an area of focal ischemia (see Fig. 14.3, p. 173). Better resolution may be obtained with a multichannel system for measuring regional cerebral blood flow (see Fig. 14.4). The patient with a neurologic deficit will often have demonstrable areas of rarefaction on a computerized axial tomogram (see Fig. 14.5). The presence of large areas of parenchymal destruction however is a strong contraindication to bypass surgery.

(c) *Size of the cortical arteries*: Our own postmortem review of 20 brains has confirmed that the distribution of cortical arteries greater than 1.0 mm in diameter is predictable. The angular artery was consistently the largest cortical branch, with a mean diameter of 1.3 mm. The posterior temporal artery (1.2 mm) and the central sulcus branch (1.1 mm) are also visible. The ascending frontal and orbitofrontal branches are usually visible, but they may be less than 1.0 mm in diameter. There is sufficient individual variation, however, so that a decision regarding the choice of a recipient vessel in any individual case should only be made after close inspection of the angiogram. Because of the error caused by magnification the angiogram is a useful indication of the relative rather than the absolute size of the cortical arteries.

(d) *Preservation of spontaneous collateral arteries*: The dural opening should be designed to spare as many spontaneously developed collateral arteries as possible. In some patients with the moya moya syndrome these may be prominent.

Often a compromise is made among the factors enumerated above when deciding which cortical artery to use. It is best to

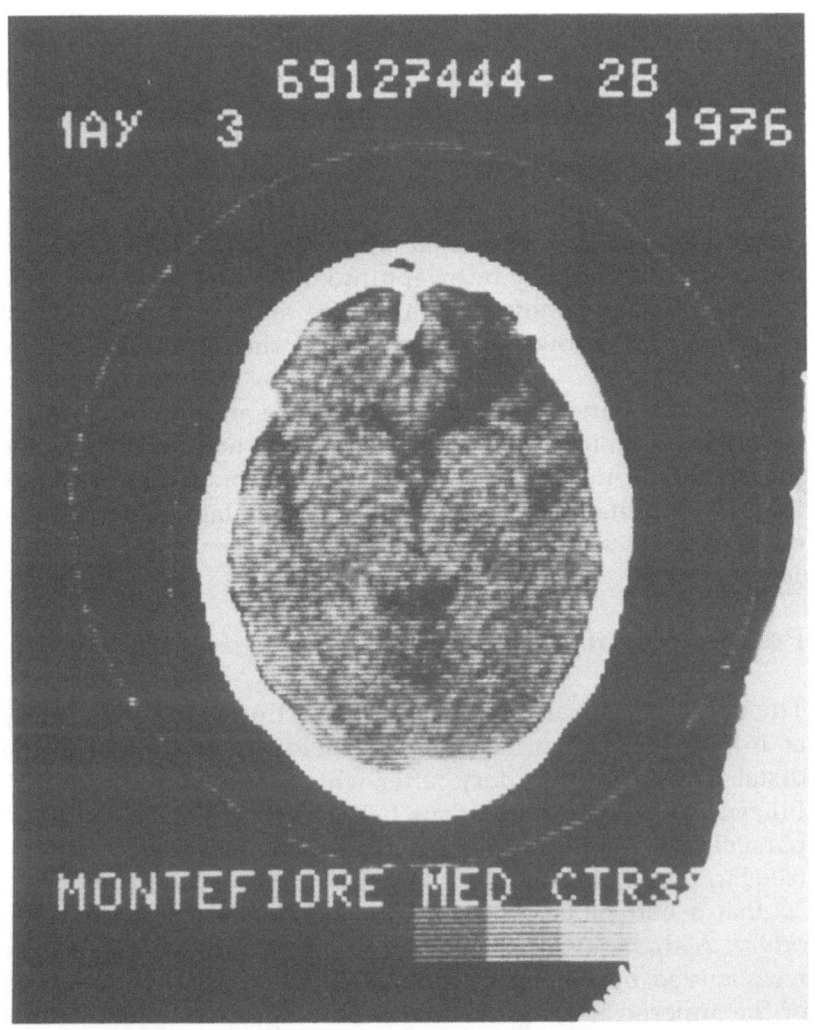

Fig. 14.5. Computerized axial tomogram 3 months after the onset and resolution of a dense left hemiparesis. A wedge-shaped area of rarefaction persists in the right fronto-temporal region.

try to graft to the primary branches of the main middle cerebral artery as they course over the gyri bordering the Sylvian fissure. In this location they are of sufficient size, whereas they rapidly narrow as they course over the surface of the cortex and dip into their respective sulci.

The Recipient Artery

It may be difficult to measure the diameter of some cortical arteries accurately without first incising the investing arachnoid. When an appropriate recipient artery is selected, the investing arachnoid is cut sharply with a #11 blade under 16× magnification. The arachnoid is stripped to expose tertiary branches and transcortical penetrating branches. This can be done most effectively by sharply cutting the milky white membrane longitudinally along the side of the artery itself. Traction on the periarterial chordae from blunt dissection perpendicular to the long axis of the artery should be avoided, as this will invariably produce mechanical vasospasm. Although transient, this may make further manipulation of the artery difficult. Should this occur inadvertently, a few drops of Papavarian solution may be applied to the vessel. Under the microscope the cotton fibers of the paddies are observed to fray and adhere to the arachnoid and may be swept into the anastomosis site. The cottonnoids are removed at this stage and small segments of absorbent paper towel are used to help suction fluid from the field.

The cortical artery segment selected for anastomosis should be at least 1 cm in length and is completely mobilized from the pial surface. One or two small perforating branch arteries less than 100 μm diameter may need to be coagulated with the micro Malis cautery forceps and cut.

Preparation of the Donor

The microscope is also used in the dissection of the scalp artery at 16× magnification. A micro Mayfield clip is applied to the distal portion of the artery, after which it is incised and mobilized from the subcutaneous tissue. After incising the galea parallel to the scalp artery its branches are coagulated and cut (see Fig. 14.6). Sharp dissection must be employed throughout, so that a cuff of fascia protects the vasa vasora of the scalp artery. A sharp jewelers forceps and a small ophthalmic scissor with curved blades are ideal for this purpose. Small branches of the superficial temporal artery are coagulated at least 2 to 3 mm away from the parent artery, so that thrombosis in branch arteries does not extend to the parent artery. Larger branches may be ligated with 6-0 silk. After the required length of the artery is dissected free the clip is opened so that the artery can bleed freely and the amount of flow can be assessed. The Mayfield clip is replaced on the most proximal portion of the artery which has been dissected free of the galea. A PE-10 Teflon tube connected through a 28-gauge needle to a tuberculin syringe is passed into the lumen. The scalp artery is then flushed clean with 1–2 cc of Heparin (5,000 μm in 25 cc of normal saline).

Under 16× magnification the distal 1 cm of the artery is stripped free of its surrounding fascia and fat by splitting the fascia longitudinally, so that the vasa varorum are not extensively interrupted. The distal lumen is then fish-mouthed to increase the size of the anastomosis.

It is important to have an adequate length of scalp artery dissected free, bearing in mind the new course of the vessel through the temporalis muscle, over the bone edge, through the dura, and to an oblique approximation with the recipient cortical artery. Adequate length must also be available so that

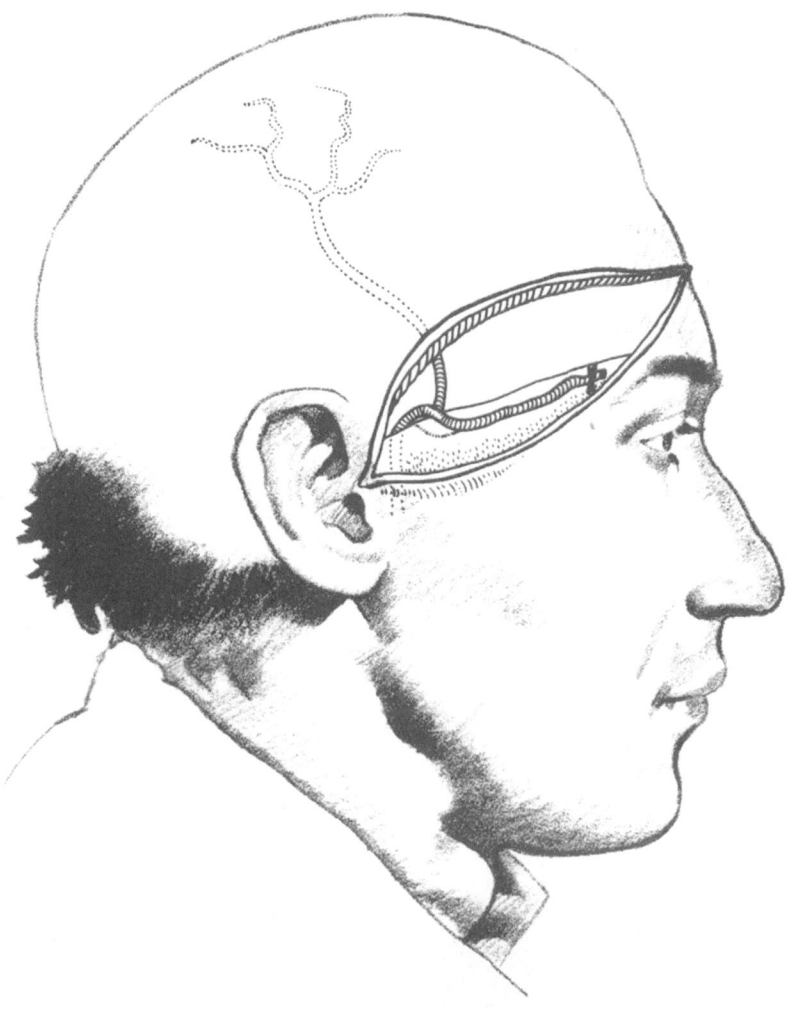

Fig. 14.6. Operative sketch showing the initial dissection of the frontal branch of the superficial temporal artery. A small Mayfield clip was applied distally, but there is sufficient circulation through small scalp branches to maintain flow in the parent vessel until this is completely dissected free from the galea.

there is no tension whatsoever on either the scalp artery or the anastomosis.

Microvascular Anastomosis

Two small rubber dams tagged with 3-0 silk suture are placed over the cortex on either side of the recipient artery. One dam has a tonguelike extension which is fitted under the recipient artery. Temporary micro Mayfield clips are applied to the cortical artery and the time is noted. A longitudinal arteriotomy incision 2–3 times the diameter of the artery is then made with a sliver of broken razor blade and is converted into an elipse using a pair of short curved microscissors.

The suturing technique must be meticulous. In larger vessel repairs, eversion, inversion, or bunching up to the wall may not significantly compromise the lumen and in fact may contribute to hemostasis. In the end-to-side microanastomosis exact placement of sutures is necessary because of the geometric

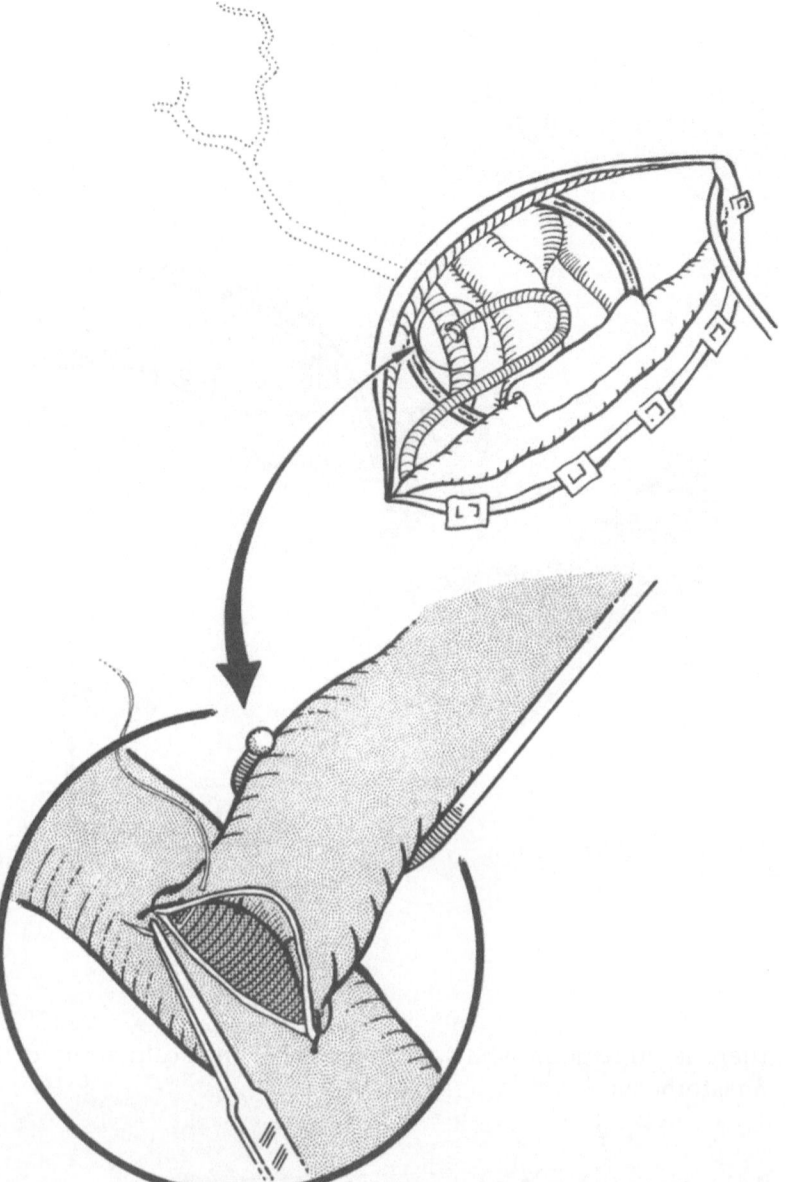

Fig. 14.7. The microanastomosis of a superficial temporal to a cortical branch has been partially completed. The enlarged sketch shows the use of a curved ball dissector to rotate the scalp artery while the second half of the anastomosis is completed.

relationship of flow to lumen diameter. The sutures are placed closely enough to the vessel edge so that the needle can be clearly seen through the vessel wall. The purpose of the suture is to bring the lumen of the scalp and cortical arteries into apposition, edge to edge. It is important not to evert the edges in an attempt to get apposition of endothelium, since this will reduce the internal diameter. A continuous suture may be more hemostatic, however, interrupted sutures will provide a better chance for long-term patency. Furthermore, hypertrophy of the graft has been documented with postoperative angiography. A continuous suture technique will limit this expansion, whereas interrupted sutures will allow the artery to expand.(5)

The 10-0 Ethicon suture (22μ diameter) on a BV-5 needle (130

Chapter 14: Contemporary Techniques of Cerebral Revascularization

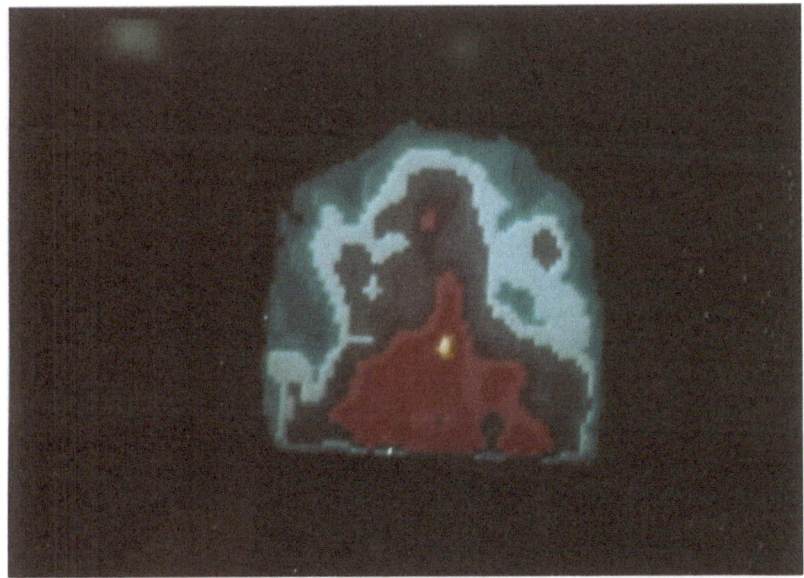

Fig. 14.3. Dynamic brain scan performed 1 month after a focal cerebral infarct indicating persistent focal ischemia in the superior temporal region on the left.

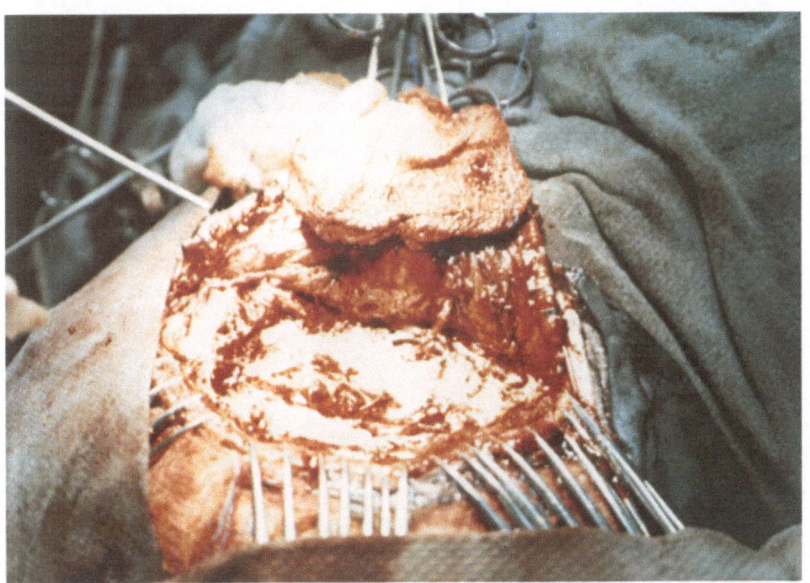

Fig. 14.8. Operative photograph taken after completion of the anastomosis and partial closure of the dura. An adequate opening must be provided in the dura for the scalp vessel to penetrate without kinking.

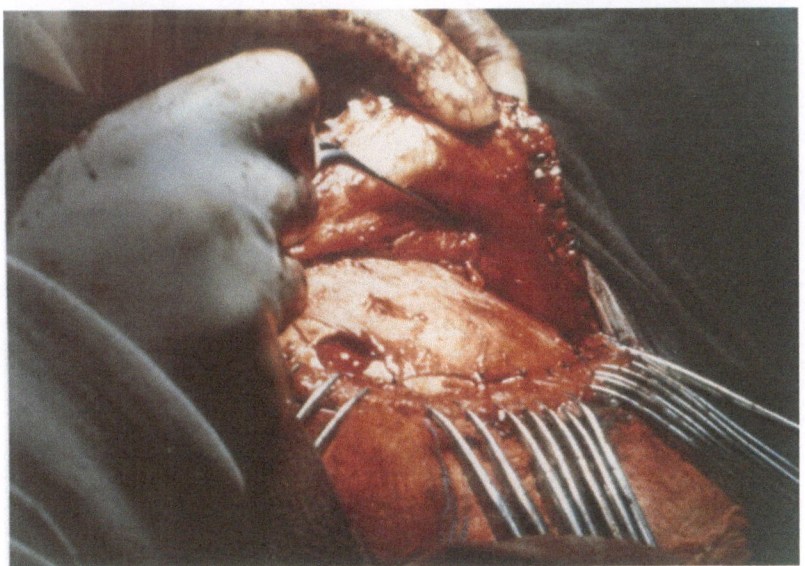

Fig. 14.9. Operative photograph after replacing and wiring the bone flap in place. The pericraneum has been partially sutured. In most cases a 2 inch trephine will be adequate.

μ diameter) is first passed through the superficial temporal artery then through the cortical artery. The sutures are precut to 4-cm lengths so that they may be tied under 25× magnification. Anchoring sutures are first placed at each end of the elliptical arteriotomy. This keeps the edges properly aligned and the lumen is reconstituted from the beginning, making it more difficult for the wrong surface to be caught in the suturing process. After the anchoring sutures are placed, tied, and cut, sutures are placed on one side and then on the other side of the anastomosis. The scalp artery may need to be rotated but should not be placed on stretch (Fig. 14.7). Generally 12–14 sutures are required depending on the size of the STA. The distal clip on the cortical vessel is then opened to allow back bleeding and this will always produce a little bleeding at the anastomosis. The clip should not be reapplied as this amount of bleeding is not sufficient to disrupt the suture line and will deposit a thin layer of platelets and fibrin along the vessel edges to promote hemostasis. When this oozing abates the proximal cortical clip and finally the clip on the STA are removed. The pulsations should ideally be transmitted from the STA toward the proximal portion of the cortical artery, however, since epicerebral arteries function as a conductive network, the portion of the vascular bed with the lowest intraluminal pressure will act as a sink to influence the direction of flow.

Closure

There may be some persistent ooze from the fascia of the superficial temporal artery and these points are identified by switching back to 10× or 16× magnification. The bipolar cautery is used, care being taken not to coagulate too close to the STA itself. Perfect hemostasis should be obtained. The dura is then closed with continuous 4-0 silk suture and an opening for the penetrating scalp artery is provided (see Fig. 14.8, p. 173). A channel is fashioned for the artery at the edge of the bone flap which is then wired in place (see Fig. 14.9, p. 173). When the muscle is closed one must be sure that the artery is not kinked. The galea and skin are closed separately and the condition of the skin edges are noted. The position of the scalp artery is again marked on the scalp for later examination. The head dressing should not be applied too tightly so that the scalp artery is not strangulated.

Postoperative Care

Rheomacrodex (Dextran 40,000 molecular weight) is infused intravenously at a rate of 50 cc/hr when the anastomosis is completed and for the first 24 hr postoperatively. The patient is nursed in the neurosurgical intensive care unit to be sure that blood pressure, pulses, and arterial blood gases are maintained at a normal level and liberal fluid replacement is employed. After 36 hr the patient is gradually elevated and may sit out of bed with careful blood pressure monitoring. The scalp will swell maximally at 3–5 days postoperatively so that the pulsation of the superficial temporal artery may be dampened temporarily. Scalp sutures are removed 5 days after surgery following which the patient may be discharged from the hospital.

Follow-up visits are scheduled so that postoperative angiography can be performed 2–4 months after the surgery.

ACKNOWLEDGMENT

This work was supported by NIH RCDA # 5 K04 NS00198-02.

REFERENCES

1. Apfelbaum R: An optical switch for improved photography through the operating microscope. Surg Neurol 6:335, 1976
2. Chou SN: Embolectomy of middle cerebral artery: Report of a case. J Neurosurg 20:161, 1963
3. Donaghy RMP, Yazargil MG, (eds): *Microvascular Surgery*. St. Louis, Mosby, 1967
4. Driesen WW: Erfolgreiche Naht der linken A cerebri media nach Verletzung bei Tumorresektion. Acta Neurochir (Wien) 10:462, 1962
5. Fein JM, Reichman OH: Assessment of graft hypertrophy after STA–MCA anastomosis. Presented at the New York Neurosurgical Society Meeting, February 15, 1977
6. Henschen G: Operative revaskularisation des zirkulatorisch geschadigten Gehirns durch Auflage gestielter Muske-lappen (Encephalo-Myo-Synangiose). Langenbecks Arch Klin Chir 264:393, 1950
7. Jacobson JH et al: Microsurgery as an aid to middle cerebral artery endarterectomy. J Neurosurg 19:108, 1962
8. Khodaddad G: Implantation of the superficial temporal artery into the brain. In Austin GM (ed): Microneurosurgical Anastomosis for Cerebral Ischemia. Springfield, Ill, Thomas, 1973
9. Lascelles RG, Burrows EH: Occlusion of the middle cerebral artery. Brain 88:85, 1964
10. Piazza G, Gaist G: Occlusion of middle cerebral artery by foreign body embolus. Report of a case. J Neurosurg 17:172, 1960
11. Rosegay H, Welch K: Peripheral collateral circulation between cerebral arteries. J Neurosurg 11:363, 1954
12. Scheibert CD: Middle cerebral artery surgery for obstructive lesions. Presented at the 27th Annual Meeting of the Harvey Cushing Society, New Orleans, May 1959

13. Shillito J: Intracranial arteriotomy in three children and three adults. In Donaghy, RMP, Yasargill, MG (eds): Microvascular Surgery, St. Louis, Mosby, 1967, pp 138–142

14. Turnbull IM: Microvascular study in experimental cerebral infarction. Surg Forum 18:437, 1967

15. Vander Eecken H, Adams RD: The anatomy and functional significance of the meningeal arterial anastomoses of the human brain. J Neuropath Exp Neurol 12:(2) 132, 1953

16. Welch K: Excision of occlusive lesions of the middle cerebral artery. J Neurosurg 13:73, 1956

17. Woringer E, Kunlin J: Anastomos entre la carotide primitive et la carotide intra-cranienne ou la sylvienne par greffon selon la technique de la sutrue suspendue. Neuro-Chir (Paris) 9(2): 181, 1963

18. Yazargil G: Microsurgery Applied to Neurosurgery. New York, Academic Press, 1969, pp 60–81

15

External carotid–middle cerebral artery bypass using free graft bypass

Mel H. Epstein

Neurology and neurosurgery have lagged behind the rest of the medical profession in vascular reconstruction procedures. Until recently, the surgical treatment of impending stroke was largely restricted to large vessel surgery in the chest and neck. However, as far back as 1955, Welch described a successful embolectomy in the middle cerebral artery which was done without the aid of the surgical microscope(5) and Henschen, in 1944, transplanted a pedicle of temporalis musce over the surface of brain in an attempt to revascularize the brain.(2) A major change in direction occurred in 1967 when Donaghy(1) and Yasargil(6) demonstrated that by using the operating microscope one could successfully anastomose a superficial temporal artery to a cortical branch of the middle cerebral artery. This procedure now appears to be the basis for reconstructing an inadequate cerebral circulation when large vessel surgery in the neck is not possible. However, on a number of occasions we have been disappointed in that a number of individuals do not have superficial temporal arteries of adequate size to anastomose to the available cortical vessels. In addition, one is limited in the number of anastomoses one can perform in a given individual by the amount of blood which can be carried by the superficial temporal artery and the occipital artery. It has appeared to us, on more than one occasion, that the amount of additional blood which can be supplied by the superficial temporal anastomosis, either with or without associated occipital artery anastomosis, was not adequate to restore normal hemodynamics to a blood starved brain.

There are also some theoretical considerations which put temporal artery bypass into question on occasion. There is an important anastomotic loop involving the anterior frontal branch of the superficial temporal artery with the supraorbital artery which ultimately supplies the ophthalmic system directing blood retrograde to the brain. By disconnecting the superficial temporal artery and then reconnecting it in a different area of the brain, one conceivably can be losing important collateral circulation in one area and simply restoring it in another. We therefore felt it worthwhile to explore the possibility of using other conduits to bring blood from the extracranial circulation to the intracranial circulation without disturbing existing collaterals.

Experimental work has been performed by Donaghy(1) using saphenous vein and arterial bypasses in animals. Lougheed et al(4) in 1971, described the use of saphenous vein grafts from the external carotid artery in the neck to the intracranial carotid artery to bypass carotid obstructions. Lazar and Clark reviewed their experience with this procedure in 1973.(3) Lougheed's procedure involves the risk of manipulating the central brain circulation. We therefore felt, if enough distal flow could be provided, that the saphenous vein might make an adequate conduit if it was connected to the carotid artery in the neck and then anastomosed end to side to a branch of the middle cerebral artery. This would avoid disturbing the carotid circulation.

Technique

The saphenous vein is removed from the leg in the standard fashion, beginning at the ankle where it is narrowest in diameter. It is anastomosed end to side to a branch of the external carotid such as the common facial artery, so there is no need to interfere with any major collateral flow into the brain during anastomosis. It is then tunneled subcutaneously over the zygoma or behind the ear and a small craniectomy is made over the basilar aspect of the sylvian fissure. The cortical artery either derives from a branch at the junction of the sylvian fissure or the sylvian fissure is dissected and a more proximal middle cerebral branch is chosen. The intracranial anastomosis is sewn with 9-0 suture material; 7-0 is used for the cervical anastomosis. The carotid artery and the graft are locally heparinized. The temporal fascia is closed in a fairly loose manner so there is no impingement on the graft, and the temporalis muscle is placed over the approximated dura. Much more data will be necessary to determine the ultimate patency rate of this type of graft; but, obviously, if one can increase the distal flow sufficiently, these grafts should stay open indefinitely. The smaller the diameter of the graft, the greater the velocity flow and the less chance of stasis and thrombosis. We have recently been working with the radial artery as a substitute conduit for the saphenous vein and feel that it is probably superior because of its smaller diameter.

Conclusion

We believe that the superficial temporal cortical vessel anastomosis is still the procedure of choice for most patients. It is possible in some difficult cases with small superficial temporal arteries, or when multiple collaterals have to be established, that free graft bypassing from the external carotid artery to the middle cerebral artery or to one of the more peripheral branches of the middle cerebral might be useful. It must be remembered, however, that there is a significant size discrepancy between the free graft and the cerebral artery. This does not make the anastomosis difficult from a technical point of view, but may ultimately make this an impractical procedure because of late postoperative clotting. Fortunately, in the four procedures done so far, there have been no significant postoperative neurologic complications and no deaths. These patients are at high risk, because of the long period of anesthesia required for the operation. At present we believe that, in spite of the more extensive surgery required for a free graft bypass, it is important to develop other methods of bypass so that vascular neurosurgeons have more flexibility in their approach to patients with cerebral insufficiency.

REFERENCES

1. Donaghy RMP: Patch and bypass in micro-angeional surgery. In Microvascular Surgery. Stuttgart, Thieme Verlag, 1967, pp 75–86
2. Henschen C: Operative Revaskularisation des zirkulatorisch geschädigten Gehirns durch Auflage destielter Muskellappen (Encephalo-Myo-Synangiose) Langenbecks. Arch Klin Chir 264:392, 1950
3. Lazar M, Clark K: Microsurgical cerebral revascularization. Concepts and practice. Surg Neuro 1:355, 1973
4. Lougheed WM, Marshall BM, Hunter M, et al: Common carotid to intercranial internal carotid bypass venous graft. Technical note. J Neurosurg 34:114, 1971
5. Welch K: Excision of occlusive lesions of the middle cerebral artery. J Neurosurg 13:73, 1956
6. Yasargil MG: Diagnosis and indications for operations of cerebral vascular occlusive disease. In Yasargil MG (ed): Microsurgery Applied to Neurosurgery. Stuttgart, Thieme Verlag, 1969, pp 95–119

16

Electromagnetic blood flowmetry in microvascular anastomosis

Harry William Stephens, Jr.

Introduction

The rapid development of microvascular surgical techniques in the last 10 years is well documented. The paucity of literature on electromagnetic blood flow studies of vessels less than 3 mm in diameter has been noted by those teaching the basics of microvascular surgery. Electromagnetic flowmeters were initially used in experimental work, but the introduction of formal teaching of microvascular surgical techniques has taken this instrument out of the purely experimental phase of microvascular surgery. The surgeon learning new techniques may now evaluate his work in the teaching laboratory and will carry this knowledge directly into the operating room.

The oldest technique to measure blood flow was to sever a vessel and permit it to bleed into a graduated cylinder over a specific period of time. As techniques were required that would provide greater accuracy and not destroy the vessel being worked on, many new instruments were introduced that measured blood flow with pitot tubes, bristle flowmeters, rotameters, and ultrasonic meters. Modification of the Fick dye-dilution technique,[2] colorimetry, and cinematography have also been used in experimental work, but these techniques have not been adapted for use in many surgical clinics because they are either too complicated, inaccurate, or cannot be safely applied to small vessels.[8] Kolin[7] and Wetterer[12] brought about the most significant advances in blood flowmetry in the United States and Germany by applying the familiar Faraday law of electromagnetic induction to accurately measure blood flow. This development and the recognition of the oscillation and shape of the pressure waves in both the arterial and the venous side of the circulation led to a better understanding of blood flow in a pulsatile system. Refinements in electronics through the introduction of miniaturization and solid-state components have made electromagnetic flowmeters sufficiently reliable and accurate so that clinicians may undertake blood flow studies in the operating room(3) with well-trained medical assistants producing accurate recordings.

Principles of Electromagnetic Measurement of Blood Flow

Poiseuille's law was originally derived to study the flow of a newtonian liquid within rigid tubes, but is generally assumed to apply to blood flow in the vascular bed as well(4):

$$\Delta P = \frac{8L\mu Q}{\pi r^4}$$

The pressure gradient (P) is directly proportional to the length of the tube (L), the viscosity (μ), and the rate of flow (Q), and is inversely proportional to the fourth power of the radius (r), and the constant π.

Electromagnetic Measurement of Blood Flow

Faraday's law of electromagnetic induction is the basis for the modern electromagnetic blood flowmeters which were developed by Kolin and Wetterer (Fig. 16.1).

$$E = (MLV) \times 10^{-8}$$

E = electromotive force (volts)
M = magnetic field (gauss)
L = lumen diameter (cm)
V = velocity of the liquid (cm/second)

Fig. 16.1. Electromagnetic induction.

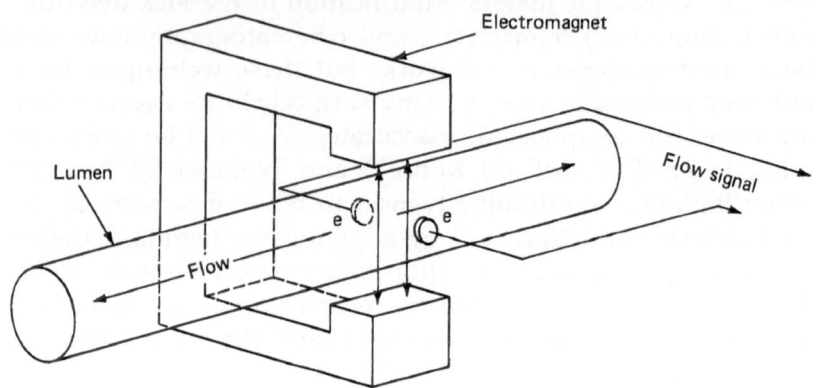

The conductive liquid (blood) is permitted to flow through a tube which is at right angles to a magnetic field, where it generates an electromagnetic force (volts) in a direction perpendicular to the magnetic field and direction of motion. Electrodes are placed 180° apart and record a voltage (emf) directly proportional to the velocity of the liquid. Kolin,[7] Wetterer,[11] Westerstein et al,[11] and Engle and Lauridson[6] demonstrated that a linear relationship exists between the velocity of the blood and the magnitude of the induced emf. These relationships hold for both laminar and turbulent blood flow in a pulsatile system.[5] Many of the initial problems limiting the accuracy of recording the emf generated in vessels were solved electronically. This was accomplished through the use of blood flow transducers that modify the magnetic field and eliminate electrode pick-up errors.[10] Square-wave signal systems were introduced with electronic damping circuits that eliminate the signal artifacts and are designed to operate at a frequency range between 400 and 1000 cps.[9] Interference from 60-cps line voltage and many of the electronic recording devices found in the modern operating room was thereby eliminated.

Miniaturized electronic systems with small blood flow transducers (probes) were developed which can measure flow in vessels as small as 1 to 2 mm. This enabled the microvascular surgeon to use probes with variable sensitivity and an accuracy of ± 5% to record flows through vascular reconstructions. These new flow transducers are small in size and cause minimal tissue displacement. There is an excellent correlation between the occluded zero blood flow signal and the zero signal obtained by electronically interrupting the current to the probe magnet. The use of electromagnetic flowmeters has become indispensable in the field of microvascular surgery and so far provides the most accurate measurement of flow through reconstructed vessels 1 to 2 mm in diameter.

Principles of Teaching Electromagnetic Blood Flow in the Microsurgical Laboratory

The student starting a basic course in microvascular surgery should be introduced to the electromagnetic blood flowmeter. He will be able to evaluate the initial vascular surgical procedures he performs and will be able to find errors that are being made and correct them prior to proceeding to other projects. He will be able to detect such early errors as suturing vessels closed and leaving intimal flaps. The introduction to the elementary principles of the electromagnetic flowmeter need not be so complex and difficult that the student is filled with apprehension. It should be considered an elementary tool to be

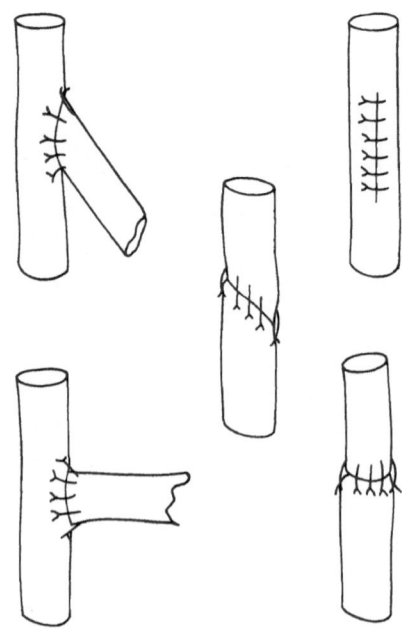

Fig. 16.2. The basic microvascular procedures used to teach application of blood flowmeter techniques.

mastered in much the same manner as were the microscope and microinstruments.

Our initial goal was to demonstrate the application of the flowmeter to the 2-mm internal carotid artery of an 800- to 900-g rat on which the student performed the basic microvascular procedures (Fig. 16.2). Blood flow was recorded using as simple a technique as possible. The 2-mm probe was placed around the vessel wall prior to each procedure. Blood flow was recorded at intervals of 5, 10, 15, and 20 minutes. Exact measurements of flow were not initially expected, but rather a rough estimate of flow was made that could be used for comparison with the postsurgical blood flows. This was done because we found that if students spent time making exact calibrations and recordings with the flowmeter, they became lost in the minute details at the expense of the surgical procedures. As the student later became more proficient with the instrument he then became involved with exact calibration and fine measurements. After the assigned surgical procedure a second series of blood flows was recorded for comparison with the first recording. A value of 100% was applied to the initial value and the second determination was compared and assigned a final value. This final flow percentage would then demonstrate to the student how well his anastomosis or vascular repair was functioning when compared to the initial flow value.

At the completion of the formal work in the course the student had a documented record of his progress as well as a recorded note of each error that caused poor blood flow in his work. This helped the student and also helped us to modify the teaching program. We were able to call attention to those problems we felt the student would encounter in learning the technique. We also discovered that if we encouraged the student to dissect the vessel and examine the blood flow values we could detect and document poor suturing as well as foreign particles sutured into the lumen of the vessel. Sketches or photographs also documented a series of technical errors which helped us develop new techniques and new instruments to eliminate such errors in the future.

Electromagnetic Blood Flowmetry Findings and Applications in the Teaching Laboratory

The basic applications of recording blood flow and the questions that were raised through our use of the flowmeter in teaching microvascular techniques in a disciplined laboratory, brought some interesting facts to our attention. We could not understand why we were recording certain flows, until by chance a visitor to the laboratory, Dr. Robert Ackland, introduced us to a technique he was using to observe the flow of blood through his vascular repairs. A small piece of plexiglass 2 mm thick and 2 mm wide was coated with black paint and a bright light was applied to one end. The end of this light conductor was applied to the side of a small 2mm vessel wall and the flow through the lumen of the vessel was then observed (Fig. 16.3). He detected an interesting phenomenon while viewing a vascular anastomosis. Around the site of the vascular repair, thrombin and platelets "piled up and then blew away like a pile of leaves after 5 to 10 minutes" (Fig. 16.4). He had observed what we had been recording with our flowmeter studies on the vessels. Our initial recordings of repaired vessels indicated that the flow through the vessel would remain at a certain level and then after 5 to 10 minutes would suddenly increase and remain at a higher value.(1) The use of both Dr. Ackland's technique and our flowmeter method solved many problems for us after that time. We recorded and sketched a

A.

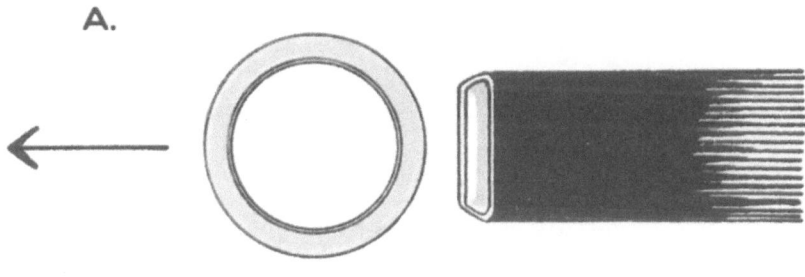

B.

2 mm. square tubing
supplying side light

LIGHT

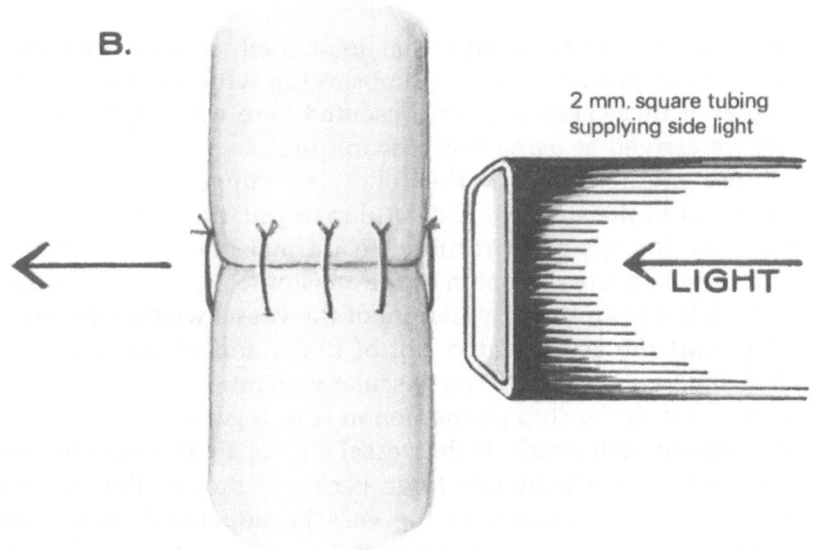

Fig. 16.3. Illumination technique using side lighting and ×25 to ×40 magnification to permit observation of surgical site and recording of the effect of surgery on the lumen of small vessels.

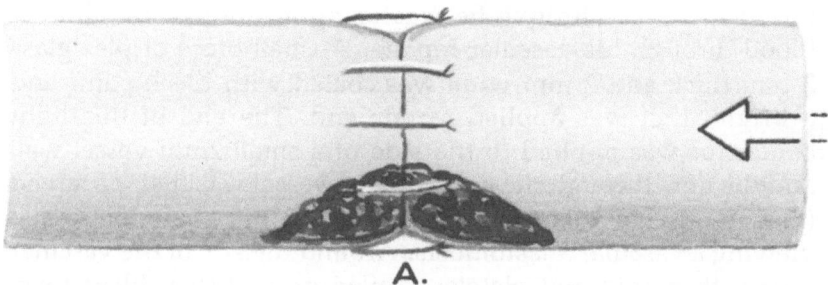

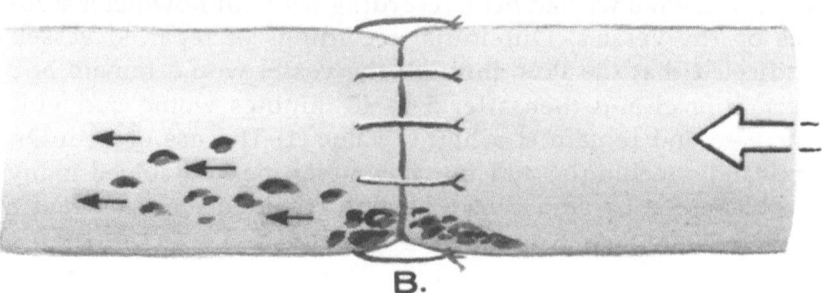

Fig. 16.4. Vessel with side lighting demonstrating the accumulation of clot and platelets around anastomosis site. The "blowing away" of clot and platelets. The cleared vessel after 5 minutes of flow. Direction of flow is indicated by arrows.

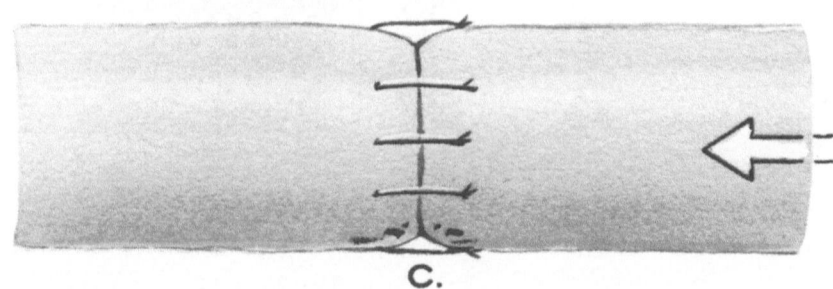

series of interesting events that explained, at least visually, some of the processes we were observing with our flowmeter. Several of these sketches are presented here with explanations that we arrived at using both techniques.

These methods led to the following suggestions that we passed on to the students. Forceful manipulations of the vessel wall with forceps often resulted in intimal injury. This led to both early and late occlusion of the anastomosis, which is probably related to an injury potential of the vessel wall which does not permit the accumulated clot of fibrin and platelets to dissolve and "wash away." The vascular wall must be treated with respect and, if the step phenomenon is observed, a functioning anastomosis will result. If the vessel shows an abnormally low flow value it is worthwhile to go back and modify the anastomosis, because in many of the vessels reoperated upon, the lumen remained open and the vessel continued to function. A

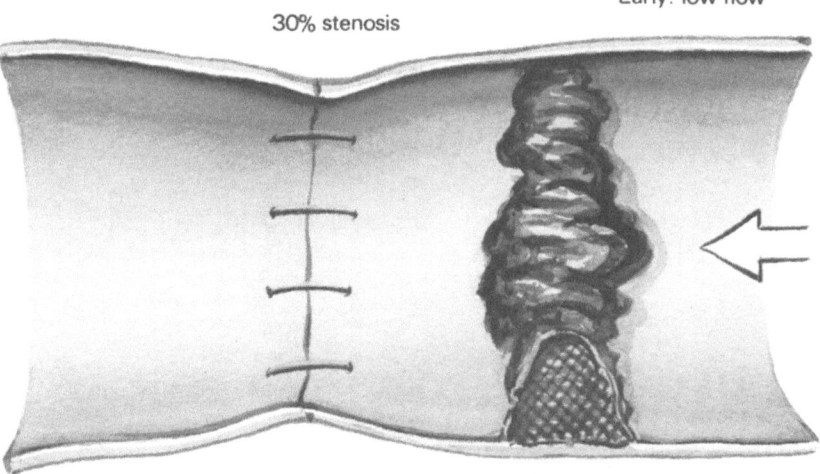

Fig. 16.5. Stenotic vessel with early low blood flow that later progressed to total occlusion. Injury to the vessel wall is also apparent.

A.

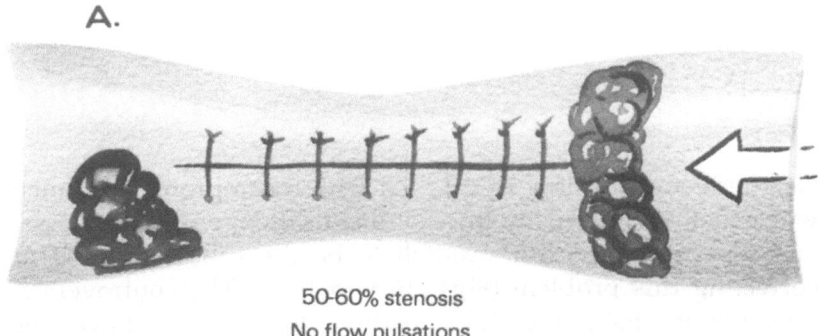

50-60% stenosis
No flow pulsations

Fig. 16.6. Vessel with 50% stenosis that had pulsations but no blood flow. Side lighting demonstrates accumulation of clot within the lumen.

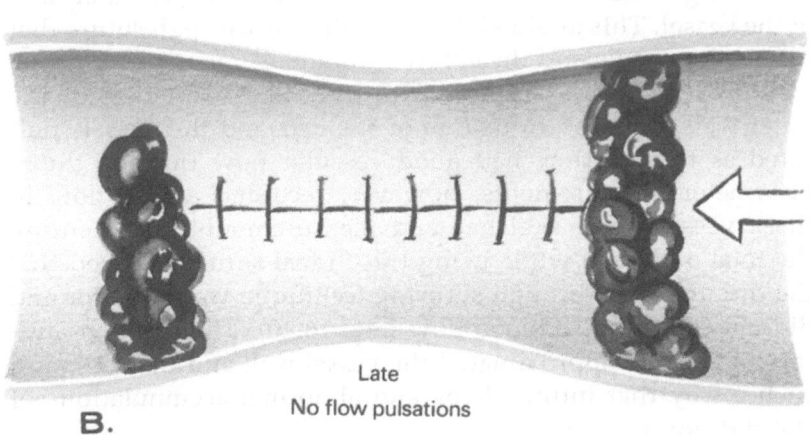

Late
No flow pulsations

B.

Electromagnetic Blood Flowmetry Findings and Applications

A.

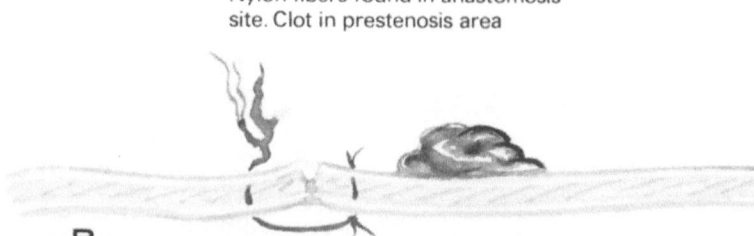

Fig. 16.7. End to end anastomosis demonstrating fibers sewn into the site of anastomosis. This vessel progressed to total occlusion with accumulation of clot at the site of anastomosis.

Sutures frayed

End-to-end 20% stenosis
Late occlusion

Nylon fibers found in anastomosis site. Clot in prestenosis area

B.

30% reduction in flow in a vessel with a compromised lumen was usually followed by total occlusion. Reopening the vessel and repairing the error was felt to be the proper method of correcting this problem (Figs. 16.4 to 16.9). The controversial question of what is the "ideal method" to suture 2-mm vessels was answered through the use of the blood flowmeter. Several of our students and many of our more experienced surgeons felt that the best method to suture these small vessels without producing a stenosis was to approximate only the outer wall of the vessel. This avoided the through-and-through suture that placed the needle and the suture through all layers of the vessel wall. Those vessels sutured with only approximation of the outer wall appeared to be free of stenosis and the vessels pulsated as though they had good vascular flow through them. Flowmeter measurements, however, recorded a zero flow in these vessels. The sketches and measurements documenting the total occlusion while using this "ideal suture" proved that the through-and-through suturing technique was superior and did not compromise blood flow (Fig. 16.10). The through-and-through suture approximated the vessel wall and the intima in such a way that intimal flaps and abnormal accumulations of clot did not develop.

Chapter 16: Electromagnetic Blood Flowmetry in Microvascular Anastomosis

Use of the flowmeter also determined the ideal number of sutures required to safely close a 2-mm vessel with little chance for injury and good postoperative blood flow. Six sutures that passed through all layers of the vessel wall parallel to the flow of blood were found to be adequate to complete a good and suitable anastomosis. After many more anastomoses, eight sutures were found to be the ideal number. If more sutures were placed in a 2-mm vessel the chances of compromised blood flow and occlusion were higher than if eight well-placed sutures were used. When this technique was adopted by the students the anastomoses proved successful and did not compromise blood flow. There was no spasm of the vessel wall and the blood clot and platelets could be observed floating away. A reduction of the step effect on blood flow was observed after the usual 5-minute period following reinstitution of flow through the vessel.

The effects of aspirin on microvascular procedures also became relevant and we observed that rats given Liquiprin (liquid

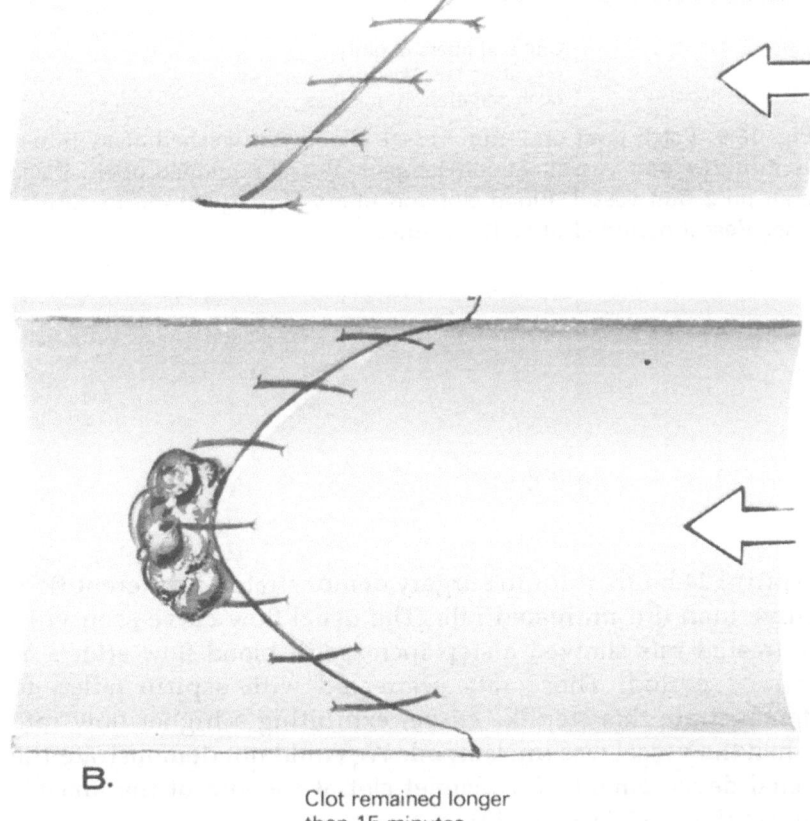

A. Beveled anastomosis

B. Clot remained longer than 15 minutes

Fig. 16.8. Anastomosis of 45° demonstrating accumulation of localized clot that reduced blood flow through the vessel.

A.

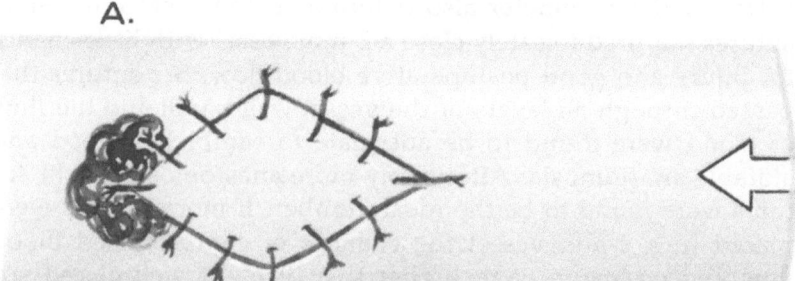

Clot washed away
after 5-10 minutes

B.

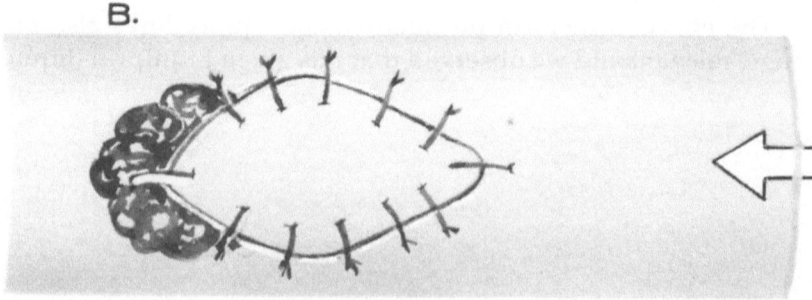

Clot and fibers of patty
on suture line. Vessel
occluded after 10 minutes

Fig. 16.9. Patch graft on 2-mm vessel. Blood clot washed away 5 to 10 minutes after vessel was unclamped. Vessel remained open. Patch graft on 2-mm vessel. Blood clot and fibers of patty affixed to suture line. Vessel occluded after 10 minutes.

aspirin) 24 hours prior to surgery demonstrated a different flow curve than did untreated rats. The usual flow curve seen with untreated rats showed a step increase in blood flow after a 5-minute period. Those rats pretreated with aspirin failed to demonstrate this steplike curve, exhibiting a higher flow rate when the vessel was unclamped. We could not demonstrate the usual development of a platelet clot at the site of the anastomosis (Figs. 16.11 to 16.13).

Fig. 16.10. Two-mm vessel cut lengthwise showing the adventitia and intima. The intima is joined only at the through-and-through suture. Two-mm vessel cut lengthwise showing the adventitia and the "ideal" suture holding only the adventitia and not joining the intima. This vessel had no narrowing and measured 2 mm after the suture line was completed. It was totally occluded and clot remained on the suture line.

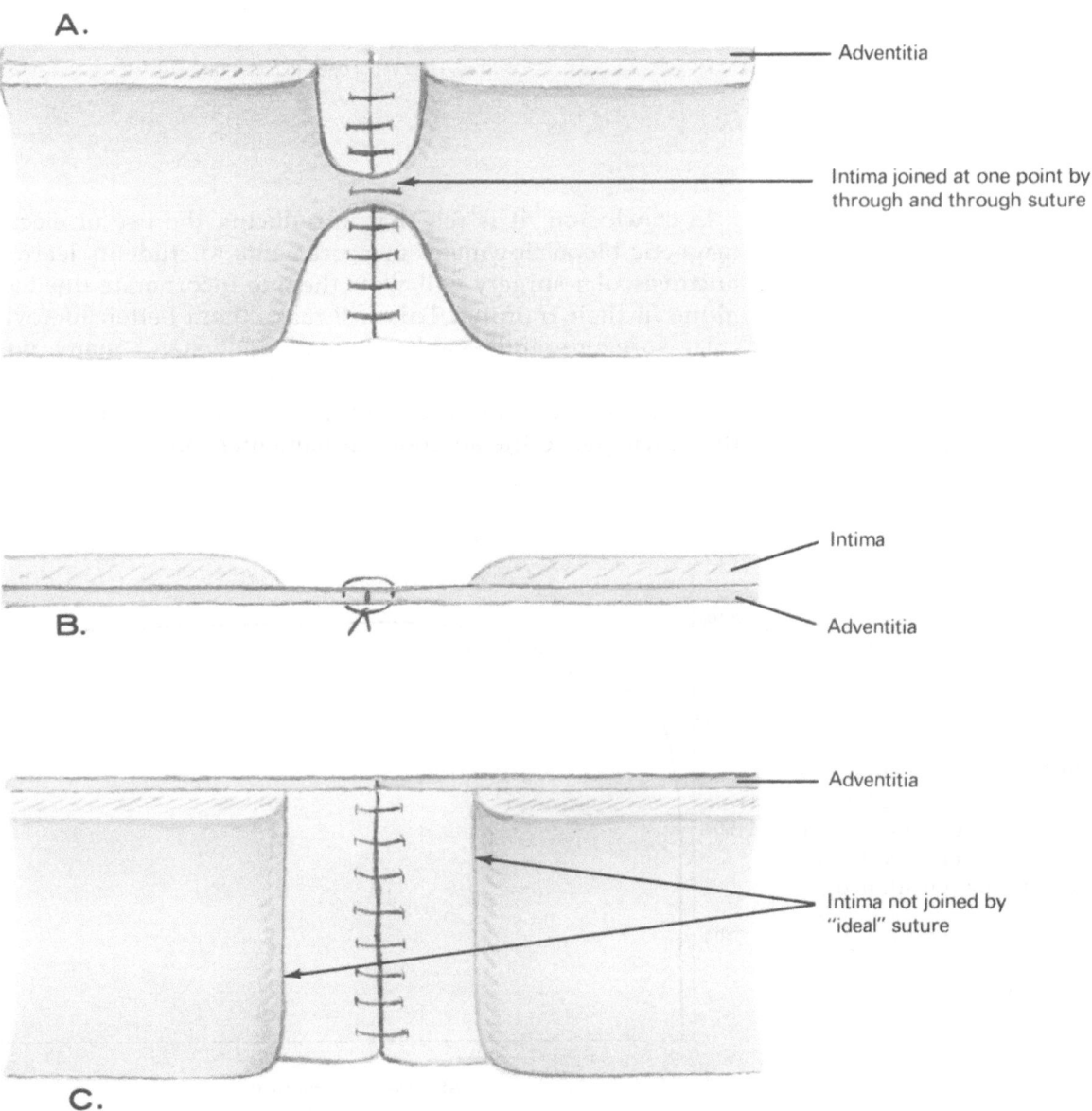

A.

Adventitia

Intima joined at one point by through and through suture

Intima

B.

Adventitia

Adventitia

Intima not joined by "ideal" suture

C.

Electromagnetic Blood Flowmetry Findings and Applications

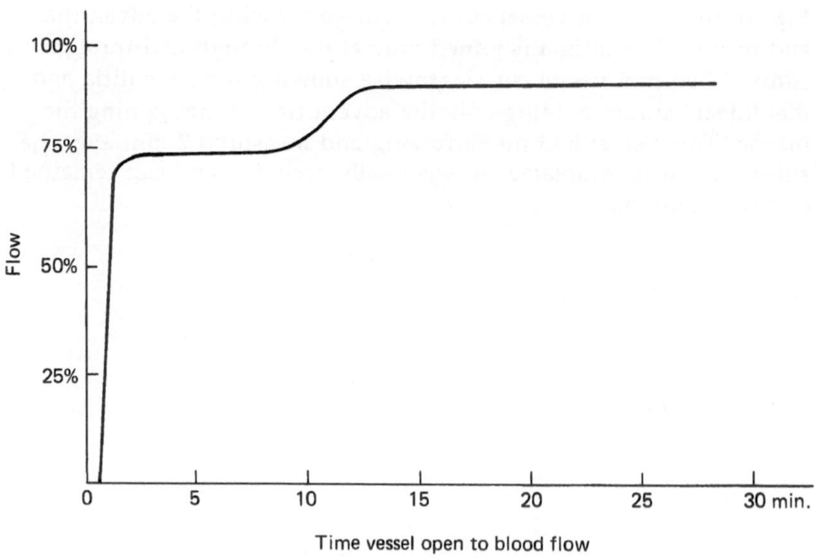

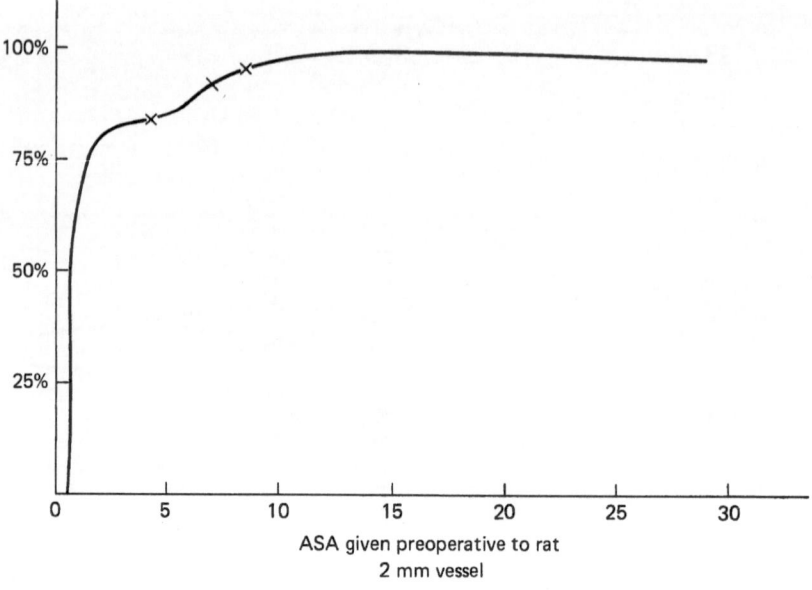

Fig. 16.11. Flow through a 2-mm vessel of rat *not* pretreated with aspirin. Zero indicates the time the clamp was removed from the vessel and flow reinstituted.

In conclusion, it is felt that introducing the use of electromagnetic blood flowmeter measurements to students learning microvascular surgery will allow them to incorporate this technique in their training. This will make them better microvascular surgeons and enable them to understand many postoperative vascular phenomena. Laboratories teaching the techniques of microvascular surgery should consider adding the flowmeter to the students' armamentarium.

Fig. 16.12. Flow through a 2-mm vessel of a rat pretreated with aspirin. Zero indicates the time the clamp was removed from the vessel and flow reinstituted.

Chapter 16: Electromagnetic Blood Flowmetry in Microvascular Anastomosis

192

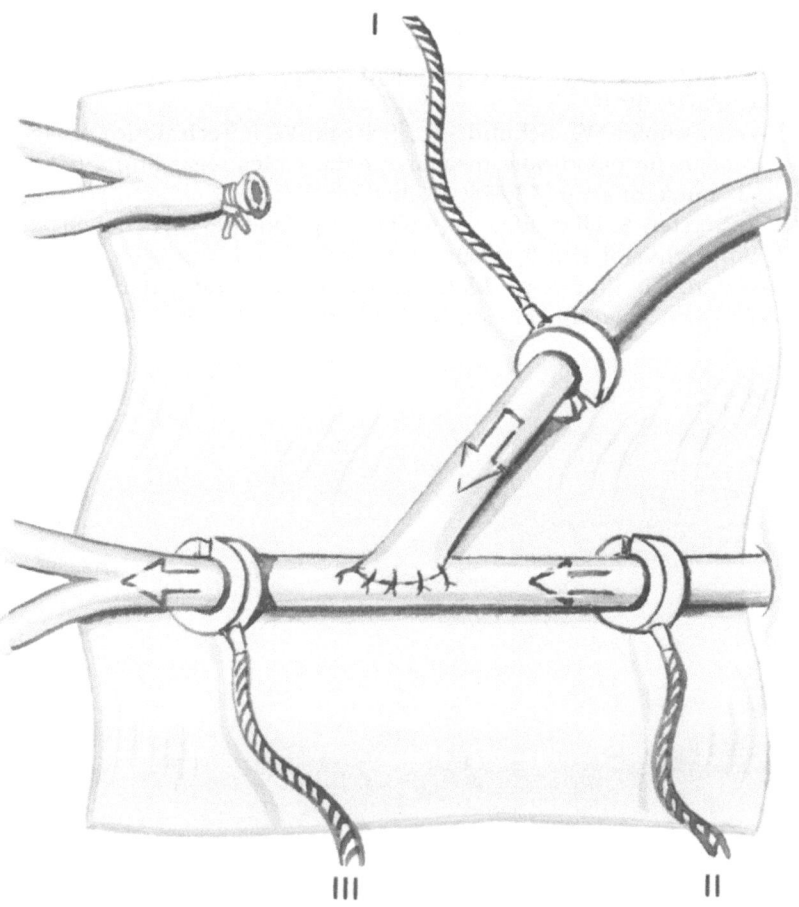

Fig. 16.13. The first teaching model for measuring blood flow through a 2-mm cross-over anastomosis. The left common carotid artery is anastomosed at a 45° angle to the right common carotid artery. Three probes are shown attached to the vessels. Probe I measures blood flow through the left common carotid artery; probe II measures blood flow through the right common carotid artery; and probe III measures blood flow through the right common carotid artery distal to the anastomosis. The student can use this rat model in the laboratory to perfect his technique. He or she will later carry out temporal artery anastomosis to the cortical branch of the middle cerebral artery with recording of blood flow at those points on the vessels that will help determine rate and direction of flow.

REFERENCES

1. Ackland R: The use of side lighting in observing blood flow in small vessels. Personal communication. June 1973
2. Arcilla R, Rowe MI: Modified dye dilution technique for cardiac output studies in tiny subjects. Am Heart J 77(6):798, 1969
3. Cannon JA, Lobpries EL, Herrold G, et al: Experience with a new electro-magnetic flow-meter for use in blood-flow determinations in surgery. Ann Surg 152:635, 1960
4. Conrad WA: Pressure relationships in collapsible tubes. Bio Eng 16(4):284, 1969
5. Denison AB, Spencer MP, Green HD: A square wave electromagnetic flowmeter for application to intact blood vessels. Cir Res 111 (1):39, 1955
6. Engell HC, Lauridsen P; The use of an electromagnetic square wave flowmeter in reconstructive vascular surgery. J Cardiovasc Surg 7:283-8, 1966
7. Kolin A: An electromagnetic flowmeter. Principle of the method and its application to blood flow measurements. Proc Soc Exp Biol Med 35:53, 1936
8. Schenk WG: Methods for measurement of blood flow. Surg Gynecol Obstet 111:103, 1960

9. Spencer MP, Denison AB: Square-wave electromagnetic flow-meters for surgical and experimental applications. Methods Med Res 8:321, 1960

10. Weissenhofer W., Schmidt, R., Schenk, WG: Techniques of electromagnetic blood-flow measurements. Notes regarding a potential source of error. 73:474, 1973

11. Westersten A, Herrold G, Assali NS: A gated sine wave flowmeter. J Appl Physiol 15:533, 1960

12. Wetterer E: Eine neue Methode zur Registrierung der Blutströmungsgeschwindigkeit am uneröffneten Gefäss. Biol 98:26, 1937

17

Brain vascularization
by transplanted omentum

M. Gazi Yasargil, Yasuhiro Yonekawa, and Elsa Pfenninger

The method of autogenous intracranial transplantation of omentum majus in the dog was previously reported.(4) This was originally conceived as an experimental method for treating hydrocephalus. Brain vascularization by transposition of omentum into the subdural space of animals was also reported.(1) Our purpose here is to show that brain vascularization has now also been observed following transplantation of omentum majus on the brain surface itself.

Method and Results

Our technique of omental transplantation using microsurgical methods has already been described (Fig. 17.1). Three dogs in our chronic experimental series had been operated upon 3 months previously.

A selective external angiogram was performed on the operated side. It showed a patent anastomosis (Fig. 17.2). The old craniotomy wound was reopened under general anesthesia and the site of anastomosis was exposed under the operating microscope. The vital transplanted omentum as well as the patency of the anastomosis of the artery and vein were examined. The artery and the vein were severed and the circulation of the transplant was isolated from the systemic circulation. On cutting the artery one could see an abundant arterial backflow. We concluded that there must be some vascular anastomosis of the omentum to the brain surface or the neighboring tissues. Small silastic tubes (0.6 mm in outer diameter) were inserted into the ends of the artery and the vein. Using the method described by Spanner(2) a carbon black solution was injected

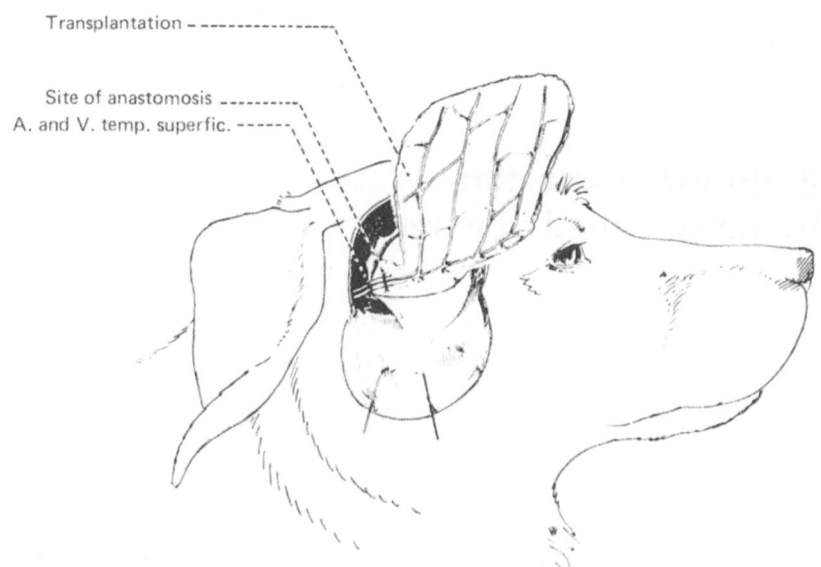

Transplantation

Site of anastomosis
A. and V. temp. superfic.

Fig. 17.1. Illustration of a completed transplantation of omentum majus, which will be placed on the brain surface.

through the tube on the arterial side into the omentum. The omentum turned black and the carbon black flowed out of the venous cannula.

Directly after the injection of carbon black, 0.3 ml/kg T61[1] was given intravenously to sacrifice the dog. The skull near the transplanted omentum was removed and the black stain in the cortical vessels was observed and photographed (Fig. 17.3).

[1]Manufactured by Farbwerke Hochst AG. Frankfurt am Main West Germany. 20% N-[2-(m-methoxy-phenyl)-2-ethyl-butyl-(1)] -2-hydroxy-butylamide; 5% 4,4'-methylene-bis-(cyclohexyl-trimethyl-ammoniumiodide); 0.5% 4'-butylaminobenzoyl-2-dimethylaminoethanol-hydrochloride.

Fig. 17.2. Angiography showing patent anastomosis.

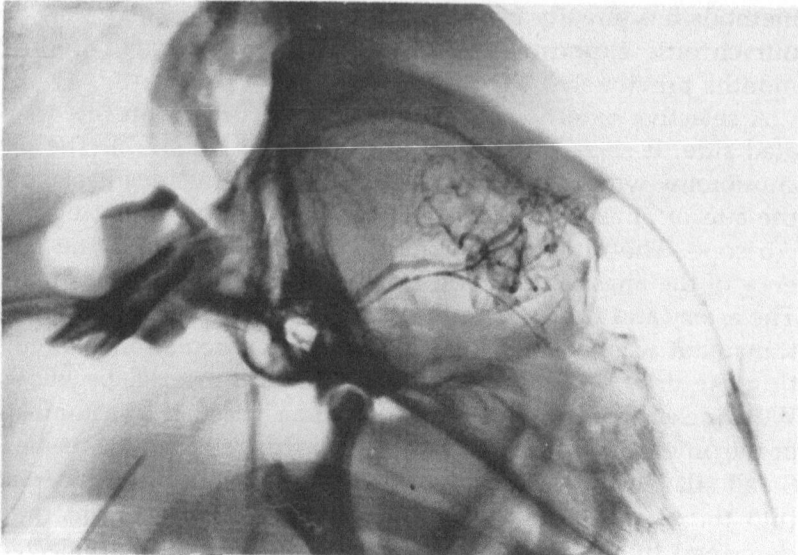

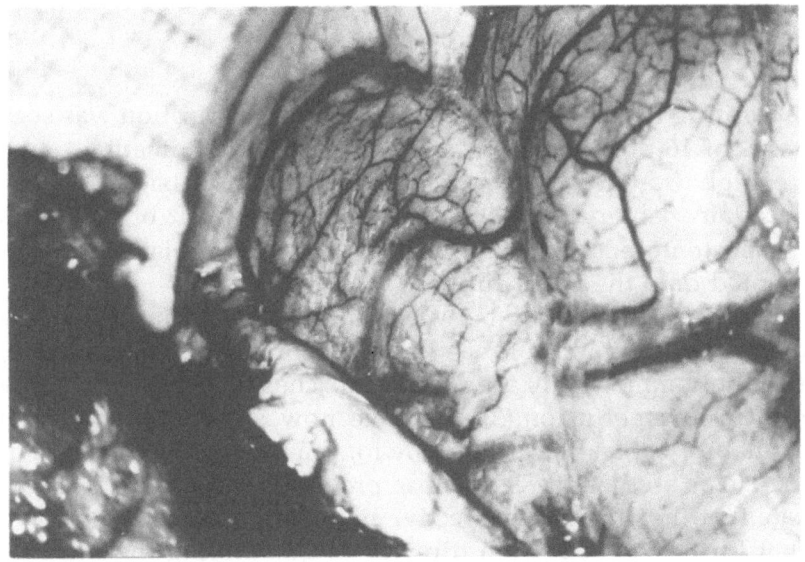

Fig. 17.3. Autopsy photograph. Black staining of cortical vessels. Omentum stained black in the lower left corner.

The staining of the cortical vessels was seen more clearly in the postmortem specimen. The brain with the omentum was fixed in 4% formalin. After adequate fixation, the brain together with omentum was cut. The penetration of dye into the cerebral vasculature was observed not only in cortical vessels but also within white matter (Fig. 17.4).

Histologically, a very vascular membrane (with arachnoid) interposed between the omentum and cortex was noted. The vascular channels of the membrane were connected with the omentum as well as the cortex. Carbon black injected from the omental artery was noted in the capillaries of cortex as well as in white matter (Fig. 17.5).

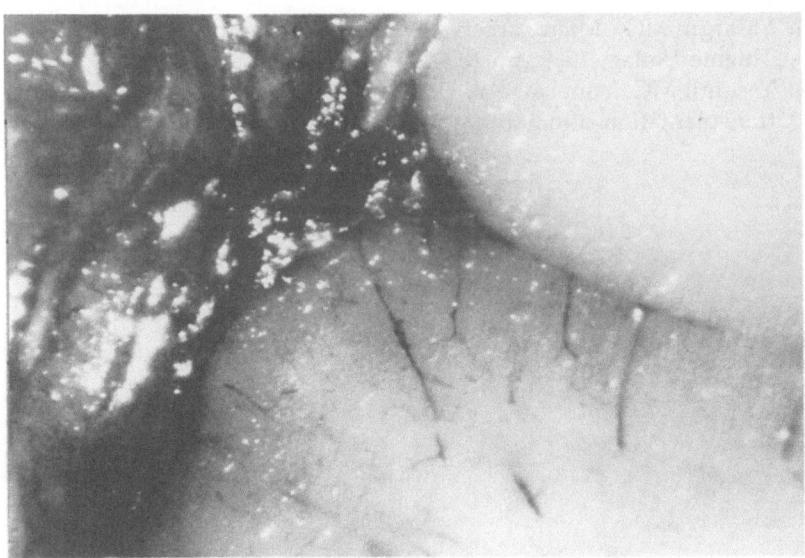

Fig. 17.4. Autopsy photograph. Staining of cortical vessels which penetrate into the white matter. Omentum, left side; brain, right side.

Method and Results

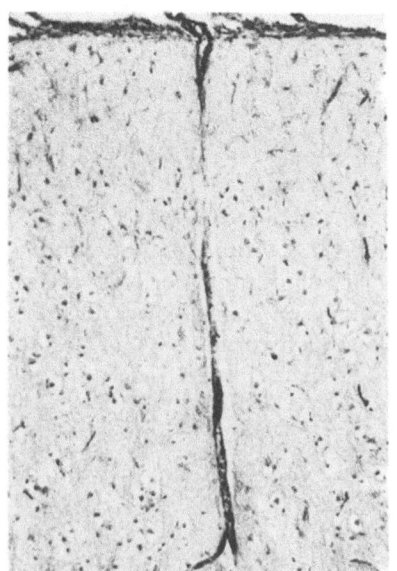

Fig. 17.5. Black staining of capillary that penetrates through the cortex into the white matter.

Discussion

According to Goldsmith et al,(1) brain vascularization was seen in 14 of 16 dogs when his method of pedicled omental transposition was used. This brain vascularization has also been ascertained by our method in which a free graft of omentum is anastomosed with superficial temporal vessels and transplanted onto the brain surface.

The bypass operation between the superficial temporal artery and a cortical branch of the middle cerebral artery is, of course, still the commonest of the new approaches to cerebral ischemia due to low perfusion.(3) We have now shown the potential availability of another procedure for the treatment of this problem. This study as well as those previously reported(1,4) indicate that this method is effective in dogs; however, we believe that further investigation directed at quantifying the increase in local circulation and the potential for generating an epileptic focus is now required.

ACKNOWLEDGMENT

This work is supported by Swiss National Funds No. 4921.

REFERENCES

1. Goldsmith HS, Chen W, Duckett SW: Brain vascularisation by intact omentum. Arch Surg 106:695, 1973
2. Spanner R: Die Entwicklung der Darmzotten der Maus durch Knospung und Spaltung untersucht am Gefassbaum. Morphol Jb 67:235, 1931
3. Yasargil MG: Microsurgery Applied to Neurosurgery. Stuttgart Thieme Verlag, 1969, pp 105–115
4. Yasargil MG, Yonekawa Y, Denton I, et al: Experimental autogenic transplantation of omentum majus. J Neurosurg 39:213, 1974

V

CLINICAL-HEMODYNAMIC
CONSIDERATIONS

18

Augmentation of collateral hemispheric blood pressure following superficial temporal to middle cerebral artery anastomosis: documentation by ocular plethysmography

Norman L. Chater, Philip R. Weinstein, and William Gee

Ocular plethysmography (OPG) is a noninvasive technique that indirectly records systolic and diastolic pressures of the ophthalmic arteries.(1) In patients with total occlusion of the internal carotid artery (ICA) proximal to the origin of the ophthalmic artery, recording of ocular arterial pressure waves may provide an accurate estimate of collateral hemispheric blood pressure (CHBP) distal to the carotid occlusion. OPG was thus considered potentially valuable for documenting augmentation of CHBP following extra- to intracranical bypass.

The technique's reliability has been established by close correlation of OPG recordings obtained with and without manual common carotid artery compression preoperatively with direct intraarterial measurements obtained before and after carotid clamping during endarterectomy for stenotic or ulcerating lesions at the bifurcation. In such cases, mean CHBP of less than 50 mmHg is considered to be an indication for intraoperative shunting; pressures of less than 60 mmHg may be associated with transient ischemic attacks.

Case Report

A 58-year-old right-handed male had a history of acute onset of left hemiplegia 10 years previously from which he recovered. He presented with progressive but fluctuating weakness and clumsiness of the left upper extremity, transient episodes of spatial disorientation, and mild confusion. Arteriogams showed total occlusion of the right ICA with poor collateral filling of right middle cerebral artery (MCA) from the left carotid injection.

Fig. 18.1. Upper left: Preoperative carotid arteriogram showing occlusion of the right ICA and 2-mm diameter of the temporal artery. Upper right: Preoperative OPG tracing showing right eye pressure of 60 mmHg. Lower left: Postoperative OPG tracing showing pressure of 76 mmHg. Lower right: Postoperative arteriogram showing middle cerebral filling through a patent temporal artery bypass.

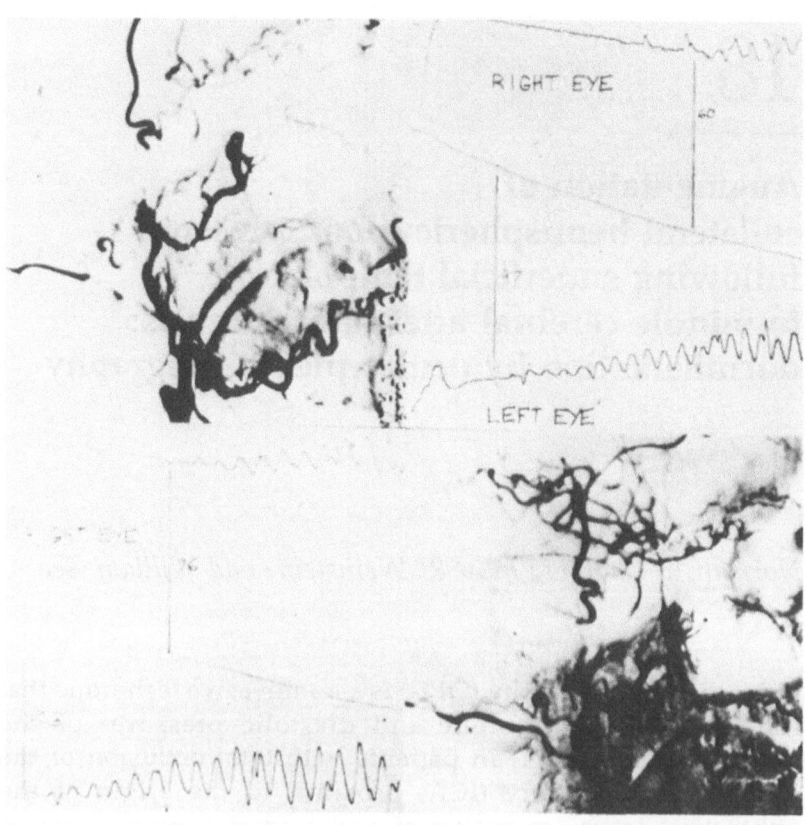

Preoperative OPG recordings showed mean pressures of 60 mmHg in the right eye and 97 mmHg in the left; systemic blood pressure was 135/80. A right superficial temporal to MCA bypass was accomplished; the patient's left arm apraxia resolved completely and his mentation improved. A postoperative arteriogram showed patent anastomosis with good filling of the distal MCA complex as well as enlargement of the superficial temporal artery (STA).

Six weeks postoperatively, his systemic blood pressure was unchanged, and OPG showed mean pressures of 76 mmHg on the right and 103 mmHg on the left, suggesting significant improvement in CHBP (Fig. 18.1). Although the slight increase shown on the left side is not as impressive as that on the right, one can hypothesize that it is related to decrease in demand for collateral flow from left to right through the circle of Willis.

One year postoperatively, the patient remained asymptomatic with the bypass patent by auscultation with a Doppler ultrasonic flowmeter. Repeat OPG determinations showed further increase in pressure on the right to a mean pressure of 95 mmHg, for an ultimate gain of over 50% with systemic blood pressure of 180/90. After the STA was manually compressed, ocular pressure dropped to 84 mmHg, confirming that CHBP was augmented through the bypass.

Conclusion

Collateral hemispheric blood pressure distal to a thrombosed internal carotid artery was improved, as measured by ocular plethysmography before and after STA-MCA bypass. Ocular pressure could be reduced transiently by compression of the STA graft. OPG may provide a useful noninvasive technique for establishing a need for microsurgical collateral augmentation procedures in patients with carotid occlusions, as well as for documenting function of the bypass postoperatively.

REFERENCE

1. Gee W, Mehigan JT, Wylie J: Measurement of collateral cerebral hemispheric blood pressure by ocular pneumoplethysmography. Am J Surg 130:121, 1975

19

Regional cerebral blood flow studies following superficial temporal–middle cerebral artery anastomosis

M. P. Heilbrun, O. H. Reichman,
R. E. Anderson, T. S. Roberts, and C. B. Powell

Introduction

Collateral circulation to the brain through anastomosis of branches of the superficial temporal artery to branches of the middle cerebral artery may remain open for long periods of time and may also enlarge with time.(3) Cerebral blood flow studies, performed to determine if this technique is of value in choosing which patients might benefit from the procedure and also to assess the value of the procedure in providing increased collateral circulation, have been reported by Schmiedek,(4) Austin,(1) and others.(6)

We have assessed the value of regional cerebral blood flow studies (rCBF) in patients undergoing STA-MCA anastomosis by measuring rCBF by the xenon clearance method during the postoperative period. The Xenon bolus was injected selectively through both the normal internal carotid input, when available, and the newly established superficial temporal input. We have combined our results with evaluation of the surgical procedure in terms of clinical and angiographic data. In this presentation, we have first considered whether the focal failure of cerebral circulation that is the cause of transient ischemic attacks (TIAs) and reversible ischemic neurologic deficits (RINDs) is due to hemodynamic causes or emboli. Skinhoj and his group have shown that patients with typical TIAs have no significant change in flow or loss of autoregulation, whereas patients with completed strokes have both focal and global flow abnormalities with evidence of loss of autoregulation and changes in CO_2 reactivity.(5) If the patients that we studied, with TIAs and RINDs, show significant changes in flow, then one might have evidence that the attacks are more often due to hemodynamic causes rather than emboli.

We next considered whether analysis of the postoperative studies alone could provide the information we were seeking. Since the internal carotid flow value represents the pathologic input channel, and the superficial temporal flow represents the newly established input channel, we concluded that use of the postoperative study alone for analysis is valid but not optimal. The xenon bolus injection method used in this study has been described(2) except for the following modifications. Rather than percutaneous catheterization of the internal and external carotid arteries in the neck, all of the studies were performed by the transfemoral method. A small-diameter polyethylene catheter was used to catheterize selectively the internal carotid artery and the external carotid artery just below the origin of the superficial temporal artery. Angiography was performed prior to the flow study, with approximately a 15-minute interval between each injection. All of the studies were performed at the University of Utah Medical Center, at an altitude of 5000 feet. Normal $rCBF_i$ (initial) values for this altitude were calculated from five patients undergoing angiography for evaluation of possible neurologic disease. The mean $rCBF_i$ for this group of patients, which we have considered normal, was 45.7 ml/100 g/minute at a mean Pco_2 of 28.6 mmHg.

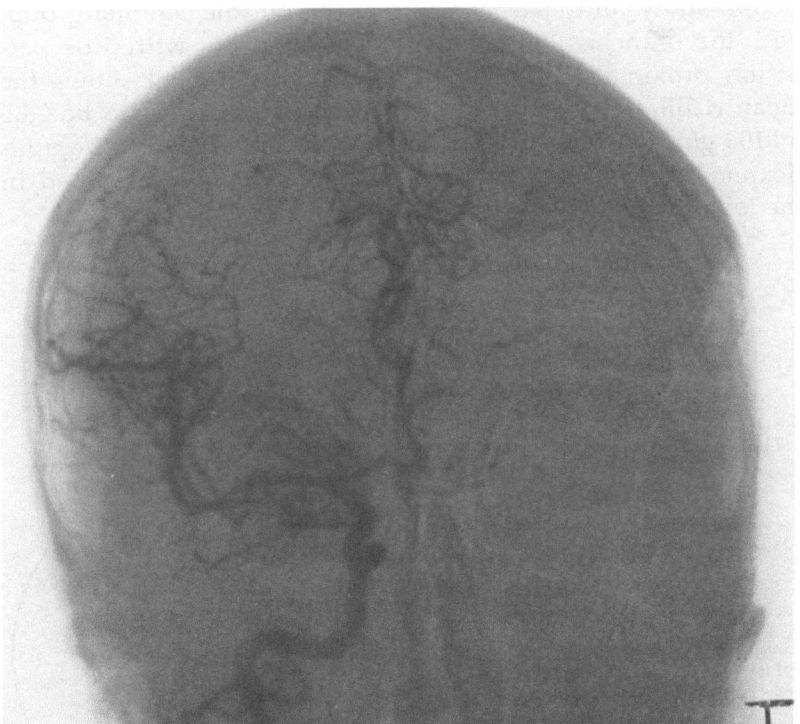

Fig. 19.1. Angiogram of contralateral side of patient with complete resolution of TIA's.

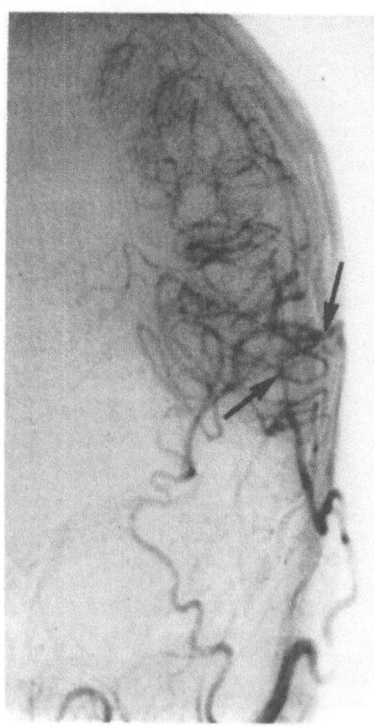

Fig. 19.2. Postoperative film of ipsilateral side with filling of whole middle group (arrows).

Results

Of the six patients with internal carotid artery occlusion, three had TIAs and RINDs and three had completed strokes. At the time of angiography, all patients demonstrated open anastomosis, although there was one late closure due to occlusion of the common carotid artery at the aortic arch. The three patients with TIAs and RINDs had a mean $rCBF_i$ of 28.5 ml/100 g/minute at a Pco_2 of 32 mmHg, while the patients with completed strokes had a mean $rCBF_i$ of 23.6 ml/100 g/minute at Pco_2 of 32 mmHg.

One patient with internal carotid occlusion showed complete resolution of TIAs (Fig. 19.1). The angiogram shows an injection on the contralateral side. Of note, there is little cross-over to the hemisphere through the contralateral anterior cerebral artery, although there is some collateral flow through leptomeningeal anastomoses. Figure 19.2 shows a postoperative film of the ipsilateral side with excellent filling of the whole middle cerebral group. Figure 19.3 shows the 2-minute xenon clearance curves with a mean $rCBF_i$ flow of 37.5 ml/100 g/minute.

The second patient with internal carotid artery occlusion, by contrast, shows good collateral filling coming from the other side, through the anterior cerebral artery as well as the leptomeningeal anastomoses (Fig. 19.4). The superficial temporal injection shows only partial filling of the middle cerebral group, with the branches being perfused distally, but with little perfusion proximally. The flow study in this patient shows the mean $rCBF_i$ through the superficial temporal artery to be 28.5 ml/100 g/minute (Fig. 19.5). The upper curves tend to be multiexponential, rather than monoexponential, as was noted in the lower curves.

INTERNAL CAROTID OCCLUSION—$rCBF_i$ STUDY—EL

Fig. 19.3. Regional cerebral blood flow determined by the 2-min Xenon clearance technique. The patient suffered from TIA's and had an internal carotid artery occlusion.

SUPERFICIAL TEMPORAL FLOW
Mean $rCBF_i$:37.5 ml/100 g/ minute
pCO_2: 43 mmHg

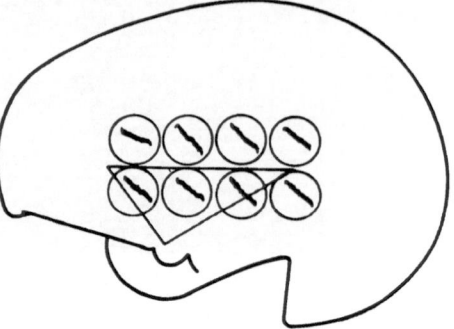

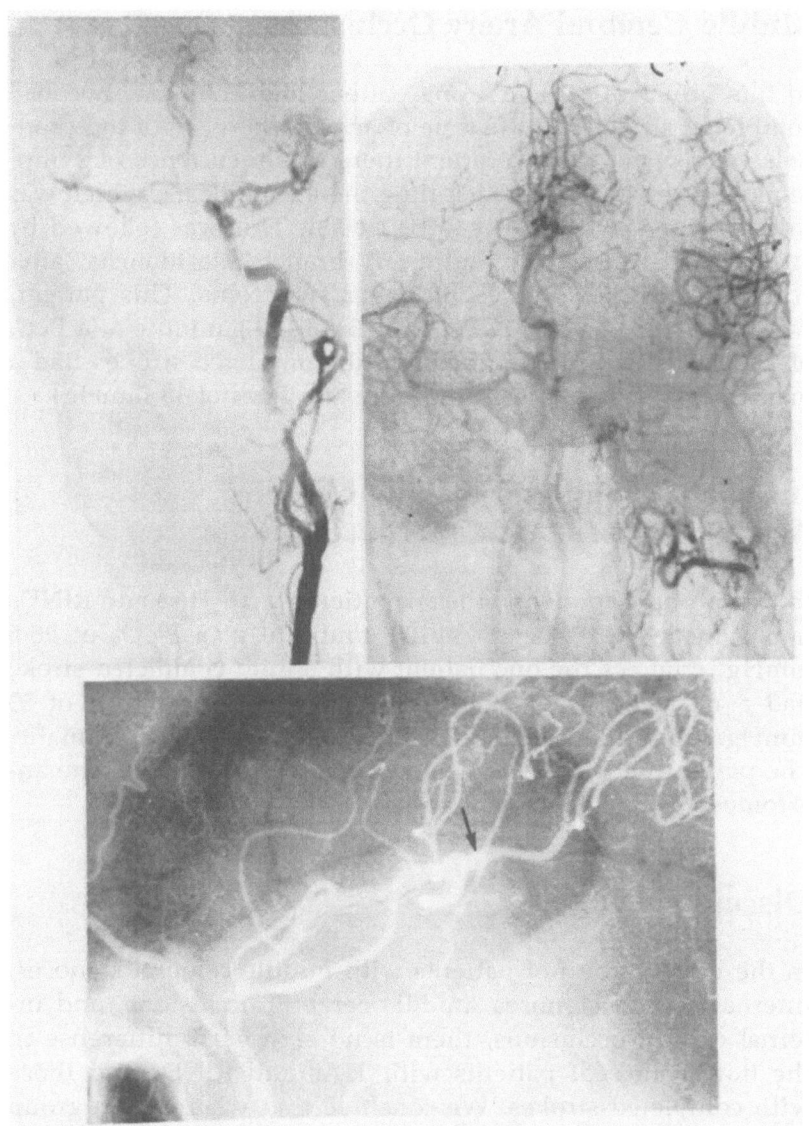

Fig. 19.4. Collateral filling in patient with internal carotid occlusion.

INTERNAL CAROTID OCCLUSION—rCBF$_i$ STUDY—CN

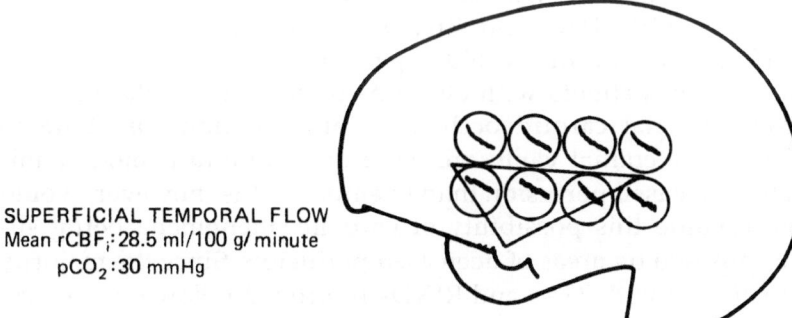

SUPERFICIAL TEMPORAL FLOW
Mean rCBF$_i$: 28.5 ml/100 g/ minute
pCO$_2$: 30 mmHg

Fig. 19.5. Regional cerebral blood flow determined by the 2-min Xenon clearance technique in the second patient.

Results

207

Middle Cerebral Artery Occlusions

In this group of patients, one patient had TIAs and two had completed strokes. At the time of angiography, all of the channels were open. In one patient there was recurrence of symptoms at 17 months, at which time the anastomosis, which was initially open, was shown to be closed. This was followed by an occipital–middle cerebral artery branch anastomosis, after which he had further resolution of symptoms. This patient, who had TIAs, had an $rCBF_i$ of 30.3 ml/100 g/minute at a Pco_2 of 27 mmHg. The two patients with completed strokes had a mean $rCBF_i$ of 26.8 ml/100 g/minute at a Pco_2 of 18 mmHg.

Internal Carotid and Middle Cerebral Artery Stenoses

In this group of patients, the six patients with TIAs and RINDs had a mean $rCBF_i$ of 31 ml/100 g/minute at a PCO_2 of 28.5 mmHg, whereas the one patient with a mild completed stroke had a mean $rCBF_i$ of 25.8 ml/100 g/minute at a PCO_2 of 23 mmHg. All of the TIA and RIND patients were asymptomatic. The patient with the completed stroke was improved. The anastomosis was patent in all patients.

Discussion

In the whole group of patients with middle cerebral stenoses, internal carotid stenoses, middle cerebral occlusions, and internal carotid occlusions, there is no significant difference in the flow values of patients with TIAs and RINDs and those with completed strokes. We conclude that whereas the group of patients studied by Skinhøj, with transient ischemic attacks, had generally normal global flow in comparison with a group of patients with completed strokes with globally decreased flow, we have found globally decreased flow in our whole group of patients, with no significant difference between the patients with TIAs and RINDs and those with completed strokes. This finding would suggest that the symptoms in the majority of patients with all forms of cerebrovascular disease, from internal carotid occlusions or occlusions or stenoses within the cranial vault, are more often due to hemodynamically decreased perfusion than to emboli. This, however, would not exclude this possibility of embolic phenomena being superimposed on areas of decreased perfusion. Since the majority of patients with TIAs and RINDs improved following surgery, this fact suggests that the neurologic deficit was based on low perfusion. This hypothesis will have to be demonstrated.

REFERENCES

1. Austin G, Laffin D, Hayward W: Physiologic factors in the selection of patients for superficial temporal artery to middle cerebral artery anastomosis. Surgery 75:861, 1974
2. Olesen J, Paulson OB, Lassen NA, et al: Regional cerebral blood flow in man determined by the initial slope of the clearance of intraarterially injected ^{133}Xe. Stroke 2:519, 1971
3. Reichman OH, Anderson RE, Roberts TS, et al: The treatment of intracranial occlusive cerebrovascular disease by STA-cortical MCA anastomosis. In Handa H, Handa J (eds): Microneurosurgery. Baltimore, University Park Press, 1975, pp 31–46
4. Schmiedek P, Steinhoff H, Gratzl O, et al: rCBF measurements in patients treated for cerebral ischemia by extra-intracranial vascular anastomosis. Eur Neurol 6:364, 1972
5. Skinhøj E, Høedt-Rasmussen K, Paulson OB, et al: Regional cerebral blood flow and its autoregulation in patients with transient focal cerebral ischemic attacks. Neurology (Minneap) 20:485, 1970
6. Spetzler R, Chater NL: Electromagnetic flow readings during superficial temporal–middle cerebral artery bypass. (in press)

20

Current status of regional cerebral blood flow measurement in revascularization microneurosurgery of the brain[1]

Peter Schmiedek, Harold Steinhoff, and Otmar Gratzl

Treatment of cerebrovascular insufficiency has advanced through introduction of the extracranial-intracranial arterial bypass technique between the superficial temporal artery and a branch of the middle cerebral artery.(1,3,4,14,15) Until now, selection of appropriate candidates as well as assessment of postoperative results have been largely based on clinical criteria and on additional findings obtained from cerebral angiography.(2,10) In previous publications, we have described the preliminary results of pre- and postoperative regional cerebral blood flow studies (rCBF) in patients that underwent extracranial-intracranial bypass surgery for cerebral ischemia.(5,6,11–13) In addition to providing a quantitative increase in cerebral blood flow following bypass surgery, our results have demonstrated that the selection of appropriate candidates could be considerably facilitated by routinely using rCBF studies during the preoperative evaluation of patients. Despite these promising results, it was felt that a more definitive assessment of rCBF studies should await further experience with its application in revascularization microneurosurgery. It is the purpose of this report to give an updated review of the present status of rCBF measurements based on a total of 154 individual pre- and postoperative flow studies in 97 patients.

Methods

Regional cerebral blood flow measurements were performed by the intraarterial ^{133}Xe injection method of Lassen and Ingvar.(7,8) Details of the method and the instrumentation used in the present study have been described in earlier reports. Therefore, only a brief summary of the technique will be given

[1]This study was supported by DFG-Sonderforschungsbereich 51: Medizinische Molekularbiologie und Biochemie.

here and mention will be made of some minor methodologic modifications as used in this laboratory. Following a percutaneous puncture of the common carotid artery, a small Teflon catheter was inserted into the internal carotid artery. Approximately 2 mc of ^{133}Xe dissolved in 3 to 5 ml of saline were injected for each measurement. The clearance of the isotope was externally monitored by 16 small collimated scintillation detectors, mounted in a honeycomblike holder, placed at a right angle to the lateral aspect of the patient's head. Pulses were recorded on magnetic tape for 2 minutes and subsequently graphically displayed on a chart recorder. For calculation of flow values, the initial slope index (ISI) was used.(9) Flow rates were expressed as ml/100 g/minute, with the normal value being 50 ml/100 g/minute ± 10%. All studies were performed in the unanesthetized patients; however, premedication was used 1 hour before the study. Every rCBF study included an arterial sample for Pco_2 determination and measurement of mean arterial blood pressure. The first baseline or control measurement was performed in the resting condition. Carbon dioxide in air (8%) was administered via a face mask 15 to 20 minutes later, and rCBF was measured again. In some cases, preferably those presenting with recent onset of cerebral ischemia, the cerebral autoregulation was tested during a short-lasting period of drug-induced hypertension. Following the completion of the rCBF measurements, the central axes of 3 detector fields were marked with small pieces of lead for later identification on a lateral x-ray of the patient's head. In patients with angiographically demonstrated occlusion of the internal carotid artery and a well-functioning collateral blood supply via the anterior communicating artery, flow measurements were performed over both hemispheres. Postoperatively, in some cases injection of isotope was made selectively into the external carotid artery, thereby allowing assessment of blood flow within the anastomotic brain region.(11)

Clinical Material

The study population consisted of 109 patients admitted to the Department of Neurosurgery with the diagnosis of cerebrovascular insufficiency during the period from January 1970 to May 1974. The mean age of these patients was 50.0 years, with the age range from 19 to 73 years. Seventy-five were men. With only a few exceptions, all patients underwent our routine protocol (including clinical and neurologic examination, cerebral angiography, and rCBF studies) in order to establish the need for a revascularization procedure. According to the history or the presenting clinical symptoms, all cases were divided into four groups. Seventeen patients presented with a history of transient cerebral ischemic attacks (TIA); 23 were classified as having prolonged reversible ischemic neurologic deficits

Table 20.1. rCBF Studies Performed in 97 Patients

	No. of Studies
rCBF Studies in 47 Unoperated Cases	51
rCBF Studies in 50 Patients with Bypass	103

Table 20.2. rCBF Studies Performed in 50 Patients with Bypass

	No. of Patients
Preoperative rCBF	50
Postoperative rCBF	39
Pre- and postoperative rCBF	29
Follow-up rCBF	14

(PRIND); 6 patients had stroke in evolution (SIE); and the remaining 63 cases had completed strokes (CS). In 62 patients an extracranial-intracranial arterial bypass procedure was subsequently performed.

A total of 154 studies were performed on these 109 patients (Table 20.1). Whereas 51 studies were performed on 47 patients that were not operated upon, 103 studies were done in the 50 patients with an extracranial-intracranial arterial bypass (Table 20.2). In the latter group there were 50 preoperative studies, 29 patients were measured pre- and postoperatively, and, in 14 patients, in addition to pre- and postoperative measurements, the study was repeated once more during the later postoperative course.

Results

rCBF Studies in 47 Unoperated Patients

In the majority of cases, ie, in 27 patients, the result of the rCBF study has been critical in the decision not to perform the bypass operation. These patients presented with one of the following rCBF patterns: In seven cases, most of whom had a history of TIAs, a normal CBF was found. In six patients only minor abnormalities of CBF were detected, and therefore these patients were considered to be inappropriate candidates for surgery. Five patients had CBF findings suggestive of acute cerebrovascular insufficiency, such as focal loss of autoregulation or paradoxical flow responses to hypercarbia. Earlier in our series three fatalities followed an extracranial-intracranial bypass operation during the acute phase of cerebral ischemia. We have therefore stopped operating on patients with signs of acute ischemia.(6) In nine patients there was strong evidence of cerebral atherosclerosis. This was reflected in a severe nonfocal reduction in CBF, usually in the range of less than 60%

Table 20.3. Results of Preoperative rCBF Studies in 50 Patients

	No. of Patients
Severe general reduction in CBF	4
Moderate general reduction in CBF	4
Relative focal reduction in CBF	24
Focal reduction in CBF	18

of normal, and a subnormal flow increase when the study was repeated during CO_2 inhalation. In the other 20 patients, which according to our present CBF criteria would have been potential candidates for bypass surgery, other factors were responsible for the decision not to operate. Of particular importance in this regard were complicating medical conditions such as a history of hypertension, coronary heart disease, or diabetes, or considerations of the patient's age.

rCBF Studies in 50 Operated Patients
(Table 20.3)

The corresponding results of rCBF measurement in 50 operated patients were divided into the following groups. Four patients had a severe general reduction (SGR) in CBF. As shown in Figure 20.1, all of these cases were operated on during the early phase of our experience with extracranial-intracranial bypass surgery. In another group of four patients, a moderate general reduction (MGR) in CBF was found, with the hemispheric mean value falling in the range of 60 to 75% of normal. In the remaining 42 patients, the preoperative rCBF measurement revealed either a relative focal reduction (RFR) (24 patients) or only a focal reduction (FR) of flow (18 patients) (Fig. 20.2). The term RFR was applied to cases with a defined area

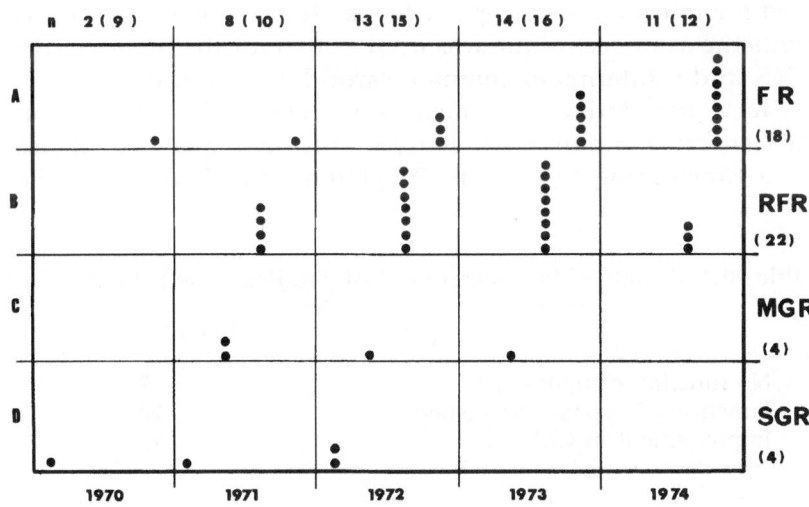

Fig. 20.1. Analysis of preoperative rCBF findings in 48 out of a total of 62 operated cases over a 5-year period. Note that during the last 2 years of this study predominantly patients presenting with FR or RFR have been operated on.

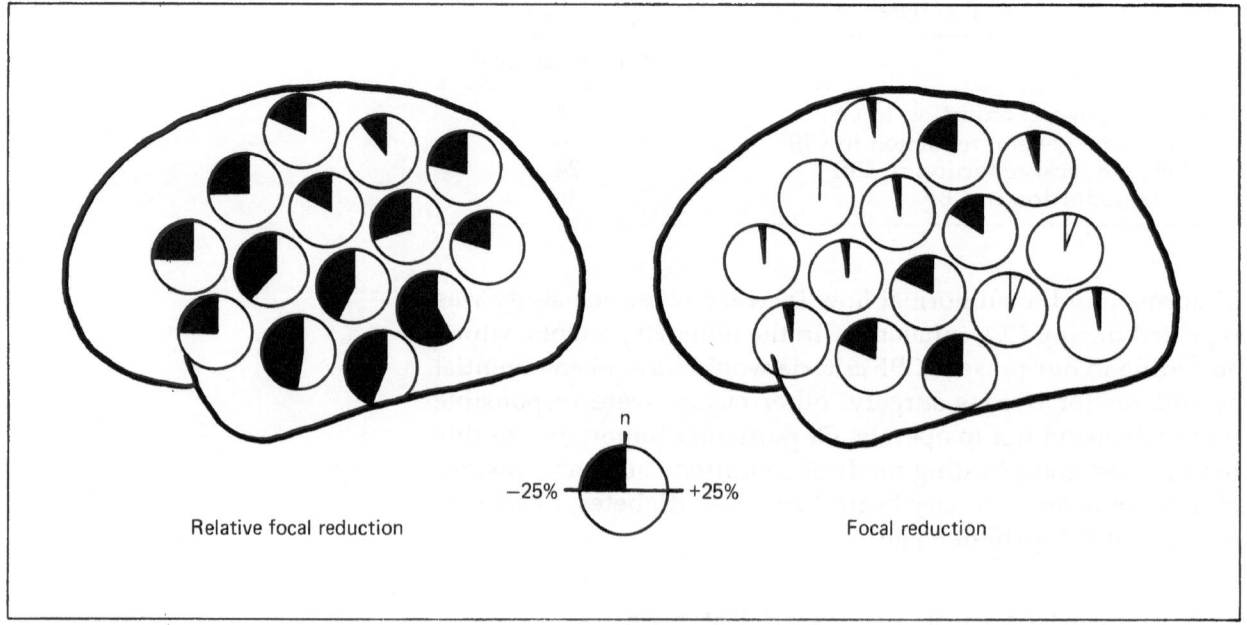

Relative focal reduction

−25% ——⊕—— +25%

Focal reduction

Fig. 20.2. Preoperative rCBF patterns thought to be most suitable for bypass surgery. Left: Relative focal reduction in CBF. In addition to a moderately reduced hemispheric CBF, flow values over the temporal region reveal a more pronounced reduction. Right: Focal reduction in CBF showing reduced flow values over the central region, whereas nonfocal flow values are within normal limits.

of ischemia, associated with nonfocal regions showing only a moderate reduction in CBF. By contrast, FR was characterized by focal ischemia within an otherwise normal CBF pattern. By definition, the focal flow values in RFR or FR were at least 10% lower than flow values in nonfocal areas.

Postoperative rCBF Studies in 39 Patients (Table 20.4)

In 39 patients the function of the extracranial-intracranial bypass was evaluated by postoperative measurement of rCBF. The CBF measurements were done within 1 week following surgery in all except six cases which were studied later in their postoperative course. In 22 patients the external carotid artery was used for injection of isotope, whereas in the remaining 17 patients the same technique was used as that for the preoperative rCBF study (internal or common carotid artery), thus allowing a direct quantitative assessment of the effect of the bypass on the ischemic brain tissue. In two patients there was no evidence for a functioning bypass. In 20 patients the function of the

Table 20.4. Results of Postoperative rCBF Studies in 39 Patients

	No. of Patients
No function of bypass	2
Function of bypass established	20
Improvement in CBF	17

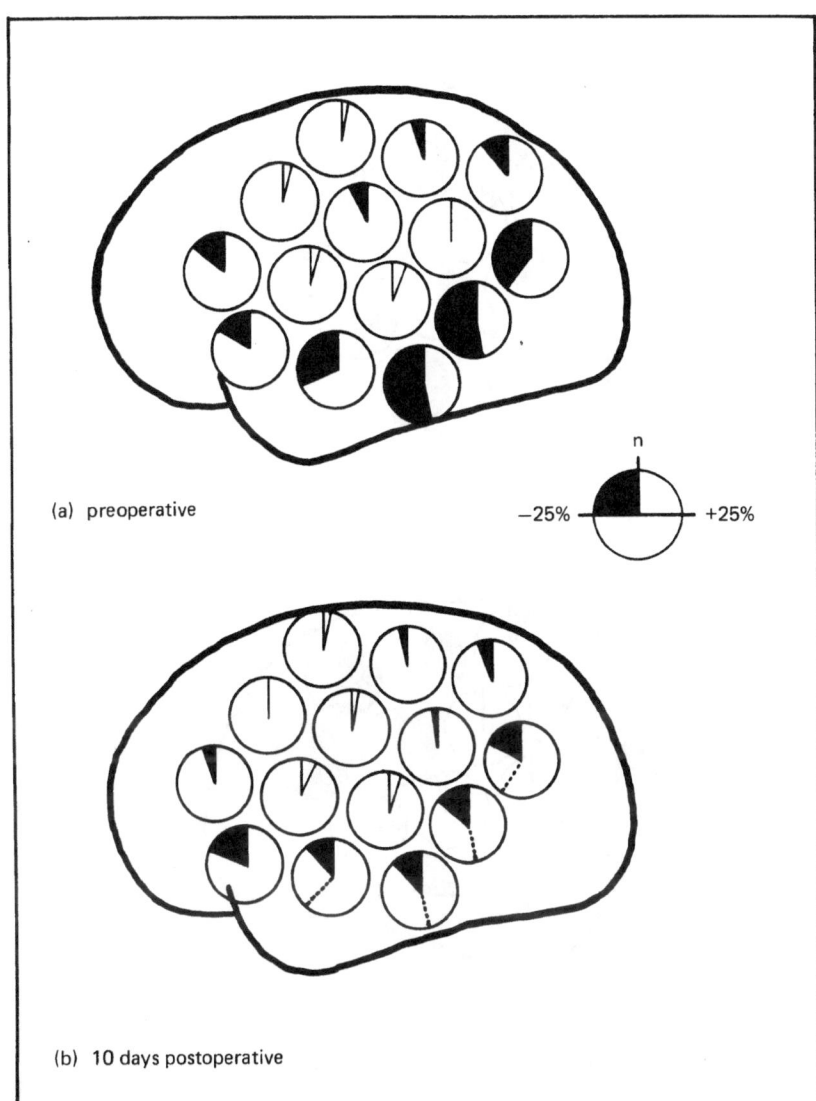

(a) preoperative

n

−25% +25%

(b) 10 days postoperative

Fig. 20.3. Comparison of pre- and early postoperative rCBF studies. Preoperatively, an area of relative ischemia is found over the temporo-parietal region. Ten days postoperatively, there is a significant improvement in rCBF values within the previously ischemic region.

bypass could by established, using criteria which have been discussed previously in greater detail.(11) In an additional 17 patients a comparative analysis of pre- and postoperative rCBF studies indicated improved flow rates postoperatively in brain areas that were shown to have impaired CBF on preoperative flow studies (Fig. 20.3). Positive and negative postoperative rCBF results were confirmed by angiographic findings.

Late Follow-up rCBF Studies in 14 Patients

A repeat postoperative rCBF study was performed in 14 patients 2 to 28 months following the first postoperative study. In three patients a delayed occlusion of the bypass was found.

Fig. 20.4. Comparison of early and late postoperative rCBF studies in a patient with internal carotid artery occlusion. The isotope was injected into the external carotid artery. Analysis of rCBF values shows good evidence of secondary improvement in CBF.

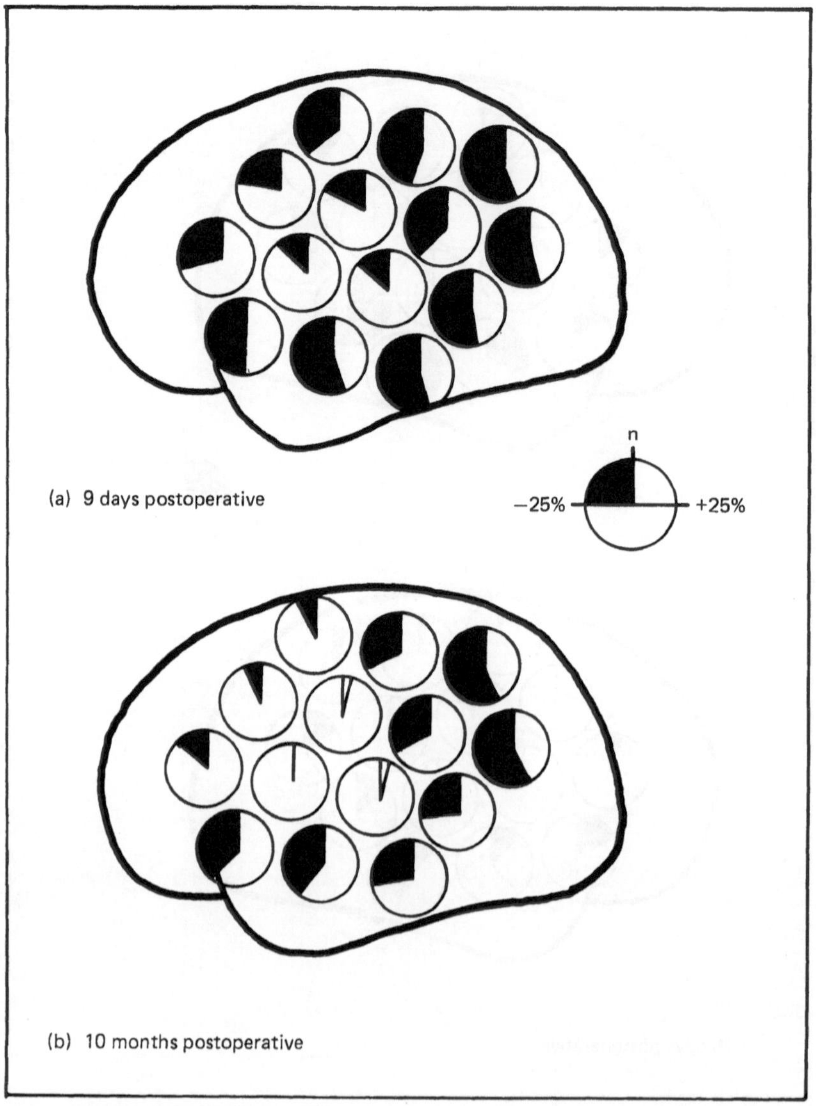

(a) 9 days postoperative

(b) 10 months postoperative

-25% $+25\%$

In six patients the early and late postoperative rCBF studies gave identical results. In five patients, however, a significant secondary improvement in flow values was found when the early and late postoperative rCBF results were compared (Fig. 20.4). The corresponding angiograms in these five patients revealed a marked enlargement in the size of the anastomosis over time.

Comment

It is well known that the natural history of cerebrovascular disease is unpredictable, thus making it difficult to evaluate the effect of any therapeutic measure. Neurologic improvement occurring in patients following bypass surgery is likely to be related to this procedure; however, it may be purely coincidental as well. It should also be emphasized that postoperative cerebral angiography will provide sufficient evidence of bypass patency and information on the function of the anastomosis by showing to what extent the distal cerebral vasculature is perfused via the anastomosis. Angiography, however, primarily demonstrates the vascular morphology but it does not necessarily permit any firm conclusion regarding the functional state of the tissue supplied by these vessels. Because of these limitations, measurement of regional cerebral blood flow was introduced as an adjunct to revascularization microneurosurgery. Initially our main interest was focused on proving that cerebral blood flow would increase quantitatively within those areas of the brain irrigated by the new collateral. Of a total of 39 patients on whom postoperative rCBF studies were performed, the comparative results of pre- and postoperative rCBF studies demonstrated a regional increase in CBF in 17 patients following surgery. In an additional 20 patients only the function of the new bypass could be ascertained. It was not possible to evaluate quantitatively the effect of the anastomosis on postoperative CBF because different methodologic approaches were used during the pre- and postoperative flow studies.

Based on the preoperative rCBF measurements, we tried to establish criteria that would allow one to predict whether a patient might be a good candidate for bypass surgery. A retrospective analysis of rCBF studies in 97 potential candidates for surgery has led us to introduce the following six CBF groups:

1. Patients with severe general reduction in CBF (SGR)
2. Patients with moderate general reduction in CBF (MGR)
3. Patients with relative focal reduction in CBF (RFR)
4. Patients with focal reduction in CBF (FR)
5. Patients with acute disorders of CBF (AD)
6. Patients with normal CBF (N)

It was concluded that only those patients presenting with either relative focal reduction in CBF or those with focal ischemia alone should be considered for extracranial-intracranial bypass surgery. The rationale for this takes into consideration the fact that the microneurosurgical approach to the treatment of cerebral ischemia is actually based on a physiologic principle. It represents an expansion by surgical means of the native collateral circulation naturally occurring in the presence of cerebrovascular occlusive disease. Moreover, the magnitude of surgical augmentation of flow is dependent on flow rates through the extracranial donor vessel. This may improve the blood supply within a limited ischemic area of the brain but should not result in an overall restoration of the generally impaired cerebral circulation. On the other hand, surgery is not indicated in patients presenting with one of the other four CBF patterns. This is supported by the poor postoperative results obtained in patients with acute onset of cerebral ischemia and by hemodynamic considerations in patients with a normal CBF or in those with severe general reduction in CBF resulting from atherosclerosis of brain vessels. It is evident that the indication for bypass surgery should be the result of a complex and careful analysis of the multiple factors involved. There is now accumulating evidence that, apart from the patient's history and his clinical condition, the preoperative rCBF study may well be the most important diagnostic aid for selection of appropriate candidates for bypass surgery.

REFERENCES

1. Austin, GM (ed): Microneurosurgical Anastomoses for Cerebral Ischemia. Springfield, Ill, Thomas, 1976
2. Chater, NL, Spetzler, RF, Mani J: The spectrum of cerebrovascular occlusive disease suitable for microvascular bypass surgery. Angiology 3:235, 1975
3. Donaghy RMP: Patch and bypass in microangeional surgery. In Donaghy RMP, Yasargil MG (eds): Microvascular Surgery. St. Louis, Mosby, 1967, pp 75–86
4. Donaghy RMP: What's new in surgery ? Neurologic surgery. Surg Gynecol Obstet 134:269, 1972
5. Gratzl O, Schmiedek P, Steinhoff H, et al: Quantitative and regional effects of microneurosurgical extra-intracranial vascular anastomosis in patients with cerebral ischemia. Eur Surg Res 6 (Suppl 1):27, 1974
6. Gratzl O, Steude U, Schmiedek P: Indications for extra-intracranial anastomosis between the superficial temporal artery and a branch of the middle cerebral artery in man. In Fusek I, Kunc Z (eds): Present Limits of Neurosurgery. Amsterdam, Excerpta Medica, 1972, pp 375–379
7. Hoedt-Rasmussen K: Regional Cerebral Blood Flow. The Intraarterial Injection Method. Copenhagen, Munksgaard, 1967
8. Lassen NA, Ingvar DH: The blood flow of the cerebral cortex determined by radioactive Krypton 85. Experientia 17:42, 1961
9. Olesen J, Paulson OB, Lassen NA: Regional cerebral blood flow in man determined by the initial slope of the clearance of intraarterially injected ^{133}Xe. Stroke 2:519, 1971
10. Reichman OH: Selection of patients and clinical results following STA–cortical MCA anastomosis. In Austin GM (ed): Microneurosurgical Anastomoses for Cerebral Ischemia. Springfield, Ill, Thomas, 1976, pp 275–280
11. Schmiedek P, Gratzl O, Olteanu V: The contribution of regional cerebral blood flow measurement to the microneurosurgical treatment of cerebral ischemia. In Austin, GM (ed): Microneurosurgical Anastomoses for Cerebral Ischemia. Springfield, Ill, Thomas, 1976, pp 244–255

12. Schmiedek P, Gratzl O, Steinhoff H, et al: Microvascular surgery of the brain and regional cerebral blood flow. In Langfitt TW, et al (eds): Cerebral Circulation and Metabolism. New York, Springer-Verlag, 1975, pp 285–288
13. Schmiedek P, Steinhoff H, Gratzl O, et al: rCBF measurements in patients treated for cerebral ischemia by extra-intracranial vascular anastomosis. Eur Neurol 6:364, 1971
14. Yasargil MG: Experimental small vessel surgery in dog including patching and grafting of cerebral vessels and the formation of extra-intracranial shunts. In Donaghy RMP, Yasargil MG (eds): Microvascular Surgery. St. Louis, Mosby, 1967, pp 87–126
15. Yasargil MG, Krayenbühl H, Jacobson JH: Microneurosurgical arterial reconstruction. Surgery 67:221, 1970

21

Estimation of
flow through STA bypass graft

O. Howard Reichman

Since the description by Donaghy and Yasargil(8), and Yasargil(22) of anastomosis between the superficial temporal artery (STA) and a cortical branch of the middle cerebral artery (MCA), there has been considerable interest in this elegant surgical procedure as a method to increase collateral circulation to the brain. Postoperative arteriography in many patients has demonstrated patency of the STA bypass graft in nearly all instances,(15,16) substantiating that this is a reliable method to develop new collateral circulation. However, a recurring question concerns the capability of this small vascular channel to provide sufficient blood flow for the support of a significant volume of brain tissue. While increased regional cerebral blood flow (rCBF)(2,9,19) is the ultimate goal of additional collateral circulation to the brain, it is essential to know the potential volume of blood flow which exists for an STA bypass graft.

Crowell(7) reported basal STA flow in three patients, measured by simple outflow collection against zero resistance, as 15 to 30 ml/minute. Several authors(1,4,7) have reported electromagnetic flowmetry readings, performed upon completion of STA–cortical MCA anastomosis, as 10 to 60 ml/minute.

Since serial arteriography has demonstrated enlargement (1,5,6,14,17,22) of the STA bypass graft in most patients and since Poiseuille's law(6) for flow in hollow tubes states that flow is directly proportional to the fourth power of the radius, it has been presumed that flow through an STA bypass graft increases beyond that measurable at the time of surgery. Therefore, a pressing need has existed for a nonsurgical method to measure flow through an STA bypass graft subsequent to the surgical procedure. An arteriographic method has been developed to determine flow through an STA bypass graft at the

Table 21.1. Calculations

$$\text{Flow} = \frac{\text{Volume}}{\text{Time}}$$

$$\text{Volume} = \pi R^2 L$$

$$R_{mag} = 1.65 \text{ mm}; \; L_{mag} = 155 \text{ mm}$$

Magnification factor:

$$\frac{45}{76} = 0.592$$

Corrected for magnification:

$$R = 0.98 \text{ mm}; \; L = 91.8 \text{ mm}$$

$$\text{Volume} = \pi (0.98 \text{ mm})^2 (91.8 \text{ mm})$$
$$= 277 \text{ mm}^3$$

$$\text{Time} = \frac{\text{\# of Frames Counted}}{\text{\# of Frames/Second}}$$

$$= \frac{17}{64}$$

$$= .266 \text{ Seconds}$$

$$\text{Flow} = \frac{\text{Volume}}{\text{Time}} = \frac{277 \text{ mm}^3}{0.266 \text{ sec}}$$

$$= 1040 \text{ mm}^3/\text{sec}$$

$$= 1040 \text{ mm}^3/\text{sec} \left(\frac{60 \text{ sec}}{\text{min}} \right) \left(\frac{\text{cc}}{1000 \text{ mm}^3} \right)$$

$$= 62 \text{ cc/min}$$

time of arteriography. This method is described, results in 20 patients are reported and compared with arteriography, and the significance of these findings is discussed in relation to other types of information concerning cerebral blood flow.

Methods

The method involved calculating the ratio produced by dividing the volume of blood contained in a cylindrical segment of superficial temporal artery by the time required for the column of blood to move from one end to the other end of the arterial segment (Table 21.1).

The formula for calculating the volume of a cylinder has been defined as follows:

$$\text{Volume} = \pi R^2 L$$

During selective external carotid arteriography with the catheter tip carefully positioned high in the external carotid artery, a magnification film from the early arterial phase was used to measure dimensions of the segment of STA (Fig. 21.1, above). R_{mag} (radius as measured with a magnification film) was one-half the diameter of the STA, measured at a position representing the average STA diameter. L_{mag} (length of the arterial segment as measured with a magnification film) was obtained

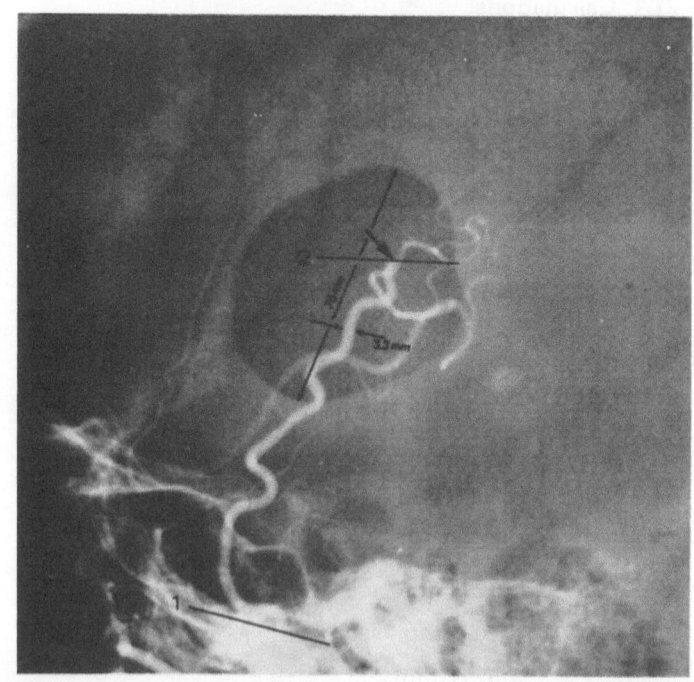

Fig. 21.1. Case 38. Method of determining flow. *Above:* Early magnification film from selective external carotid arteriogram. Site of STA–cortical MCA anastomosis is indicated by heavy arrow. Measured segment of STA lies between line 1 and line 2. Diameter of STA measured 3.3 mm (R_{mag} = 1.65 mm). Diameter of craniectomy measured 76 mm. Below: Unmagnified film obtained with craniectomy placed adjacent to x-ray cassette and focal spot of x-ray tube at a distance of 72 inches from film. Same diameter of craniectomy measured 45 mm on unmagnified film. Magnification factor: 45/76 = 0.592.

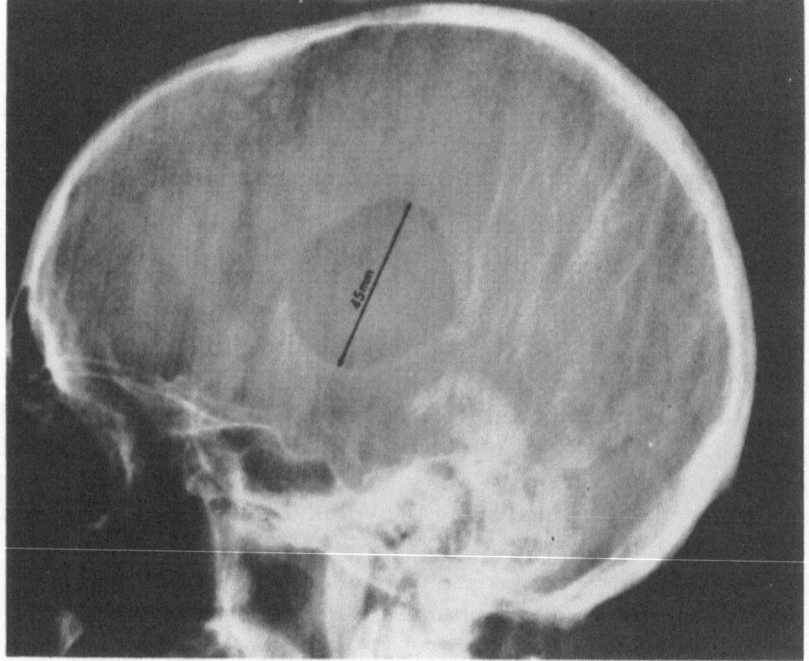

by tracing the segment of STA on a piece of translucent paper (Fig. 21.2) and conforming a piece of malleable wire (electricians' solder) to the exact contour of the artery, after which the wire was cut to exact length, carefully straightened, and measured. Correction for magnification was accomplished by multiplying the measured values by a magnification factor. The magnification factor was derived from the ratio produced by dividing a measured diameter of the craniectomy on a film placed 72 inches from the focal spot of the x-ray tube with the craniectomy adjacent to the film (Fig. 21.1, below), by the same diameter as measured on the magnification film (Fig. 21.1, above). The value of R (actual radius) was obtained by multiplication of R_{mag} by the magnification factor. The value for L (actual length) was obtained by multiplication of L_{mag} by the magnification factor. These values were then substituted into the formula and the volume of blood in the cylinder calculated as shown by the example of Case 38 in Table 21.1.

Time was determined utilizing cinearteriography (at a calibrated rate of 64 frames/second). The number of frames required for movement of the leading edge of contrast material through the STA segment (Fig. 21.3) was divided by 64 frames/second to obtain the actual time required for the volume of blood contained within the cylinder to pass through the STA segment.

Having values for volume and time, flow was calculated and converted into appropriate units to express blood flow through the STA bypass graft.

Results

Figures 21.4 to 21.24 document the STA bypass graft flow as determined in each of the first 20 patients that were studied by this method with its accompanying arteriogram. This ma-

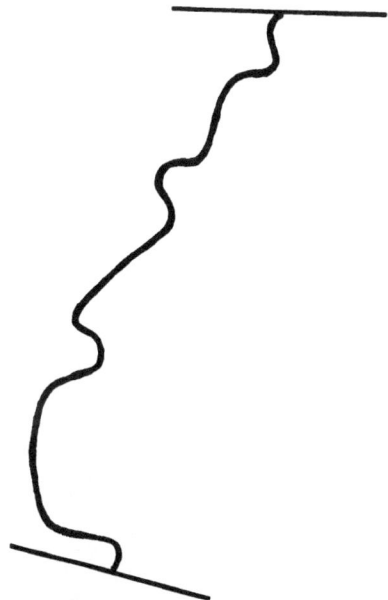

Fig. 21.2. Case 38. Method of determining flow. Segment of STA traced on translucent paper for measurement of length. A piece of malleable wire (electricians' solder) was conformed to the contour of STA, cut to exact length, carefully straightened, and measured (L_{mag} = 155 mm).

Table 21.2. Estimation of STA Flow

Case no.	cc/min	Weeks after surgery
31	50	25
33	44	29
36	160	24
38	62	7
39	77	61
40L	110	28
42	47	45
43	28	25
44	130	14
46	48	27
49	42	29
50	39	68
54	82	24
55	120	55
64	53	56
68	62	29
69	39	28
72	120	26
78	170	25
82	240	17
Average	86	32

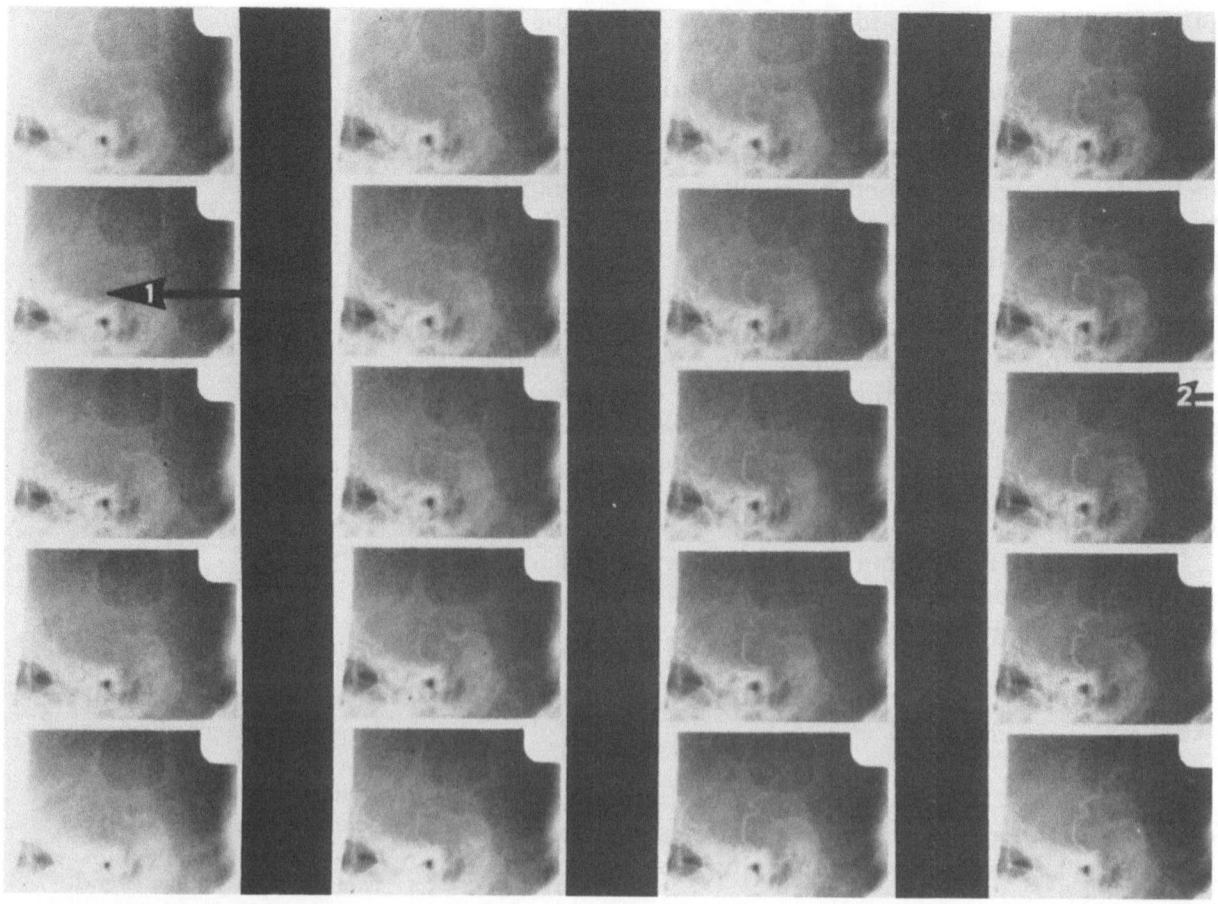

Fig. 21.3. Case 38. Method of determining flow. Cinearteriography exposed at 64 frames/second. Arrow 1 points to the leading edge of contrast material as it entered the STA segment. Arrow 2 indicates that the leading edge of contrast material has reached the distal end of STA segment. The transit time for passage of the volume of blood contained within the cylindrical arterial segment was derived as the number of frames between arrows 1 and 2 divided by 64: 17/64 = 0.266 seconds.

terial is summarized in Table 21.2, which includes the number of each case as it relates to the total series, the flow determination, and the duration in weeks between surgery and the arteriographic study (average, 32 weeks). Flows ranged between 28 and 240 ml/minute with an average of 86 ml/minute. The calculated flow generally correlated directly with the extent of perfusion demonstrated by arteriography. The lowest flow of 28 ml/minute with filling of the operculofrontal artery occurred in the presence of a recanalized internal carotid artery (ICA) occlusion in Case 43 (Fig. 21.11). Patients with flow determinations in the range of 30 to 50 ml/minute filled a single major division (ascending frontal complex, posterior parietal, angular, or posterior temporal)(21) of the middle cerebral artery during arteriography. Patients with flow determinations in the range of 80 to 160 ml/minute had filling in all major divisions of the middle cerebral territory. Case 78 with bilateral ICA occlusion had a calculated flow of 170 ml/minute and demonstrated filling of the ipsilateral MCA territory with perfusion extending into both anterior cerebral arteries and into the contralateral MCA trunk (Fig. 21.22 and 21.23). The exceptionally high flow of 240 ml/minute in Case 82 (Fig. 21.24 and 21.25)

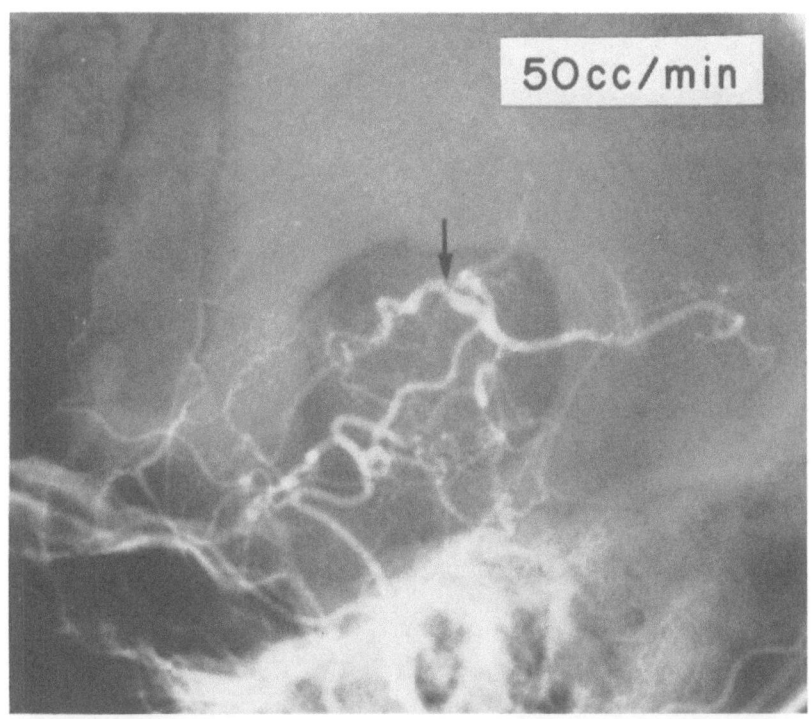

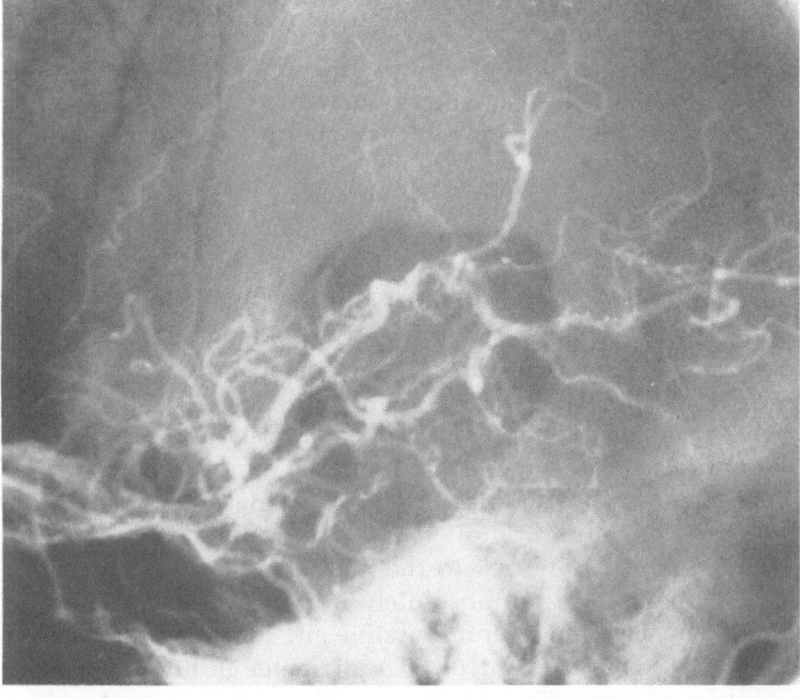

Fig. 21.4. Case 31. Cerebrovascular "moyamoya" disease. Above: Early phase of selective external carotid arteriogram shows STA–cortical MCA anastomosis (arrow) with distal filling of angular artery. Below: Later phase shows retrograde flow into proximal portion of angular artery with perfusion along the sylvian region.

occurred in the presence of ipsilateral ICA occlusion and contralateral ICA stenosis, but without other explanation.

Three patients (Cases 42, 54, and 72) with double-branch anastomosis had flow determinations that spanned the range of the study. The duration between surgery and determination of flow did not seem to influence the magnitude of flow.

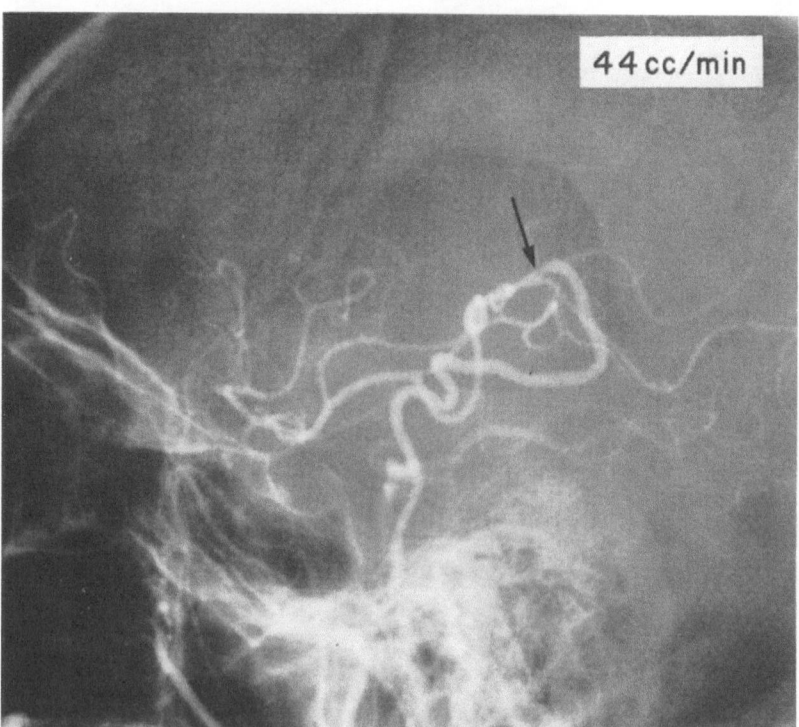

Fig. 21.5. Case 33. STA–cortical MCA anastomosis (arrow) with proximal and distal filling of the angular artery and a few of the operculofrontal branches.

The flow determinations and extent of perfusion during arteriography were appropriate for the observed balance with other sources of input (primary anatomic pathway and other sources of collateral circulation) as noted previously.(14,17)

Discussion

This method for determining the volume of blood flow through an STA bypass graft has two important advantages: it can be performed at any time during the postoperative period and compared with the extent of perfusion demonstrated by arteriography; and it is simple and does not rely upon theoretical assumptions such as adequacy of mixing of a tracer substance, containment of a tracer substance, determination of a partition coefficient, or calibration of complex equipment.

The principle drawback to the method is lack of precision: (1) STA diameter is not absolutely uniform and a decision is required in selecting a representative site for measurement; (2) accuracy in measurement of STA diameter is limited by the resolution of x-ray film, yet the resulting expression of radius is used as a squared function for calculation; (3) measurement of STA length considers only two dimensions; (4) limited resolution of cinearteriography restricts accuracy in determining the exact number of frames required for passage of contrast material through the STA graft; (5) transit time for contrast material within the STA segment is influenced by the pulsation of flow resulting from the cardiac cycle; and (6) determinations were made in awake patients breathing room air but, unfortunately, arterial P_{CO_2}(20,23) was not measured during arteriography in this study.

Because of these limitations, the term "estimation" has been preferred over "measurements" in commenting upon flow through the STA bypass graft. However, this method is con-

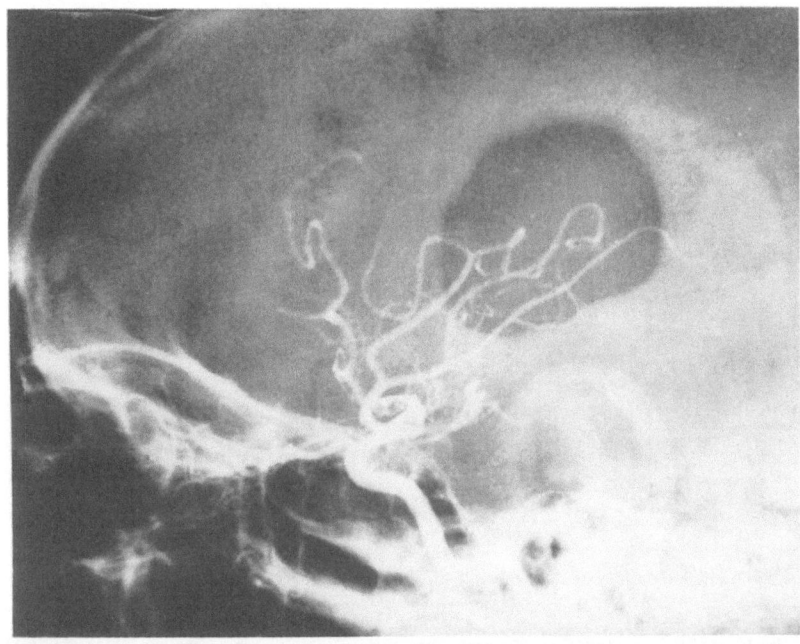

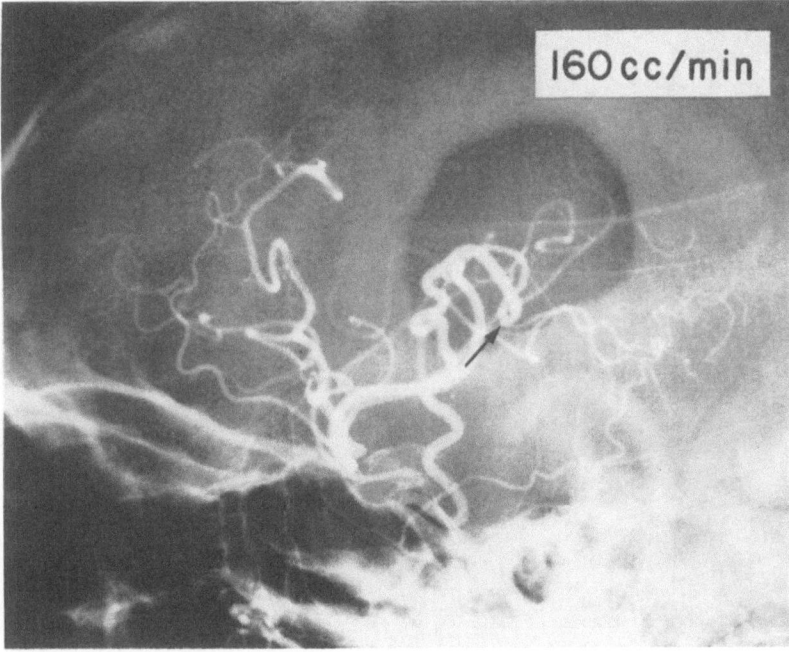

160 cc/min

Fig. 21.6. Case 36. Above: Selective internal carotid arteriogram shows some filling of the ascending frontal complex through a tight ICA stenosis (supraclinoid portion). Below: Selective external carotid arteriogram. STA–cortical MCA anastomosis (arrow) with retrograde flow to MCA trifurcation and perfusion of the entire MCA territory demonstrated during later films.

Discussion

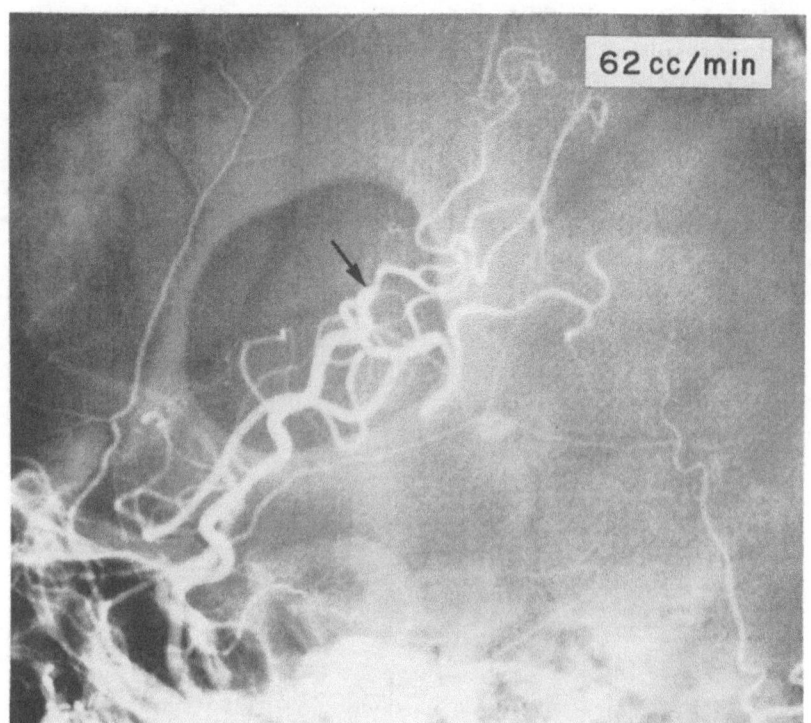

Fig. 21.7. Case 38. Selective external carotid arteriogram demonstrates STA–cortical MCA anastomosis (arrow) with filling of the posterior parietal and angular MCA branches.

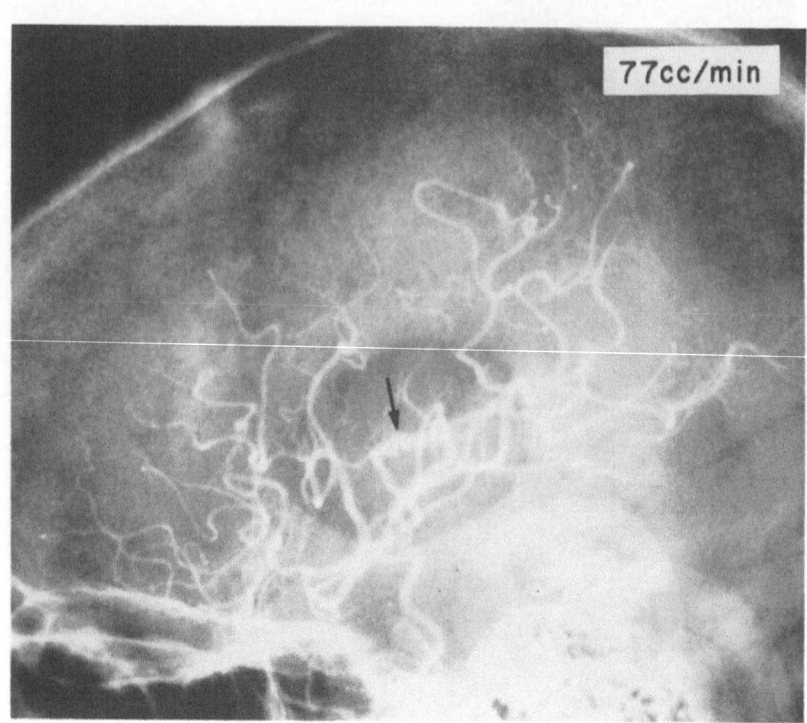

Fig. 21.8. Case 39. Selective external carotid arteriogram demonstrates perfusion of entire middle cerebral circulation by STA bypass graft. Site of anastomosis is indicated by arrow.

Chapter 21: Estimation of Flow Through STA Bypass Graft

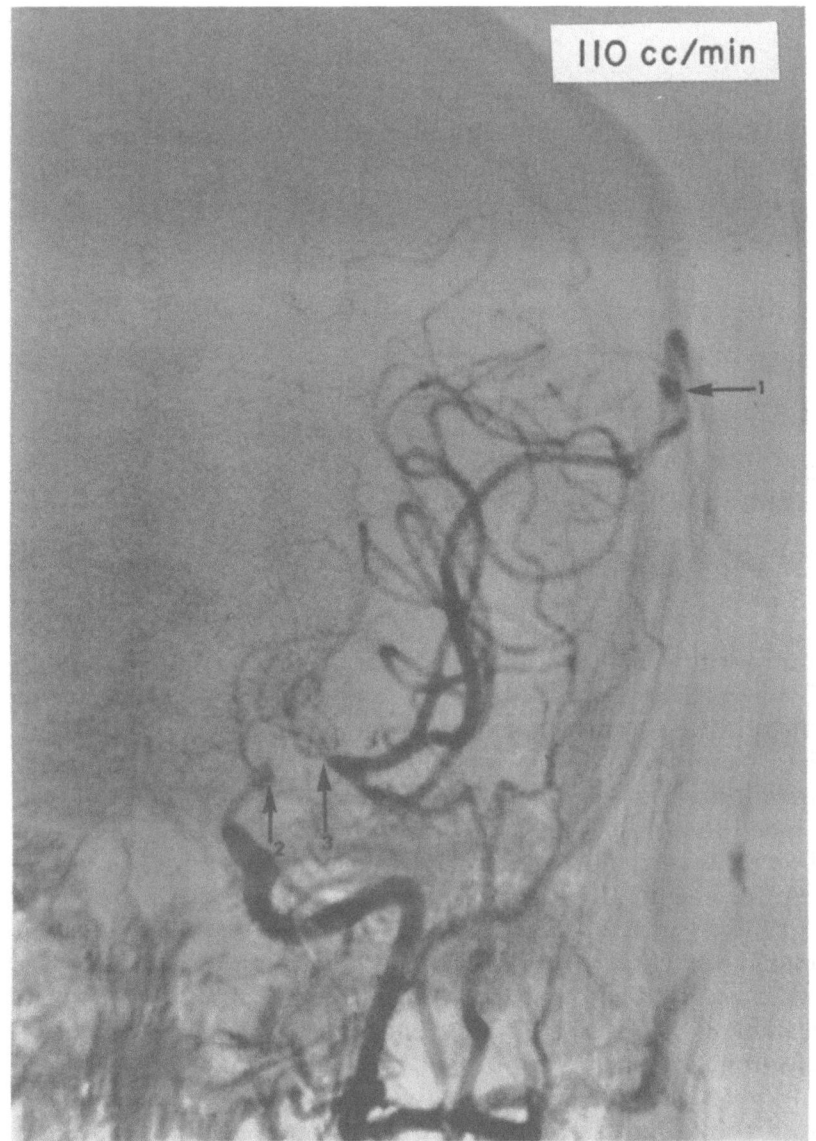

110 cc/min

Fig. 21.9. Case 40. Frontal projection (subtraction version) of left carotid arteriogram demonstrates perfusion of entire MCA territory by STA bypass graft through anastomosis (arrow 1). Filling extends retrograde to the trifurcation with perfusion of several lenticulostriate branches (arrow 3). Contrast material from ICA irrigates only a few lenticulostriate branches (arrow 2). The segment of MCA between arrow 2 and arrow 3 has become occluded.

sidered sufficiently reliable to assign an order of magnitude to the collateral flow that has been developed by STA–cortical MCA anastomosis and draw some important conclusions.

The volume of STA bypass graft flow and the extent of perfusion depend upon a balance between flow through the primary anatomic pathway, other sources of collateral circulation, adequacy of the STA as a conduit, and the peripheral cerebral vascular resistance.(14,17) The observation of STA perfusion confined to a single branch of the MCA (Fig. 21.11, above) and an STA flow determination in the range of 30 to 50 ml/minute were found in the presence of considerable flow through the primary anatomic pathway (Fig. 21.11, below) or through collateral channels, serving other portions of the MCA territory

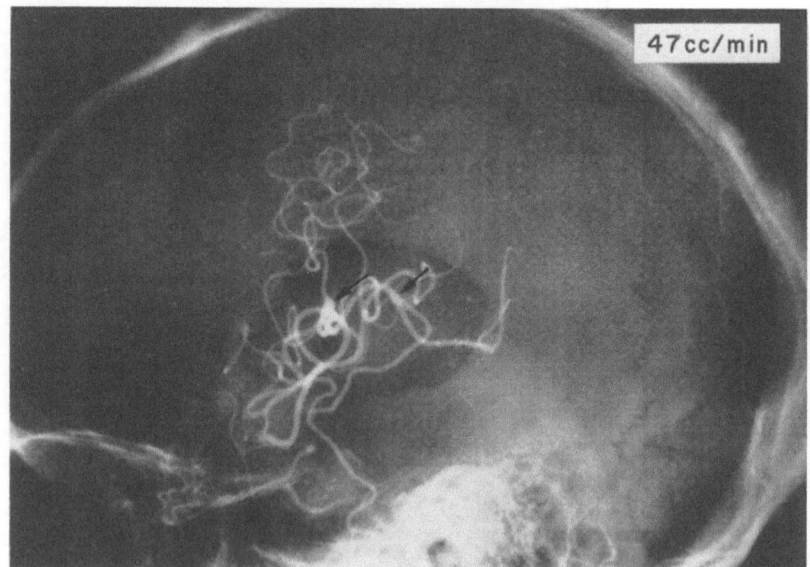

47cc/min

Fig. 21.10. Case 42. Selective external carotid arteriogram with double-branch anastomosis (arrows) shows filling of the ascending frontal complex with some filling in the angular region.

but not that major branch perfused by the STA bypass graft. Since the STA bypass graft flow, alone, usually filled all of the major MCA branch (ascending frontal complex, posterior parietal, angular, or posterior temporal),(21) a range of 30 to 50 ml/minute is considered the magnitude of flow normally assigned to each major MCA branch. Perfusion of a major MCA branch must be an important supplement to middle cerebral territory circulation.

When perfusion from the STA bypass graft filled the four major branches of the MCA, the determination of flow was within the range of 80 to 160 ml/minute. This finding is consistent with observations by Nornes.(11,12) Using miniature electromagnetic flow probes, he found direct and indirect flows in the MCA trunk ranging between 90 and 125 ml/minute and in the anterior cerebral artery (ACA) ranging between 70 and 120 ml/minute in a few patients undergoing craniotomy for trapping of an aneurysm. These patients were under general anesthesia, ventilated to maintain a relatively normal Pco_2, and mildly hypotensive, with surgery occurring usually 2 to 4 weeks after subarachnoid hemorrhage.

If normal MCA flow has a magnitude of approximately 150 ml/minute and ACA flow a magnitude of 100 ml/minute, these together equal 240 ml/minute. While the literature contains a rather wide variation for ICA electromagnetic flowmetry, (3,13,18,20,23) rCBF,(2,3,9,10,19,23) and total cerebral blood flow(10,23), it seems reasonable to accept 250 ml/minute as the order of magnitude for normal ICA blood flow. If each ICA contributes 250 ml/minute and the vertebrobasilar system contributes another 250 ml/minute, the total input of 750 ml/minute

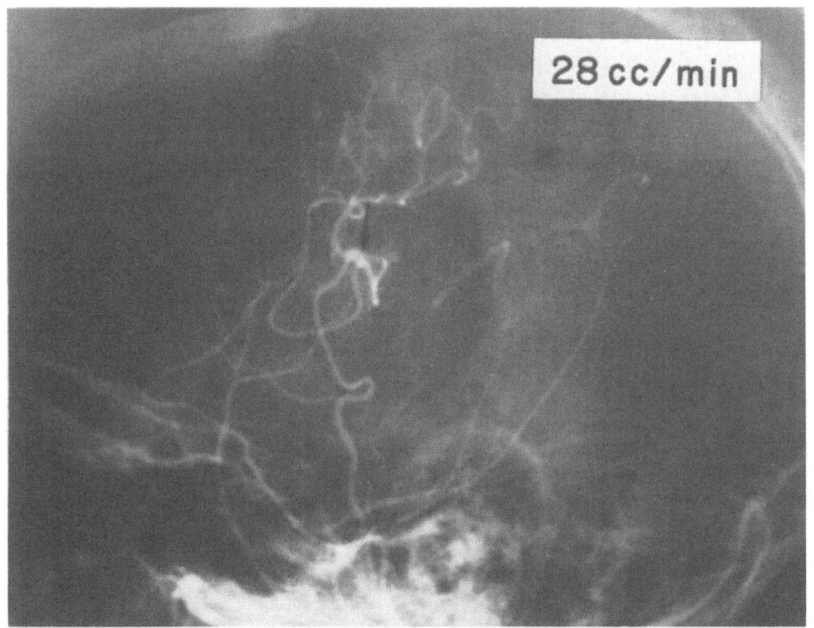

28 cc/min

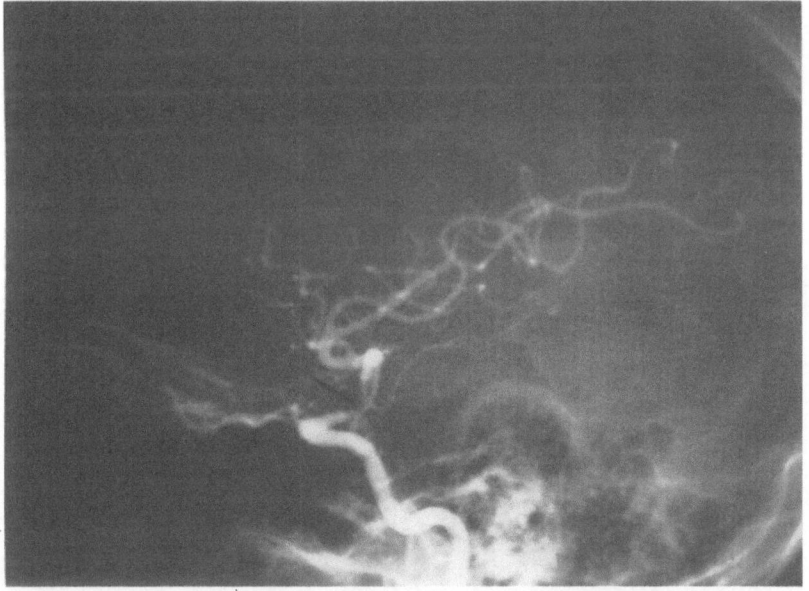

Fig. 21.11. Case 43. Above: Selective external carotid arteriogram shows filling of operculofrontal region through anastomosis (arrow). Below: Selective internal carotid arteriogram shows recanalization of internal carotid above the anterior clinoid process (arrow) with perfusion of the entire middle cerebral artery territory exclusive of the operculofrontal branch.

is equivalent to the total cerebral blood flow(23) for a brain weighing 1400 g as derived from the average flow of 54 ml/minute/100 g reported by Kety and Schmidt.(10)

Discussion

231

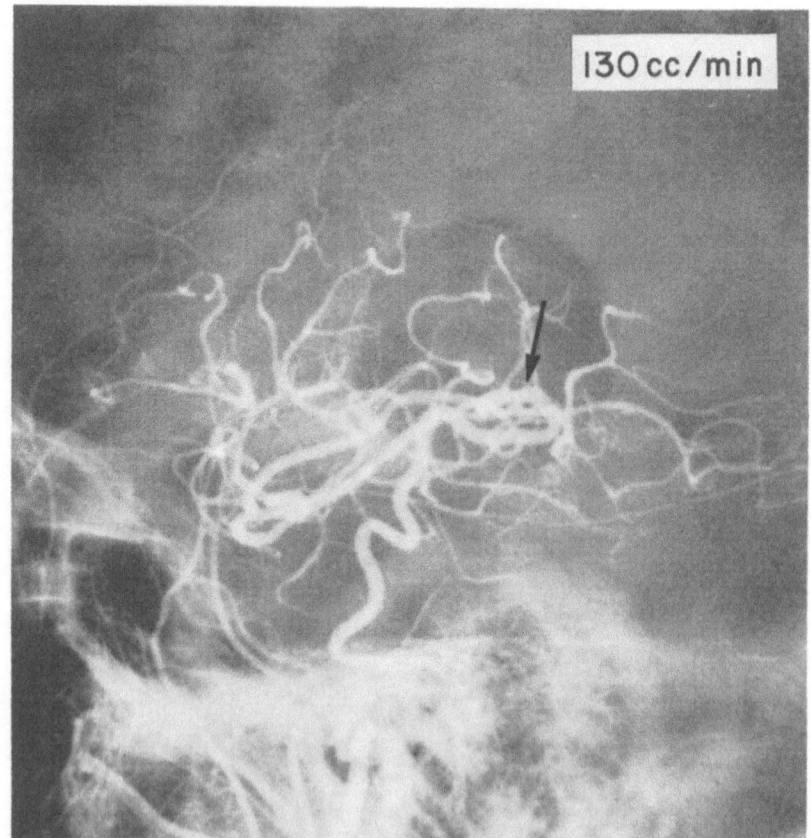

Fig. 21.12. Case 44. STA-cortical MCA anastomosis (arrow) with perfusion of entire middle cerebral territory.

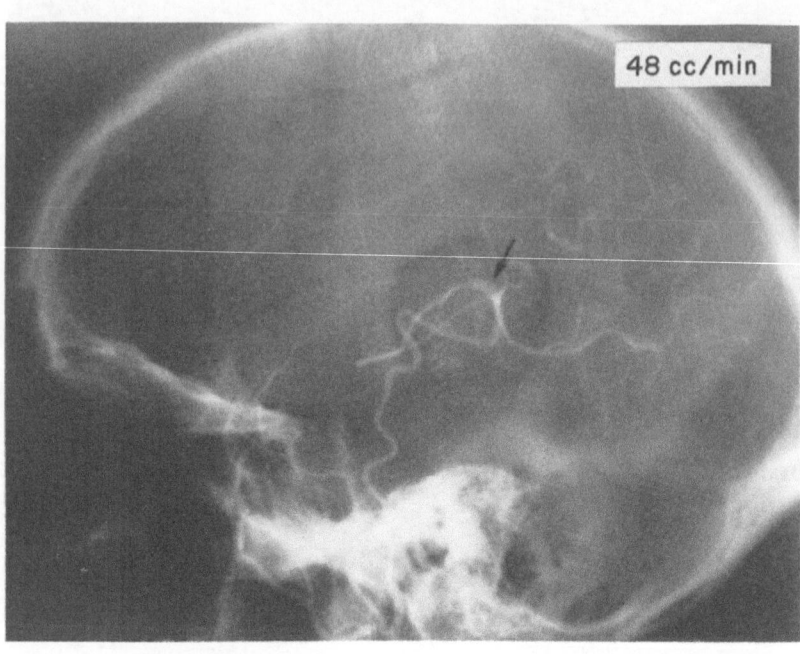

Fig. 21.13. Case 46. STA–cortical MCA anastomosis (arrow) with perfusion limited to the angular branch of MCA.

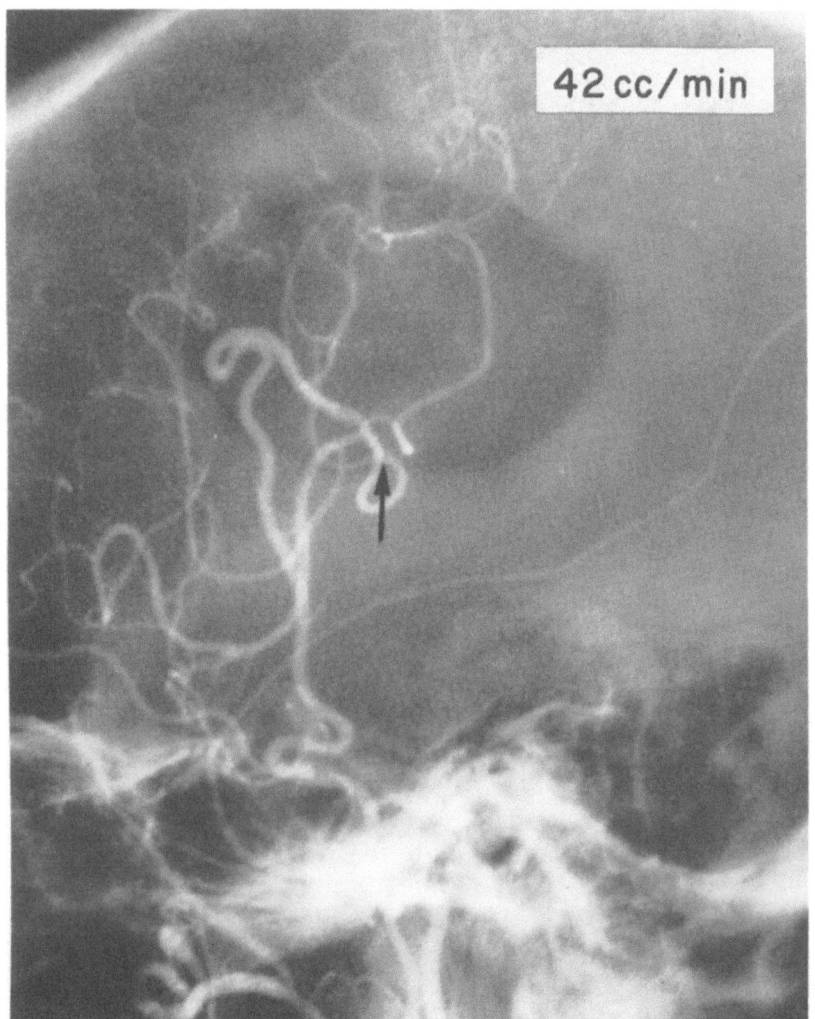

Fig. 21.14. Case 49. STA–cortical MCA anastomosis (arrow) with filling of entire ascending frontal complex.

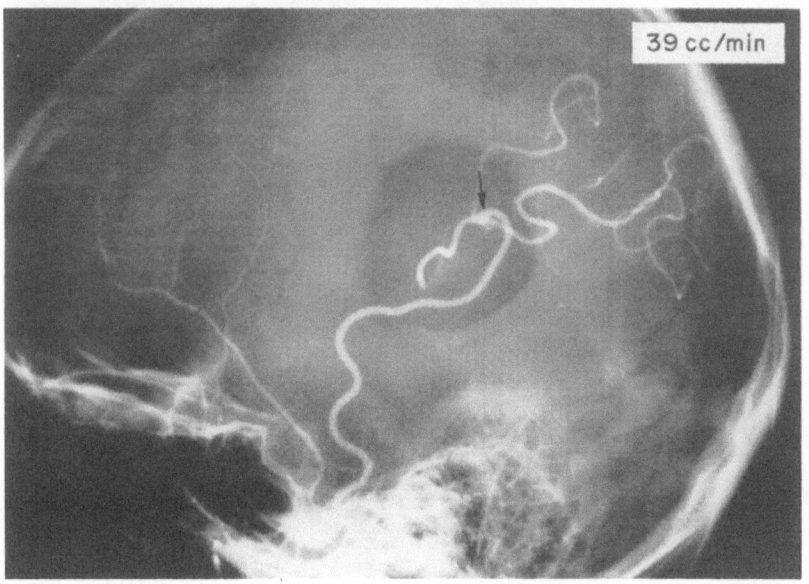

Fig. 21.15. Case 50. STA-cortical MCA anastomosis (arrow) with filling limited to posterior parietal region.

Discussion

233

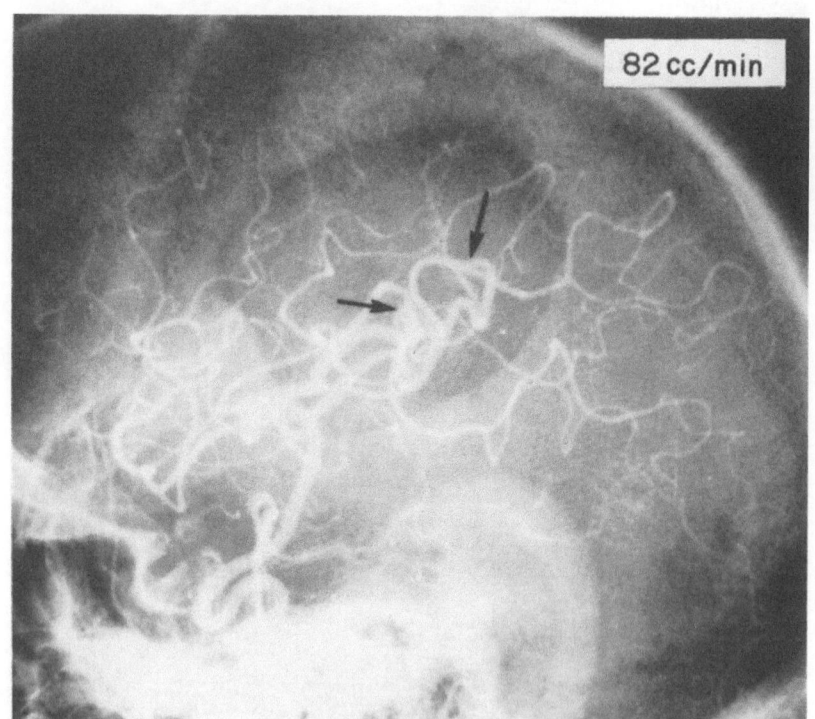

Fig. 21.16. Case 54 STA bypass graft with double-branch anastomosis (arrows) fills entire MCA territory.

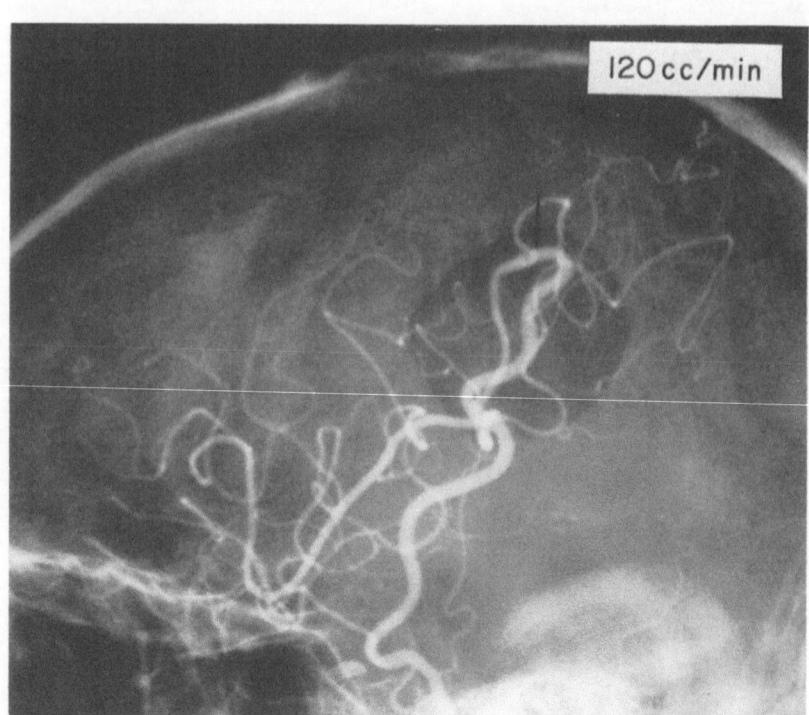

Fig. 21.17. Case 55. STA-cortical MCA anastomosis (arrow) with filling of entire middle cerebral artery territory.

Chapter 21: Estimation of Flow Through STA Bypass Graft

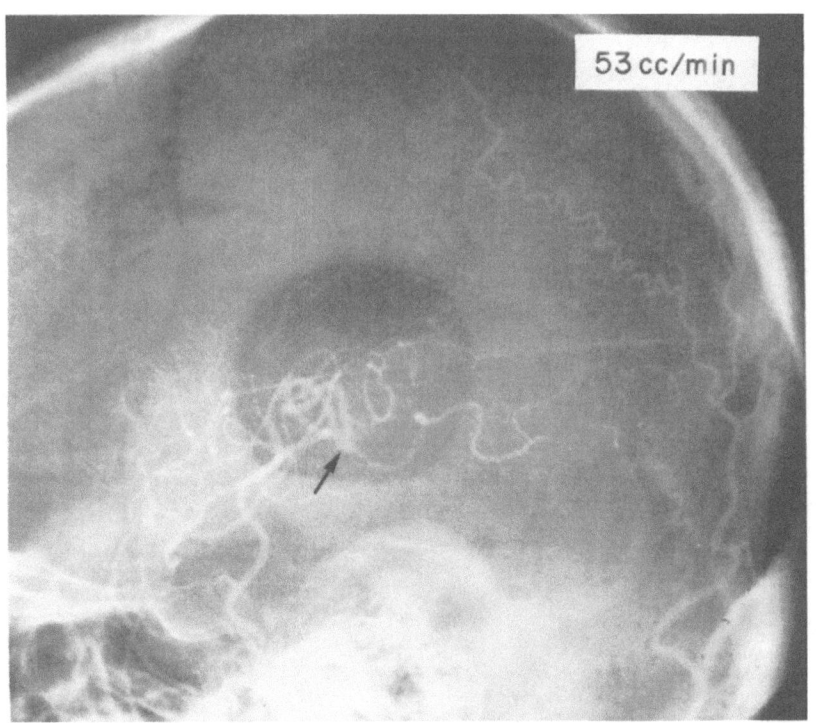

Fig. 21.18. Case 64. STA-cortical MCA anastomosis (arrow) with perfusion of vessels in the angular and operculofrontal regions.

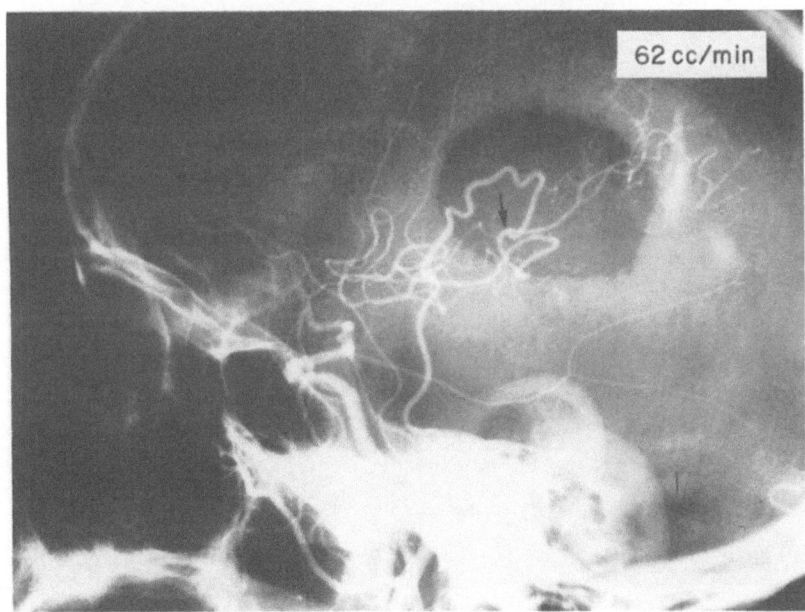

Fig. 21.19. Case 68. STA–cortical MCA anastomosis (arrow) with filling of the posterior parietal and operculofrontal regions.

Discussion

235

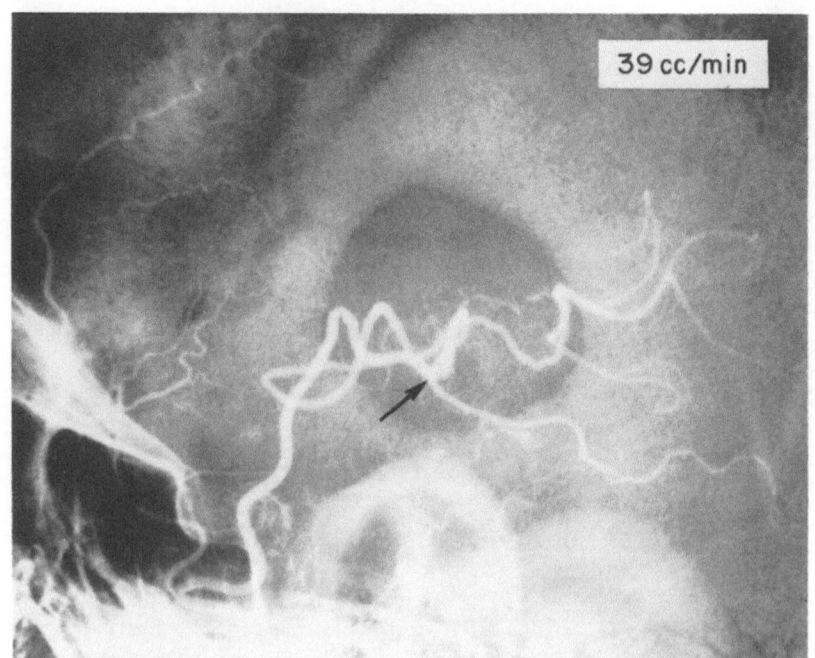

Fig. 21.20. Case 69. STA–cortical MCA anastomosis (arrow) with filling of the angular and posterior temporal regions.

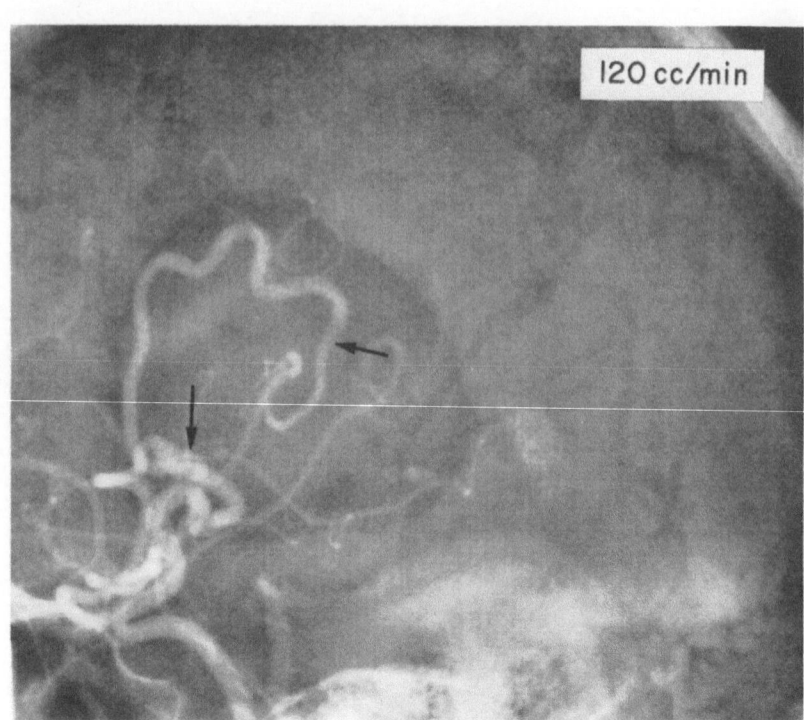

Fig. 21.21. Case 72. Early phase of arteriogram showing STA bypass graft with double-branch anastomosis (arrows) which demonstrated filling of entire MCA territory on later films.

Chapter 21: Estimation of Flow Through STA Bypass Graft

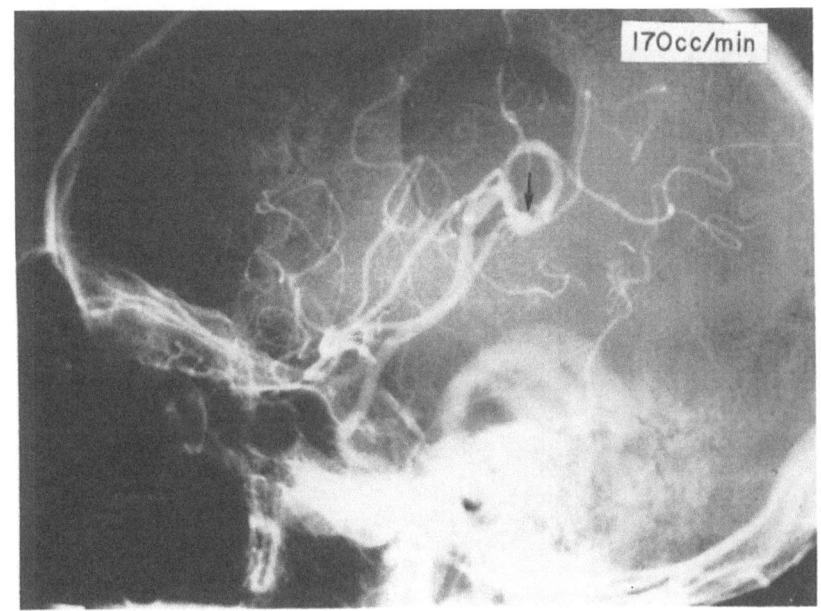

Fig. 21.22. Case 78. STA–cortical MCA anastomosis (arrow) with filling of entire middle cerebral territory.

Fig. 21.23. Case 78. Frontal view (subtraction version) of selective right external carotid arteriogram. Left: Early phase shows STA–cortical MCA anastomosis (arrow 1) with perfusion of entire right middle cerebral territory and filling beyond ICA bifurcation (arrow 2) into proximal segment of anterior cerebral artery. Right: Later phase shows retrograde filling of distal ICA stump and extension of filling into both anterior cerebral arteries and the proximal trunk of the left MCA.

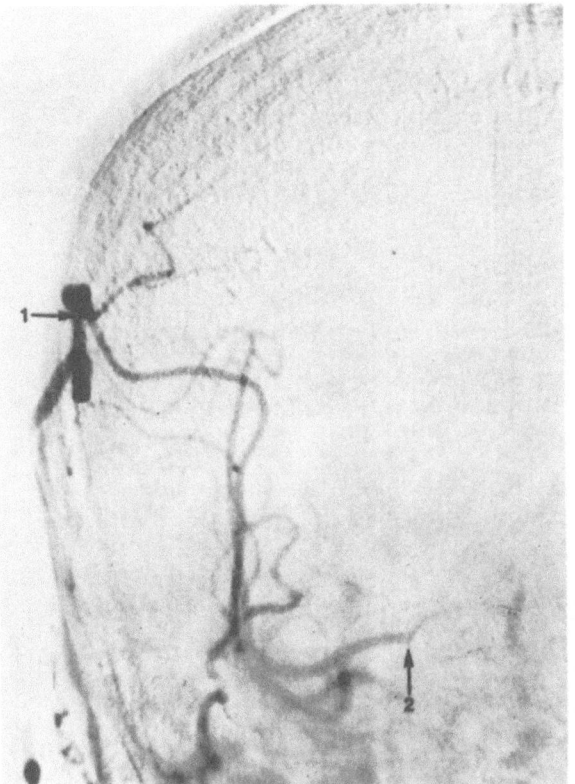 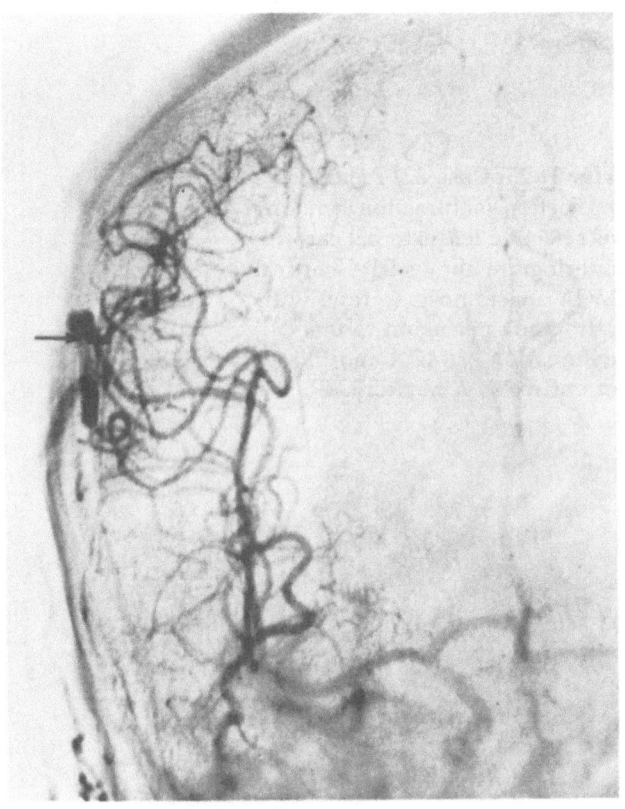

Discussion

237

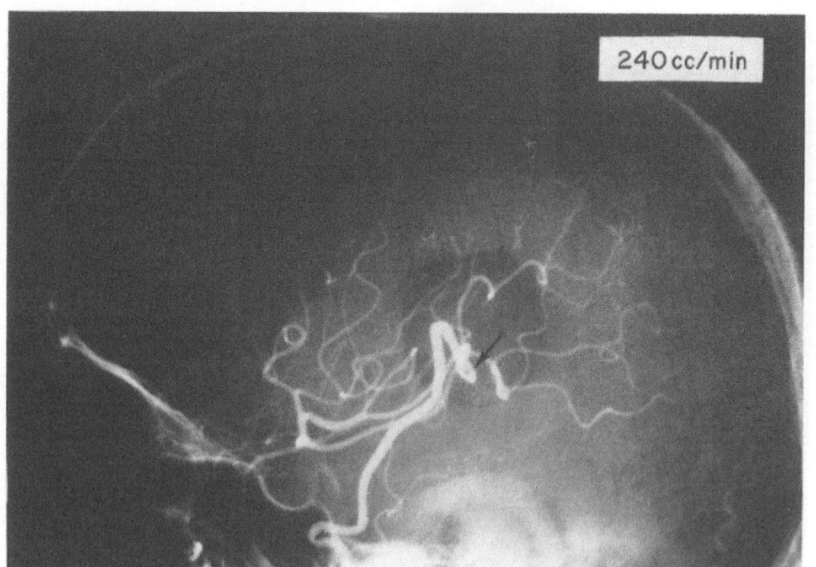

Fig. 21.24. Case 82. STA–cortical MCA anastomosis (arrow) with filling of entire middle cerebral territory.

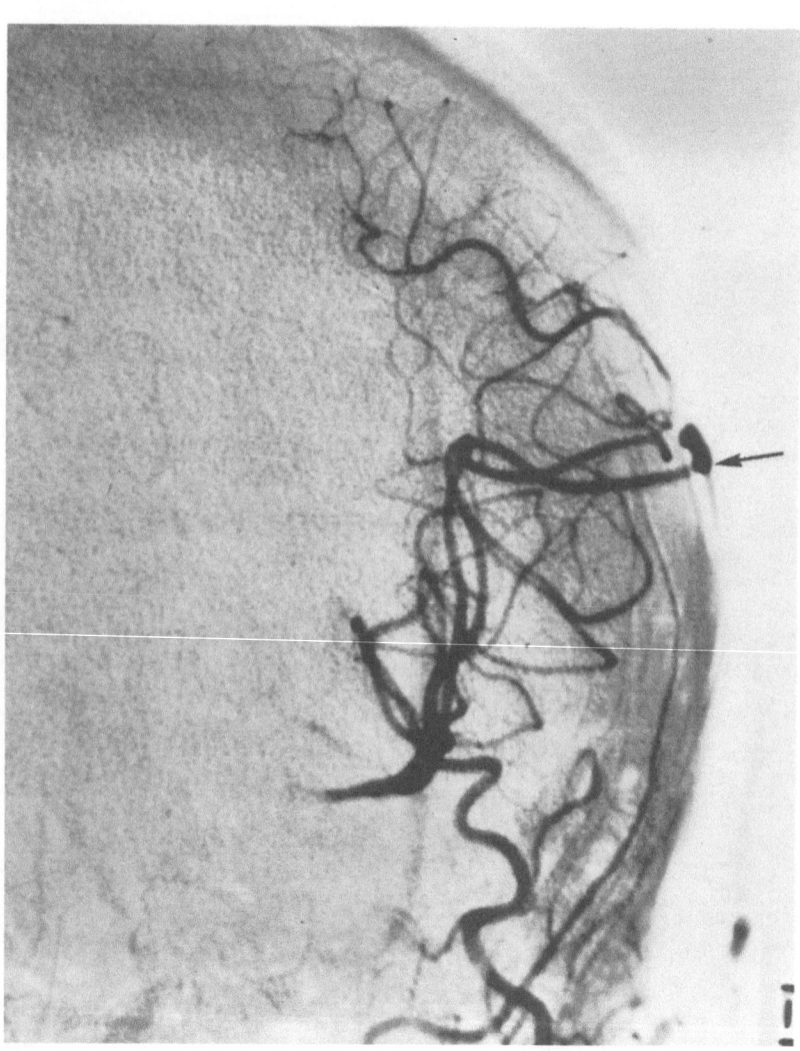

Fig. 21.25. Case 82. Frontal projection (subtraction version) of selective left external carotid arteriogram shows STA–cortical MCA anastomosis (arrow) with retrograde perfusion to the trifurcation of MCA and filling of entire MCA territory.

Summary

An arteriographic method has been devised for estimating the volume of blood flow through a superficial temporal artery (STA) bypass graft to a cortical branch of the middle cerebral artery (MCA). The average flow, determined in 20 representative patients, was 86 ml/minute with a range of 28 to 240 ml/minute. The calculated flow in each patient correlated well with the extent of perfusion observed during arterial and venous phases of selective external carotid arteriography.

REFERENCES

1. Ausman JI, Latchaw RE, Lee MC: Results of multiple angiographic studies on cerebral revascularization patients. Presentation before the Third International Symposium on Microneurosurgical Anastomoses for Cerebral Ischemia, Rottach-Egern, West Germany, June 30, 1976
2. Austin G, Hayward W, Laffin D: Use of cerebral blood flow for selection and monitoring of patients. In Austin GM (ed): Microneurosurgical Anastomoses for Cerebral Ischemia. Springfield, Ill, Thomas, 1976, pp 327–338
3. Boysen G, Ladegaard-Pedersen HJ, Valentin N, et al: Cerebral blood flow and internal carotid artery flow during carotid surgery. Stroke 1:253, 1970
4. Chater N: Surgical results and measurements of intraoperative flow in microneurosurgical anastomoses. In Austin GM (ed): Microneurosurgical Anastomoses for Cerebral Ischemia. Springfield, Ill, Thomas, 1976, pp 295–304
5. Chater N, Mani J, Tonnemacher K: Superficial temporal artery bypass in occlusive cerebral vascular disease. Calif Med 119:9, 1973
6. Chater N, Spetzler R, Tonnemacher K: Anatomical localization of optimal middle cerebral branch for anastomosis. In Austin GM (ed): Microneurosurgical Anastomoses for Cerebral Ischemia. Springfield, Ill, Thomas, 1976, pp 39–51
7. Crowell RM: Electromagnetic flow studies of superficial temporal artery to middle cerebral branch artery bypass graft. In Austin GM (ed): Microneurosurgical Anastomoses for Cerebral Ischemia. Springfield, Ill, Thomas, 1976, pp 116–124
8. Donaghy RMP, Yasargil MG: Extra-intracranial blood flow diversion. Presentation before the American Association of Neurological Surgeons, Chicago, Illinois, April 11, 1968 (Abstract 52)
9. Heilbrun MP, Reichman OH, Anderson RE, et al: Regional cerebral blood flow studies following superficial temporal–middle cerebral anastomosis. J Neurosurg 43:706, 1975
10. Kety SS, Schmidt CF: The nitrous oxide method for the quantitative determination of cerebral blood flow in man. Theory, procedure, and normal values. J Clin Invest 27:476, 1948
11. Nornes H: Monitoring of patients with intracranial aneurysms. Clin Neurosurg 22:321, 1975
12. Nornes H: Personal communication, June 25, 1976

13. Nornes H: The role of the circle of Willis in graded occlusion of the internal carotid artery in man. Acta Neurochir (Wien) 28:165, 1973

14. Reichman OH: Arteriographic flow patterns following STA–cortical MCA anastomosis. In Austin GM (ed): Microneurosurgical Anastomoses for Cerebral Ischemia. Springfield, Ill, Thomas, 1976, pp 338–358

15. Reichman OH: Extracranial-intracranial arterial anastomosis. In Whisnant JP, Sandok BA (eds): Cerebral Vascular Diseases. Ninth Princeton Conference. New York, Grune, 1975, pp 175–185

16. Reichman OH: Neurosurgical microsurgical anastomosis for cerebral ischemia. Five years' experience. In Scheinberg P (ed): Cerebral Vascular Diseases. Tenth Princeton Conference. New York, Raven Press, 1976, pp 311–330

17. Reichman OH, Davis DO, Roberts TS, et al: Anastomosis between STA and cortical branch of MCA for the treatment of occlusive cerebrovascular disease. In Mérei FT (ed): Reconstructive Surgery of Brain Arteries. Budapest, Akadémiai Kiadó, 1974, pp 201–218

18. Roberts B, Hardesty WH, Holling HE, et al: Studies on extracranial blood flow. Surgery, 56:826, 1964

19. Schmiedek P, Gratzl O, Spetzler R, et al: Selection of patients for extra-intracranial arterial bypass surgery based on rCBF measurements. J Neurosurg 44:303, 1976

20. Tindall GT, Craddock A, Greenfield JC Jr: Effects of the sitting position on blood flow in the internal carotid artery of man during general anesthesia. J Neurosurg 26:383, 1967

21. Waddington MM: Atlas of Cerebral Angiography with Anatomic Correlation. Boston, Little, Brown, 1974

22. Yasargil MG: Diagnosis and indications for operations in cerebrovascular occlusive disease. In Yasargil MG (ed): Microsurgery Applied to Neurosurgery. Stuttgart, Thieme Verlag, 1969, pp 95–119

23. Youmans JR, Albrand OW: Cerebral blood flow in clinical problems. In Youmans, JR (ed): Neurological Surgery, Vol. 2. Philadelphia, Saunders, 1973, pp 651–697

22

Cerebral blood flow in stroke-type patients

G. Austin, D. Laffin,
R. Vasudevan, E. Lichter, and W. Hayward

Few factors in the genesis of the occlusive type of stroke lend themselves to quantitive assessment. The most critical factors are tissue oxygen availability(tO_2) and regional cerebral blood flow (rCBF). These are critically related by the fact that tissue O_2 availability is proportional to the product of arterial Po_2 (aPO_2) and CBF.(27) Only in animals or under special surgical conditions in man can tO_2 be measured or approximated.(2,10) However, rCBF can be quantitated in stroke-type patients, by noninvasive techniques. The original work of Kety and Schmidt in 1946 first showed that mean CBF could be quantitated in man by the application of the Fick equation and the inhalation of certain gaseous indicators.(21,23) They originally used nitrous oxide and more recently, radioisotopes have been used.(16,18,19,22) Originally, radioisotopes were injected into the internal carotid artery and the radioactive decay was measured over regions of the head and brain. This represents clearance of isotope by blood flow. Since recirculation of isotope was negligible by this technique, a simple exponential equation resulted for each of two compartments (fast and slow, or gray and white matter).

Unfortunately, the carotid injection technique results in occasional complications and, therefore, is not suitable for outpatient use or for repeated monitoring of hospital patients. Subsequently, an inhalation technique was developed by Mallet and Veal and later by Obrist.(14,24,28) More recently, an IV bolus technique was developed by Austin et al. This proved to be accurate and as reproducible as the internal carotid injection method.(4,6,9) Thereafter, studies in stroke patients have usually shown a regional reduction.(5,7) However, in some acute patients, a vasodilation was found to exist in the region

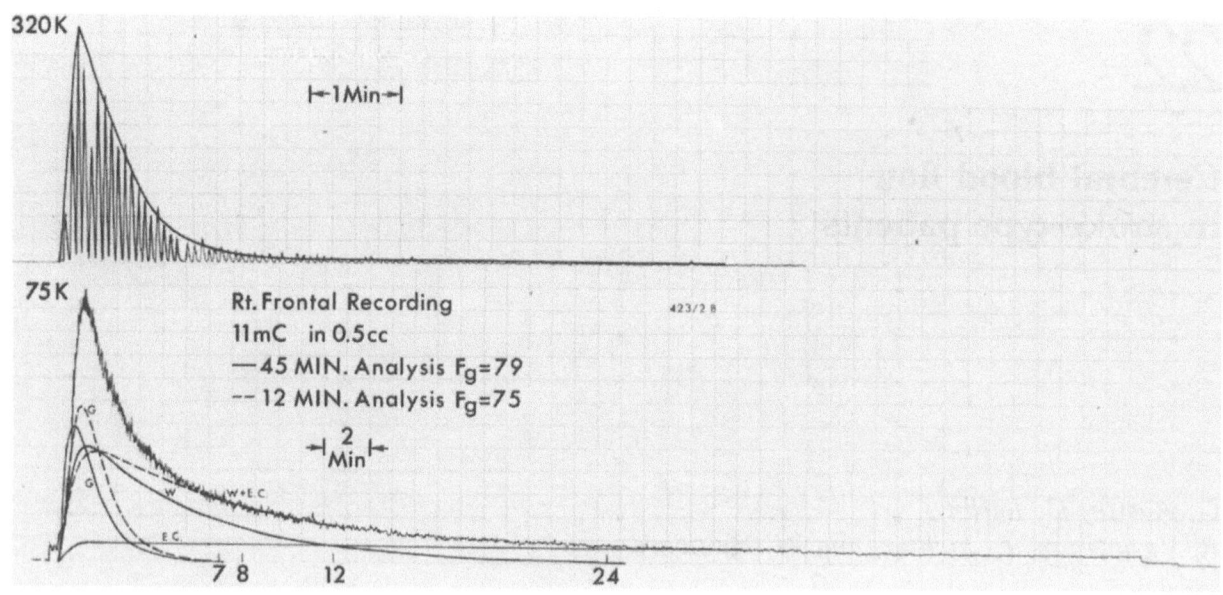

Fig. 22.1. Top: End-expired air curve following IV injection of ^{133}Xe. Bottom: Recording from single probe in right frontal region. Control patient showing comparative results of 45-minute analog analysis versus those of 12-minute analysis. Note the significant difference between gray matter flows in the two forms of analog analysis.

of mild injury or infarctions. In addition, it was observed that intracranial steal phenomena could develop in these patients with the use of vasodilators such as CO_2 or papaverine.(17,25) These were shown to occur because of diffuse vasodilation in the remainder of the brain which drained blood away from the already maximally dilated blood vessels in the region of an acute infarct. Stroke-type patients are those having transient ischemic attacks (TIAs), reversible ischemic neurologic deficits (RINDs), minor strokes, or major completed strokes. In minor or major strokes, the neuronal damage is usually complete in the region of cerebral involvement. In patients with TIAs or RINDs, the damage is transitory, incomplete, or in evolution. These patients usually have regions of decreased CBF, except in the occasional case of acute infarct with maximum regional vasodilatation. In the present concept of TIAs, RINDs, or strokes, the neurologic deficit is assumed to occur because of a critical reduction in brain Po_2 (bPo_2) to a threshold level. At that level O_2 utilization is impaired with a resultant decrease in oxidative phosphorylation.(2,10) The latter results in inadequate maintenance of the neuronal ion pumps and is manifest clinically by the signs or symptoms of TIAs.

Theoretically, one should be able to measure significant changes in background rCBF in many of these patients, and especially in those with TIAs. These values of depressed rCBF might be used to predict the increased likelihood of stroke. In the case of RINDs or minor strokes, repeated monitoring of rCBF might be used to measure response to therapy, regression of neuronal damage, or the degree of natural improvement. In all cases, a correlation of the neurologic findings and the angiographic results is necessary to achieve maximum usefulness of the measured rCBF. In this chapter we describe the technique and results of measuring rCBF in stroke-type patients by the noninvasive IV bolus method using ^{133}Xe.

Methods

Patients were selected for study from among those admitted with TIA, RINDs or minor strokes. Many of these were in the process of being prepared for a possible microanastomosis for cerebral ischemia. The common symptoms of TIAs have been previously described.(4,10) Regional cerebral blood flow was measured in assumed gray and white matter (fast and slow components) by a 3-compartment system using a 45-minute period of measurement;(4,9) or rCBF in gray matter was measured in an assumed 2-compartment system using a 12-minute period of measurement.(6) In both cases flow is assumed to remain steady during the period of recording (Fig. 22.1 and 22.2). In the early portion of this work, an analog computer was used and for the past year a digital computer program was used to solve the Fick equation in the form of its convolution integral as shown below:

$$C_i = \frac{dc_i}{dt} = fi \left[A(t) - \frac{C_i}{\lambda_i} \right] ; \text{ or } C_i = W_i\lambda_iK_ie^{-K_it} \int_0^t A(\tau)e^{K_i\tau} d\tau \quad (1)$$

(Fick equation)   (convolution integral form of the integrated Fick equation)

where:

C_i = concentration of the injected isotope in the i_{th} compartment

C_1 = the fast compartment (gray)

C_2 = the slower compartment (white) (in the case of inhalation or intravenous injection, C_3 = the extracerebral compartment, which is assumed to have only one slow component with a half-time of about 30 minutes)

In the case of an internal carotid injection, the isotope ^{133}Xe is injected directly and, hence, recirculation is negligible and the arterial concentration A(t) approaches 0. Under these conditions,

$$\frac{dC_i}{dt} = \frac{-fi}{\lambda_i}, C_i = -K_iC_i; \text{ where } K_i = \frac{fi}{\lambda_i}$$

and the solution becomes

$$C_i = C0_ie^{-K_it}$$

where C0 is the concentration.

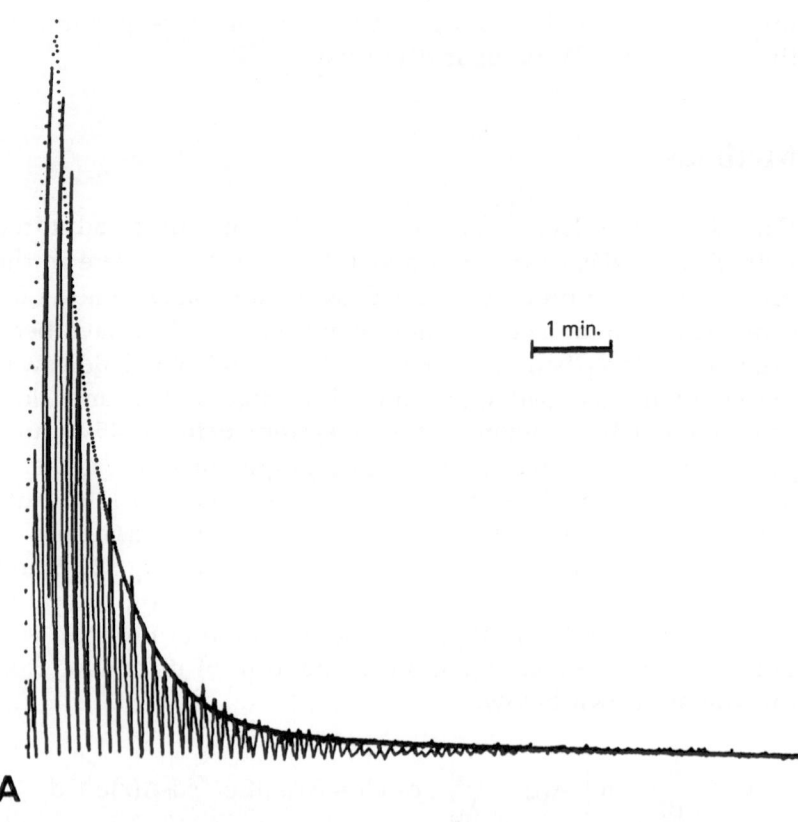

1 min.

Fig. 22.2. A. Expired air curve following IV injection of ^{133}Xe. Envelope of this curve is used to approximate the arterial concentration. This curve forms the basis of the digital computer analysis in Figure 2B and 2C. 2B. Twelve-minute digital analysis of cerebral blood flow by IV ^{133}Xe technique. Analysis started on third point following peak of curve. Injection of 30 mc. ^{133}Xe made at t = 0. $K_1 = F_1/\lambda_1$ and $K_2 = F_2/\lambda_1$. A_1 and A_2 have same meaning as W_1 and W_2 in the mathematical analysis, ie, the relative weight of the tissue compartment combined with a proportionality factor. 2C. Forty-minute digital analysis of same curve as that in 2B. This shows a 3-compartment analysis as compared to the 2-compartment and 12-minute analysis in 2B. Numbers on abscissa are the times in minutes. Values on ordinate are the relative concentrations of isotope in brain tissue expressed in counts per minute.

A

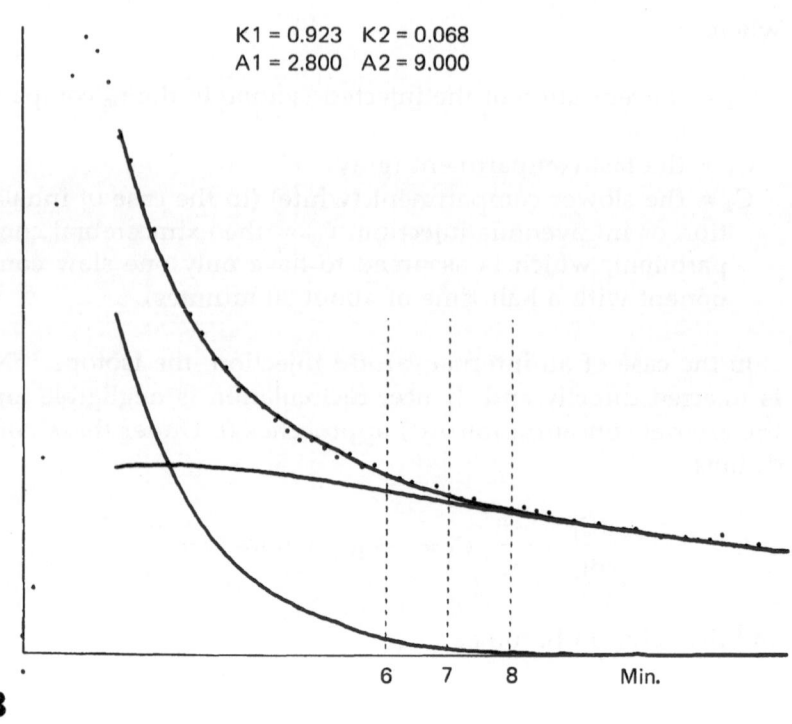

K1 = 0.923   K2 = 0.068
A1 = 2.800   A2 = 9.000

6   7   8   Min.

B

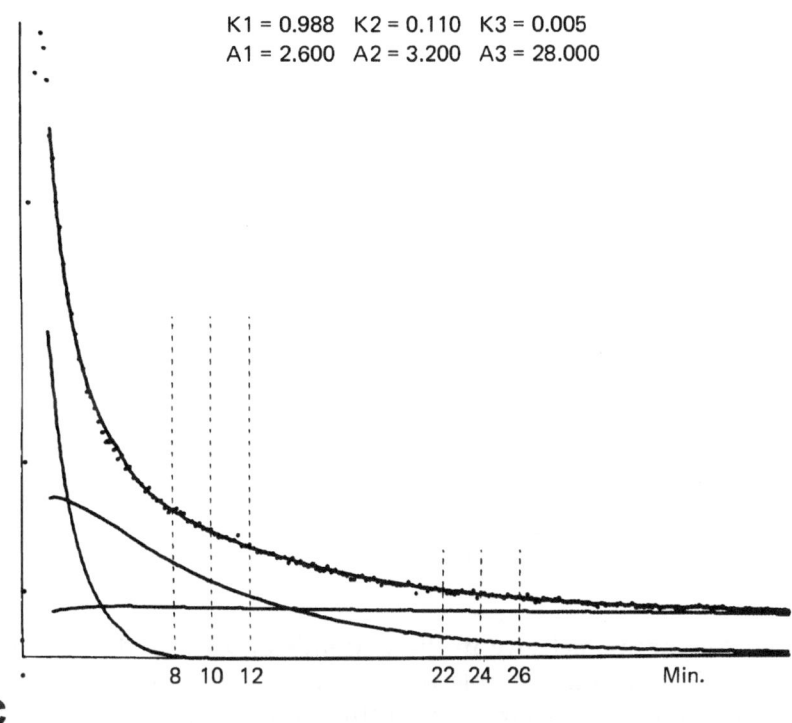

K1 = 0.988   K2 = 0.110   K3 = 0.005
A1 = 2.600   A2 = 3.200   A3 = 28.000

8 10 12   22 24 26   Min.

c

In this case the results of the radioactive decay over the head from each probe are plotted on semilog paper and a double exponential curve is obtained. The slower component is representative of the white matter compartment and the faster component is representative of the gray matter compartment. By the process of "peeling off" the experimental curves, the slopes and individual values of K and, therefore, flow are obtained.

When the isotope is given by inhalation or by IV bolus, the situation is different and recirculation of isotope must be considered. The full Fick equation with time-varying arterial coefficients (equation 1) must be solved. This can be done for each compartment directly by analog computer (Fig. 1 and 2),(8,9,13) or its corresponding convolution integral can be solved by a digital computer program. Since the IV bolus method and inhalation method are both noninvasive and carry no morbidity, they are very useful for measuring rCBF in outpatients or repeated monitoring of hospital patients before and after therapy. In Appendix II, for convenience, the full details of the digital computer solutions are described. A full description as well as the advantages and rare limitations of the IV bolus method are given in Appendix I, since these have not been described in detail elsewhere. Briefly, a bolus of 30 mc of ^{133}Xe dissolved in 0.5 ml of saline is injected into any convenient arm vein. Four collimated sodium iodide scintillation detectors are used over each hemisphere to count the radioactive decay. In addition, another detector 5 feet from the patient's body is used to meas-

Table 22.1. Mean cerebral blood flow values in patients with verified pathologic conditions

Group[a]	CBFg (ml/100g/minute)	CBFw (ml/100g/minute)
Control (10)		
Aged 21 to 56 years	75±9	25±2
Aged 48 to 77 years	75±5	25±2
Small vessel disease (6)	53±5	23±3
Carotid occlusion (8)	44±18	25±5
Brain tumor (19)	42±10	22±3
Pathologic (6)		
Internal carotid method	58±15	19±4
IV method	55±13	22±2
Reproducibility of IV method	±14%	
Variation (different computer operator)	±7%	

[a]Number of cases are in parentheses.

ure the gamma activity in the patient's end-expired air. Since xenon is so highly soluble in air, the concentration in the patient's end-expired air is proportional to the patient's arterial concentration and forms the basis of the A(t) function in the Fick equation. This is shown in Figure 1 which depicts the shape of the concentration curves for each compartment, as well as the shape of the expired air curve for both the 45-minute, 3-compartment model and the 12-minute, 2-compartment model. In the latter, only the gray matter flow is used, since the white and extracerebral compartments are taken together.

Results

Normal control values are given in Table 22.1 for two age groups. There was no significant difference in CBF between younger and the older age groups tested. Table 22.1 shows the reproducibility (±14%) of the method (ie, rCBF repeated in one week on the same patient) as well as the accuracy of the analog computer method, when determined by different members of the team (±7%). Table 22.1 gives the published reductions in CBF obtained by the IV method(4,8) for various pathologic groups. Table 22.2 shows a comparison of the results obtained by the IV method with those obtained by the inhalation technique and the carotid injection method. Figures 22.3 to 22.5 show the comparative results of 12- to 45-minute flows, and relate the analog computer solution technique to the digital solution technique, as well as the accuracy of the digital computer analysis.

In essence there was no significant difference between the analog and digital computer solutions.

Table 22.2. Comparison of grey matter and white matter flows by IV technique, common carotid injection, inhalation, and internal carotid injection: using [133]Xe

Method	F^g (ml/100 g/minute)	F^w (ml/100 g/minute)
Internal carotid injection (19) (N = 7)	79.7±10.7	20.9±2.6
Inhalation (28) (N = 15)	74.5±9.9	24.8±3.5
Common carotid injection (34) (N = 18)	93.5±18	24.4±4.3
IV Injection 15 mc (4) (N = 22)		
3-compartment analysis	75±9	25±2
2-compartment analysis	70±10	—

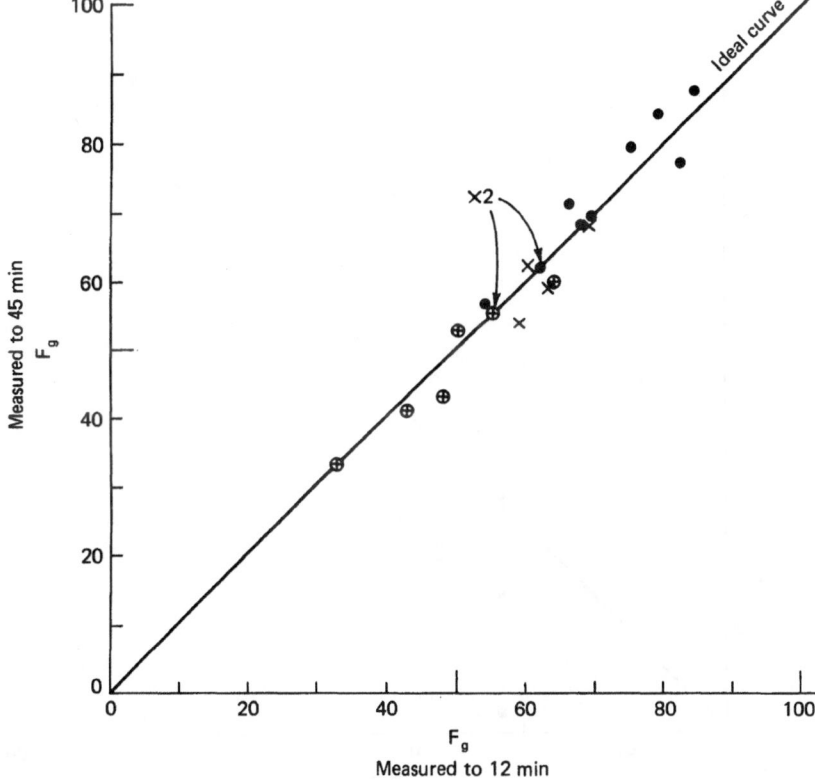

Fig. 22.3. Gray matter flow measured by 12-minute, 2-compartment method on abscissa and compared with 45-minute, 3-compartment method on ordinate. Note the insignificant difference between gray matter flows as measured in controls, mathematically generated curves, or in pathologic patients. Note: 12-minute flows do not provide values for white matter flow. Normal controls, $n = 10$, × generated curves, $n = 4$; pathologic patients, $n = 7$.

Results

Table 22.3. Preoperative depression of cerebral blood flow according to the distribution of lesions

Region	No. of Patients	Mean (ml/100 g/minute)	SD	Percentage Depression	P
Left internal carotid occlusion	15	62.07	15.55	−17.33	<0.015
Right internal carotid occlusion	12	57.62	11.59	−23.17	<0.001
Middle cerebral stenosis	8	53.94	17.16	−28.1	<0.005
Bilateral internal carotid occlusion	6	57.77	20.83	−23.0	<0.11
High internal carotid stenosis	6	51.87	12.91	−30.84	<0.001

Preoperative rCBF

Primarily, in the majority of patients being studied, rCBF was reduced more in the distribution of the middle cerebral artery. These patients had had TIAs or minor strokes. Also, they all had angiographically visualized lesions showing inaccessible pathology in the internal carotid artery or middle cerebral artery. In accordance with the present theory of a hemodynamic or embolic etiology, one would expect a background decrease in rCBF in the majority, but not necessarily in all patients. Table 22.3 shows the average reductions in rCBF that were found in association with pathology in the middle cerebral artery(MCA) or internal carotid artery. In each pathologic group,

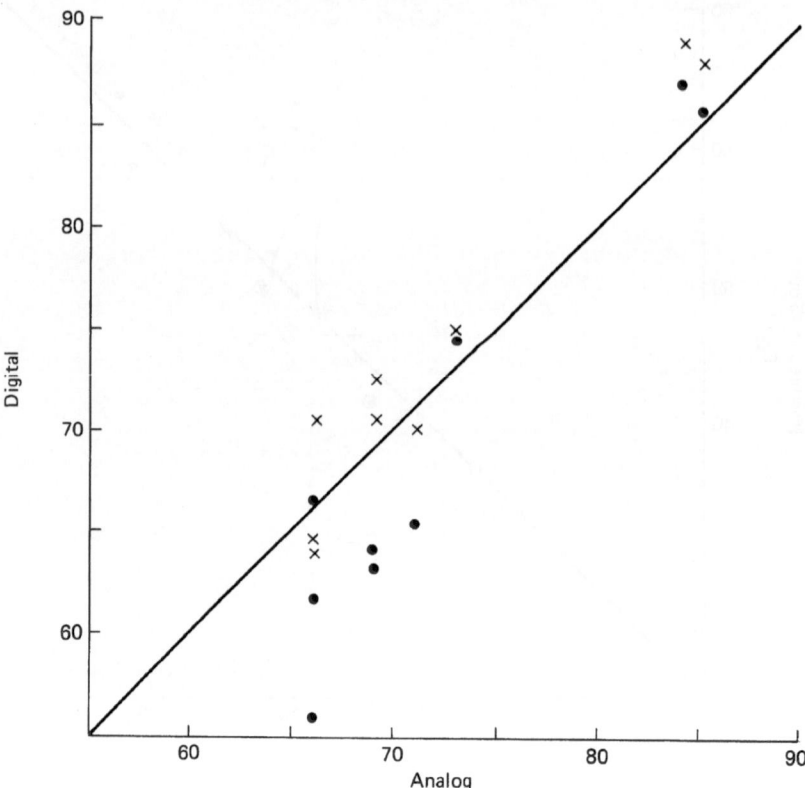

Fig. 22.4. Comparison of digital versus analog methods of computing rCBF after IV bolus injection of ^{133}Xe. Note that in 12-minute (λ) analysis a slight underestimation of gray matter flow by digital computer calculations occurs. In 40-minute (λ) analysis there is no significant difference between digital and analog computer methods.

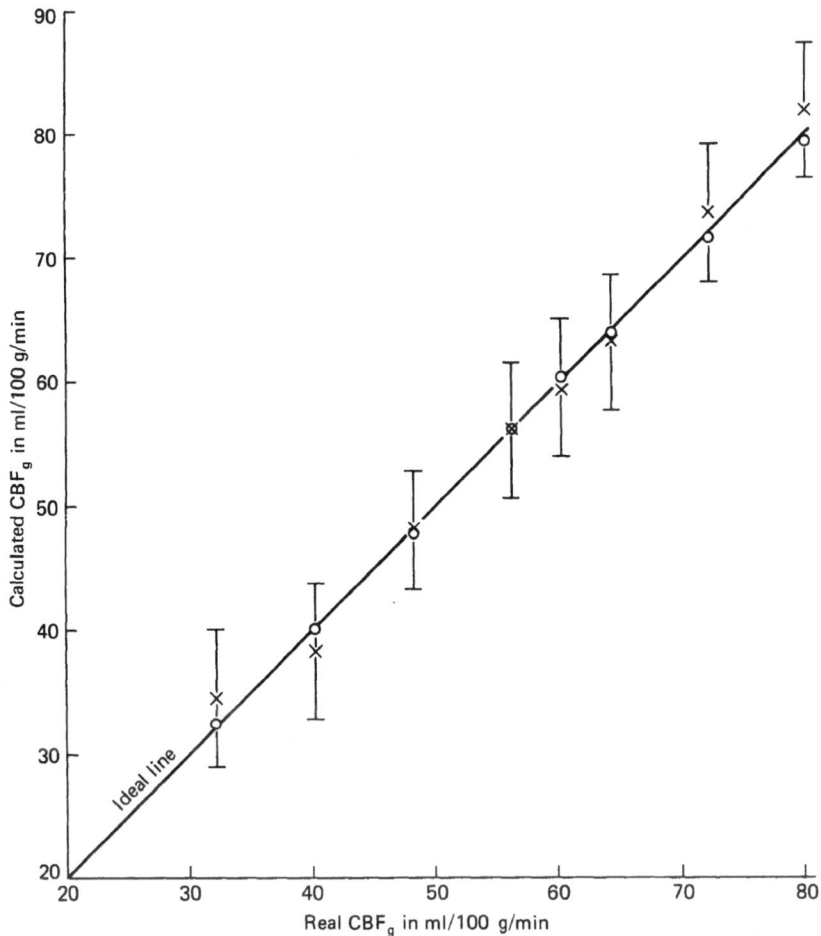

Fig. 22.5. Accuracy of a digital 2-compartment analysis. For each selected K_1 (or CBFg),ten different 40-minute curves were mathematically generated by a computer, with different K_2, K_3, W_1, W_2, and W_3. Each point represents the mean CBFg obtained by 12-minute analyses of these ten curves. Make almost perfect fit (n = 0.999) mathematically generated curves in absence of noise (o). In the presence of noise, (x), spread is indicated by bars.

a minor percentage had normal rCBF as shown in Table 22.4. Reasons for this are not clear, but possible explanations will be considered in the discussion. The average increase in rCBF following microanastomosis was most significant over the parietal-temporal distribution of the middle cerebral artery. This is shown in Tables 22.5 and 22.6. It is not surprising that the parietal-temporal region shows the maximum increase in rCBF since this is the actual site where the anastomosis of the superficial temporal artery (STA) to the MCA occurred. These rec-

Table 22.4. Percentage of patients in each pathologic group showing normal rCBF as measured by IV bolus injection technique (^{133}Xe)[a]

Pathologic Lesion	Percentage
Right internal carotid occlusion	25
Left internal carotid occlusion	44
Bilateral internal carotid occlusion	33
High internal carotid stenosis	0
Middle cerebral stenosis	11

[a]Normal cerebral blood flow ±1 SD.

Table 22.5. Results of 3-compartment analysis using IV bolas technique of measuring rCBF pre- and postoperatively[a]

No. of Patients	Region	Flow Preoperatively (ml/100 g/minute)	Flow Postoperatively (ml/100 g/minute)	P
16	Operated frontal	47±10	55±18	0.16
13	Operated parietal	46±9	57±13	0.04
11	Opposite frontal	47±8	58±19	0.19

[a]Results calculated by analog computer based on 40-minute recording following injection.

ords were originally analyzed by the analog computer solution of the full arterial time-varying Fick equation. In another, later group of randomly selected patients undergoing microanastomosis for cerebral ischemia a digital computer program was used and the results, in terms of improvement, were about the same. Again, these patients had a marked depression in rCBF preoperatively. The results suggest that in the majority of patients with a decreased rCBF preoperatively, a significant increase in rCBF could be expected following microanastomosis. These results also infer that there was usually a preoperative deficit in the tissue oxygen availability, since none of the pa-

Table 22.6. Improvement in rCBF following microanastomosis

No. of Patients	Region	Flow Preoperatively (mg/100 g/minute)	Flow Postoperatively (ml/100 g/minute)	Flow Change (Ml/100 g/min) (%)	P (× 10⁻²)
		Side of Operation[a]			
12	Frontal	42.09	48.16	6.07 (14.4)	8.9
12	Parietal	39.88	46.06	6.18 (15.5)	1.7
11	Temporal	40.38	48.82	8.44 (20.9)	4.7
12	Occipital	40.41	43.98	3.57 (8.8)	17.5
12	Mean	40.36	46.59	6.23 (15.4)	3.1
		Side Opposite Operation			
10	Frontal	43.52	48.25	4.73 (10.9)	5.8
11	Parietal	43.28	49.37	6.09 (14.1)	0.56
10	Temporal	42.22	53.70	11.48 (27.2)	1.0
10	Occipital	44.15	46.03	1.88 (4.3)	24.4
12	Mean	42.22	47.98	5.76 (13.6)	0.56
		Total Brain			
12	Total Mean	41.28	47.31	6.03 (14.6)	0.65

[a]rCBF measured by IV injection of ^{133}Xe and digital computer analysis of 2-compartment system. All results given in gray matter flow and for a 12-minute period of recording.

tients showed an elevated aP_{O_2} and many had a significant reduction in aP_{O_2} due to chronic obstructive pulmonary disease or mild chronic congestive heart failure.

Discussion

Validity of rCBF

The noninvasive IV bolus method of measuring rCBF has now been checked many times for accuracy. It has been used in approximately 800 patients flow studies at Loma Linda University Hospital. First, it has been compared against normal values for gray and white matter obtained by the internal carotid injection method and later against values reported for the inhalation method. There was no significant difference in control values. Also, when the analog computer method or digital computer method of analysis was used on artificially generated curves (by computer), the values of rCBF obtained were very close to those employed to generate the curves. Lastly, in cases of known brain pathology, including severe cerebrovascular stenosis, cerebral vasospasm, and brain tumors with increased intracranial pressure, there was usually a significant depression of rCBF, as might be expected. The ease and rapidity of the IV bolus injection method are advantageous and exceed these aspects of other methods. Similar to the inhalation method, it is completely safe and may be repeated multiple times with impunity. Its drawbacks are few, as related in Appendix I, the chief drawback being the inability to use it in patients with severe respiratory disease or Cheyne-Stokes respiration.

Patients With Cerebrovascular Pathology and Normal rCBF

There are several reasonable explanations for the occurrence of normal rCBF in patients with cerebrovascular pathology. First, originally only two probes, and more recently, for the past year and a half, only four probes, were used for hemispheric determinations. Thus, a scintillation detector could miss detecting a relatively small region of abnormality. Second, despite there being a significant cerebrovascular occlusive abnormality demonstrated by angiography, a significant and adequate collateral flow may have developed with increased flows through the opposite internal carotid and also through the vertebrobasilar system, with subsequent dilatation of the ipsilateral posterior communicating artery branch of the circle of Willis. Additional major sources of collateral flow include the ipsilateral ophthalmic artery and the epicerebral system of pial collaterals between the anterior, middle, and posterior cerebral arteries. TIAs, however, might still occur in the presence of normal background rCBF, on a hemodynamic or embolic basis. With reference to the hemodynamic etiology, an abrupt drop in blood pressure due to decreased cardiac output could trigger the TIA, if the blood flow decreased enough to critically lower the tO_2. This could occur readily in patients with loss of autoregulation. In fact, recent studies report that more than 90% of patients studied with TIAs show a loss of autoregulation.(32,33)

Patients with Cerebrovascular Pathology and Decreased rCBF

In patients with TIAs or strokes one would normally expect a background decrease in rCBF(8,10). The amount of regionality would depend on how far toward the peripheral resistance the occlusive lesion occurred. In other words, one would expect more regional decrease in CBF with a branch occlusion of the middle cerebral artery than with an occlusion of the internal carotid artery. This is suggested by the results of Table 22.3. The degree of depression of rCBF would depend on the following factors relative to the time of measurement of rCBF:

1. Acuteness of onset
2. Amount of collateral blood supply
3. Arterial O_2 saturation
4. Intactness of chemical vasodilatory response to tissue hypoxia
5. Impairment of autoregulation
6. Symmetry of the circle of Willis

Others(30,31) have also observed a decrease in rCBF with occlusive cerebrovascular disease. If one assumes a symmetric circle of Willis, then approximately 34% of the total blood input enters the brain through the basilar artery. In terms of output from the circle of Willis, approximately 62% effluxes through the middle cerebral artery. It has been estimated in animals and man that symptoms of ischemia first occur when the rCBF is reduced by 25 to 50%. This explains why the symptomatology is so varied with an internal carotid artery occlusion. If there is a small anterior communicating or posterior communicating artery on the side of carotid occlusion, the damage may range from mild to a complete hemispheric infarction. Since together these anomalies are present in approximately 50% of all circles of Willis, it can be estimated that a patient has roughly a 50% chance of surviving a carotid occlusion without resultant neurologic deficit. Although the degree of collateral blood flow is the key factor in determining neurologic deficits in patients with occlusive disease, the outcome of embolic insults is not so logically predictable. There is little relationship between measured rCBF and the neurologic deficit produced by embolic occlusion of such critical small vessels as the ganglionic branches of the middle cerebral artery or the artery of the central sulcus.

Improvement in rCBF Following Microanastomosis

Blood flow through the superficial temporal artery before and following anastomosis has been estimated to be between 10 and 120 ml/minute).(5,11,29) Within a matter of 1 to 2 weeks the diameter of this artery often doubles, thus providing a much larger flow than that measured intraoperatively.(1a,15) Schmiedek et al have reported significant postoperative increases in rCBF.(30,31) Blood has also been shown to flow both proximally and distally from the point of anastomosis.(5) This changes the direction and degree of preexisting collateral flow, which explains the postoperative improvements in contralateral rCBF following microanastomosis. The increase in rCBF which we have reported previously as well as in this chapter amounts to approximately 20% over the preoperative level in the middle cerebral artery distribution. In the random sample of 12 patients analyzed by digital computer (Table 22.6), rCBF was decreased to approximately 57% of normal preoperatively, but rose to approximately 67% of normal postoperatively. This increase appears larger over the parietal region because the site of anastomosis most frequently involves a middle cerebral artery recipient in this region. The relief of TIA symptoms or the improvement in the neurologic deficit in minor stroke victims is attributed to the measured change in cortical Po_2 following anastomosis.(2,3) This has been shown to be accompanied by an increase in the oxidized level of cortical cytochrome a,a_3 measured intraoperatively. In the absence of a decrease in substrate input to the mitochondrial respiratory chain, an increase in the oxidized level of cytochrome a,a_3 means an increase in O_2 utilization. In the absence of uncoupling, this implies an increase in oxidative phosphorylation and ATP formation. Currently, we conclude that this is associated with an increase in membrane resting potential. The raised threshold for abnormal neuronal discharge and, in some instances, the increased membrane resting potential to a level where revived neuronal activity is possible are the probable causes of clinical improvement.

Appendix I: Regional CBF measurement by intravenous isotope injection technique

The intravenous bolus injection technique is somewhat similar to the inhalation technique, originally proposed by Mallet and Veal(24) and subsequently modified by Obrist.(28) However, in a number of ways it appears to have advantages over the inhalation technique which will become clearer during the discussion. It is a simpler method of injection and requires less equipment. Also, it is less likely to cause isotope contamination of the frontal sinuses.

Four scintillation detectors are used over each hemisphere in the prefrontal, rolandic, temporal, and parietal areas. An additional detector is used to record the gamma activity in the end-expired air by means of a plastic tube leading from a face mask to a scintillation detector 5 feet from the patient's body. From this point the air is evacuated to an outside vent by a constant suction pump. The end-expired air is recorded because it has been shown to be proportional to the arterial concentration of isotope. This is due to the fact that the gaseous isotope ^{133}Xe is extremely soluble in air. The recording from all scintillation detectors is continued for 35 to 40 minutes for analysis of a 3-compartment system or for 12 minutes for analysis of a so-called 2-compartment system. Each recording channel is permanently stored on a computer disk. In addition, the record from the end-expired air curve and from all eight head probes is visualized on a cathode ray tube (CRT) at the time of the test to monitor the injection and subsequent activity. The isotope concentration curves recorded from each probe are analyzed for computing cerebral blood flow by assuming that the Fick equation holds individually for each compartment. In the long recording (35 to 40 minutes) a 3-compartment system is assumed. This consists of an initial fast (gray matter), slow (white matter), and slower compartment from the extracerebral tissue. The latter is comprised of blood flow in the dura, bone, and scalp. For the purpose of analysis, it is considered to be a single compartment showing one component in the recorded head curve. In the brief 12-minute flow technique, the white matter and extracerebral components are lumped together and only the gray matter flow is assumed to be salvageable. In its analysis, however, gray matter flow by the 12-minute method is virtually the same as that recorded by the 35- 40-minute method. Rather than solving the integrated form of the Fick equation, ie, the convolution integral, by digital means, it has sometimes been appropriate to compute the cerebral blood flow by solving the Fick equation individually for each compartment by analog computer. This was the technique used for analysis in the first 500 patients. Subsequently, digital computer analysis has been adopted because of its speed and the fact that it does not require an analog computer operator. Nevertheless, in the Loma Linda University laboratory, the analog technique, in modified form for digital computer analysis as described below, is still retained. When any discrepancy arises in the routine digital computer flow analysis, the analog method is used to check possible sources of error. There is no significant difference between the two methods of analysis in terms of gray matter flow.

Analog Computer Analysis

For analog computer analysis, the Fick equation is first converted to its voltage-simulated form for solution, where the voltage is proportional to the isotope concentrations. The Fick equation is slightly rearranged to become more appropriate for analog computer evaluation. The solution is first carried out by trial-and-error fit of the extracerebral component by making the simplifying assumption that, after 24 minutes, the gray matter and white matter have completely cleared of isotope. Therefore, after 25 minutes, the remainder of the curve is extracerebral and it is assumed that this can be fitted by a monexponential form.(4,8,9) It is known that clearance of the gray matter is concluded by 4.5 minutes in normals. It is assumed, on the basis of experience with the internal carotid technique, that even in pathologic cases the gray matter will have cleared by 10 minutes. Thereafter, the Fick equation is solved and fitted to the white matter component since the head curve is assumed to consist of only extracerebral plus white matter clearance curves after the 10-minute point. Finally, the remaining early portion of the head curve is fitted for the gray matter component by summing the first part, ie, the gray matter solution, to the sum of the white and extracerebral components. By projecting the solutions of the analog computer through a cathode ray oscilloscope and down through a lens system onto the recorded inkwriter curve from each of the scintillation detectors, it is possible to obtain an exact fit by adding on and fitting each component successively.(8) Control and pathologic values for flows compare favorably with those of the internal carotid method.

Relative tissue weights may also be obtained with the IV analog method through a modification of Obrist's equation.(28) By taking the point where the gray and white matter curves cross, a considerable simplification is introduced. This provides the particular time at which the gray matter and white matter are equal, thus simplifying the computation.

12-Minute IV Method Using Analog Computer Analysis

It can be seen that in the first 10 minutes, both the IV bolus method(6) and the inhalation method(28) preferentially saturate the intracranial contents with isotope in comparison to the extracerebral components. This forms the basis for a 2-compartment analysis. Following brief IV injection of ^{133}Xe, the gamma activity is monitored for 12 minutes by four probes over each side of the head. An additional probe monitors the end-expired air curve used to approximate the arterial function. One assumes a 2-compartment system of gray matter flow lasting up to 8 minutes, and white matter plus extracerebral flow continued after 8 minutes. The analog method is used to solve and fit the Fick equation for each of the two compartments, with a function generator input for the A(t) curve.

Digital Computer for Analog-type Analysis

Since the digital computer simultaneous solution method of obtaining flows for the three compartments has been developed (see Appendix II for the mathematical derivation) the analog technique has been modified as follows. The envelope of the expired-air curve is displayed on a CRT and fitted with a multiple exponential function generator to obtain A(t). Instead of three successive solutions of the Fick equation, we now successively solve and fit its integrated form, ie, the convolution integral, for each compartment; first, for the extracerebral component, then for the white matter, and finally the gray matter component. The fitting is done by trial and error, with initial guesses for the values of K_1 (f_1/λ_1); and W_1, the relative weights. By adjusting these values for each compartment, a perfect fit is finally obtained for the head curve recorded from each probe. This can be used for either a 2- or 3-compartment model.

Digital Computer for Simultaneous Solution of Flow Values

The digital computer method for simultaneously obtaining the flow values for each compartment is based on the use of a least squares minimization technique. (Appendix II) This involves the simultaneous solution of six equations in six unknowns, ie, the values of K_1 and W_1 for each component of an assumed 3-compartment system. Initial guesses are selected in the mid-range for each value of K_1 and W_1. By an iteration technique, the error term is gradually reduced to a minimum, and the correct values for K_i and W_i are obtained. A similar procedure is used for simultaneous solution of a 12-minute, 2-compartment model.

Originally, 5 to 10 mc of ^{133}Xe dissolved in 0.5 ml of saline were injected as a bolus. In the past 2 years, the injection has been increased to 15 to 20 mc of ^{133}Xe since this still remains well within the safe limits of dosimetry, but provides a much higher count rate over the head, ie, a peak head count of at least 60K.

The head probes, 18 mm in diameter, are positioned as follows. The prefrontal probe is placed 6 cm anterior to the tip of the ear, 6 cm above the zygoma, and parallel to the base of the skull. This minimizes possible contamination from the air sinuses. Probes have cylindric collimation. Parietal probes are placed at the level of the top of the ear, but 2.5 cm posteriorly. The rolandic or central probe is placed at the midpoint of nasion-inion line and 5 cm from the midline. The temporal probe is placed 2 cm above the zygoma and just anterior to the exterior auditory canal. These are reproducible positions, but in sick, hospitalized stroke patients the sites of probe position are marked with indelible ink in order to reproduce the head probe position.

Basic Assumptions

The following are the main basic assumptions involved in the IV isotope injection method for measuring rCBF.

1. The gaseous isotope ^{133}Xe is freely diffusible and is not metabolized
2. The analysis of rCBF is conducted on blood flows occurring through a 3-compartment system in parallel: gray matter (fast), white matter (slower), and extracerebral (slowest)
3. The extracerebral compartment is assumed to consist of only one slow component with a half-time of approximately 30 minutes
4. The envelope of the end-expired air recording is proportional to the arterial concentration of isotope
5. The Fick equation, or its integrated form, the convolution integral, is assumed to hold for each compartment

Possible Sources of Error in the Measurement of CBF by IV Isotope Method

Inadequate Isotope in Brain

Approximately 80 to 90% of isotope is released through the lungs after intravascular injection. Since only 15 to 20% of the cardiac output of isotope goes to the brain, there could be an insignificant amount of isotope in the brain following an IV bolus injection to give a satisfactory signal-to-noise ratio. To test this theory, the authors have made CBF measurements with internal carotid injections of as little as 25 μc in several patients. This seems to provide an adequate signal-to-noise ratio and is probably close to the limits of resolution of our instrument.

Contamination of Head Count from Air in Sinuses

It is possible that air in the frontal or sphenoidal sinuses could contribute to the overall head count due to the high partition coefficient for air compared to blood. This would depend on the size of the air sinuses and the probe position. Since the frontal and sphenoidal sinuses are located in the frontal part of the skull one would expect the frontal count to be considerably higher than that of the parietal probe. We have not found this to be so. To avoid this type of contamination we position probes well above (2.5 cm) the line of the zygoma and 3 cm back from the frontal sinuses.

Contamination from Radioactivity in Expired Air

Agnoli and his colleagues(1,1a) mentioned radioactive contamination from expired air as a possibility for explaining their high count in the first few seconds. By comparing simultaneously the peak head count and expired air count on the same scale, this appeared to be unlikely. There is a lag of 30 to 40 seconds between the expired air peak and the head count peak. In two cases we measured CBF by the IV technique in patients who had had tracheostomy. Since the expired air is evacuated from the tracheostomy tube and does not pass through the mouth or nose from the lungs, there should be a significant drop in initial head count if the expired air in the mouth or nasal pharynx was making an important contribution to the initial part of the head curve. This did not appear to be true.

Recirculation of Isotope

Recirculation of isotope is inconsequential after the internal carotid injection method, but must be considered after a bolus injection. This is because the isotope is taken up and released at different rates by tissues other than the brain. For this reason the arterial concentration becomes a function of time. This factor is taken into consideration by deconvolution of the head curve, and generating electronically the envelope of the end-expired air curve.

The End-expired Air Curve is Not Always a True Approximation of the Arterial Isotope Concentration

In patients with normal pulmonary function, it has been demonstrated that with xenon inhalation the concentration of ^{133}Xe in the end-expired air is virtually proportional to the concentration in the arterial blood. There is a time lag of 6 to 9 seconds. We have been impressed with the ease of monitoring the end-expired air in stuporous patients as long as Cheyne-Stokes or any other severe respiratory irregularity was not present. In these instances, the approximation is not suitable and should not be used in cases of severe pulmonary disease.

Error Due to Extracerebral Component

When recording over the head after an IV bolus injection of ^{133}Xe, there is an extracerebral component in addition to the fast and slow cerebral components (average gray and average white matter). We assume that because of its small amplitude, the extracerebral component may be reasonably fitted by a monoexponential having a $t_{0.5}$ of 25 to 30 minutes. However, it is known from the work of others that the extracerebral component also has a small faster portion with a $t_{0.5}$ of 2 to 3 minutes. This could lead to a small error which would decrease the gray matter slope, and lead to a slower gray matter flow. The average gray matter flow (Fg) in controls of 77 ± 11 ml/100 g/minute compares favorably with the internal carotid values of 80 ± 11 and lead us to believe that the extracerebral component results in no major error. Furthermore, the manner in which Fg is decreased in pathologic cases appears consistent with results in the same patient as determined by an internal carotid measurement.

Estimation of Dosimetry

The number of rads absorbed by the tissue, following a 10 mc IV injection, is quite small. We estimate this as follows:

$$D = \frac{A}{m} \qquad \text{(dosimetry equation)}$$

where:

D = dose in rads
A = mc=hours
m = mass of tissue exposed
ϕ = specific absorbed fraction
Δ = equilibrium dose constant—rads/mc=hour (specific for ^{133}Xe)

Now,

$$A = N\lambda$$

where:

λ = effective disintegration rate = $0.693/t_{0.5}$
N = number of mc
$t_{0.5}$(effective) = $t_{0.5}$ (Biol.). When $t_{0.5}$ (Biol.) is $<<$ $t_{0.5}$ (physical), $1/\lambda$ + t (average time in lung) = $1.44\ t_{0.5}$ (effective)
A = mc $\times$ 1.44 (effective)
Av. Lung 1,000 g
d(lung) = $10^4 \times 1.44 \times 0.5 \times \Sigma\Phi\Delta$
$\Sigma\Phi\Delta$ = 0.01
D = 0.072 rads (for 10 mc injection ^{133}Xe)

and

D (brain) = 1.5 mrads
D (total body) = 5 mrads

The total body dose is negligible. The lung dose is about the equivalent of one chest x-ray. The brain dose is the equivalent of about one-eighth of an angiogram.

Appendix II: Derivation of Digital Computer Analysis

Assume that cerebral blood flow following an intravenous (IV) isotope injection is measured through three compartments in parallel, consisting of a fast (gray matter), slow (white matter), and slowest (extracerebral) component. Assume also that extracerebral flow occurs in a single slow compartment.

Let C_i = concentration of isotope in the ith compartment and, from the Fick equation,

$$\frac{dC_i}{dt} = f_i (A - C_i/\lambda_i) \qquad (1)$$

where

A = arterial concentration of isotope as a function of time

f_i = perfusion flow through the ith compartment in ml/100 g/minute

λ_i = tissue-to-blood partition coefficient of isotope (^{133}Xe) for the ith compartment

t = time in minutes

$K_i = f_i/\lambda_i$

Equation 1 is a first-order linear differential equation. Transposing and multiplying by the integrating factor e^{Kt}, integration then yields

$$C = W\lambda Ke^{-Kt} {}_0\!\int^t A(\tau)e^{K\tau} \, d\tau$$

where τ = a dummy variable, or

$$C_i = W_i \lambda_i K_i e^{-K_i t} {}_0\!\int^t A(\tau)e^{K_i\tau} \, d\tau = f(t,K_i,W_i) \qquad (2)$$

W_i = relative weight of the ith compartment combined with a proportionality factor

Now express as a Taylor series the function $f(t,K_i,W_i)$ as it takes on the values of $f(t,K_i + \epsilon K_i, W_i + \epsilon W_i)$ when(26),

1. K_i has a value $K_i + \epsilon K_i$ near to a given fixed value K_i
2. W_i has a value $W_i + \epsilon W_i$ near to a given fixed value W_i

Then, omitting the subscript i and dropping terms of second and higher order,

$$T = f(t,K + \epsilon K, W + \epsilon W) = f(t,K,W) + \epsilon K \frac{\delta f}{\delta K} + \epsilon W \frac{\delta f}{\delta W} \qquad (3)$$

Expanding Equation 3, one obtains

$$\frac{\delta f}{\delta K} = \lambda We^{-Kt}\!\int Ae^{K\tau}d\tau - W\lambda Kte^{-Kt}\!\int Ae^{K\tau} \, d\tau +$$

$$W\lambda Ke^{-Kt}\!\int \tau Ae^{K\tau} \, d\tau = \text{``B''}$$

$$\frac{\delta f}{\delta W} = \lambda Ke^{-Kt}\!\int Ae^{K\tau} \, d\tau = \text{``D''}$$

and

$$f(t,K,W) = C$$

Then the difference between the theoretical and observed values at each point becomes

$$T - [C + \epsilon KB + \epsilon WD]$$

In order to minimize the difference between the observed and calculated results, we proceed as follows. Assume that the most likely values of the small constants ϵK and ϵW are those for which the sum of the squares of the differences between the observed and calculated results are minimal. Proceeding with the least squares formula,(26)

$$S = [T - (C + \epsilon KB + \epsilon WD)]^2 \qquad (4)$$

Then

$$S = T^2 + C^2 - 2CT - 2\epsilon KBT + 2\epsilon KBC - 2\epsilon WDT \qquad (5)$$
$$+ 2\epsilon WCD + 2\epsilon K\epsilon WBD + (\epsilon KB)^2 + (\epsilon WD)^2$$

Minimizing Equation 4 by equating the partial derivatives of Equation 5 with respect to ϵK and ϵW to zero gives(12,26)

$$\frac{\delta s}{\delta \epsilon k} = -2BT + 2BC + 2\epsilon WBD + 2\epsilon KB^2 = 0 \qquad (6)$$

$$\frac{\delta s}{\delta \epsilon W} = -2DT + 2CD + 2\epsilon KBD + 2\epsilon WD^2 = 0 \qquad (7)$$

or

$$BB\epsilon K + BD\epsilon W = B(T - C) \qquad (8)$$
$$BD\epsilon K + DD\epsilon W = D(T - C) \qquad (9)$$

In matrix formulation Equations 8 and 9 can be written

$$\begin{bmatrix} BB & BD \\ BD & DD \end{bmatrix} \begin{bmatrix} \epsilon K \\ \epsilon W \end{bmatrix} = \begin{bmatrix} B(T - C) \\ D(T - C) \end{bmatrix}$$

or

$$A_{ij} \cdot X_i = Y_j$$
$$X = A^{-1}Y$$

Similar equations to Equations 6 and 7 are formulated for each of the three compartments giving six equations in the six unknown error terms. In practice, initial values for K_i and W_i are selected in the middle of the expected range of each parameter. Since second- and higher-order terms have been dropped in the Taylor series expansion, the initial values obtained for the error terms are only approximations. The computation procedure is, therefore, reiterated using updated values of K_i and W_i until no further significant improvement is obtained. The digital computer program for this was written by one of the authors (Laffin) and is one component of a software system that is obtainable on request. In a subsequent article, the effects of number of counts per minute, duration of recording, added noise, and significance of the expired air curve envelope will be discussed. The programs were written in Fortran and are run on a PDP 11/10 computer. Analysis of the 3-compartment, 40-minute recording curves requires 120 seconds per curve, whereas analysis of the 2-compartment, 12-minute recording curves takes only 20 seconds per curve.

REFERENCES

1. Agnoli A, Prencipe M, Priori AM, Bozzao L, Fieshchi C: Measurement of the rCBF by intravenous injection of 133-Xe. A comparative study with the intraarterial injection method. In: Brock M, Fieschchi C, Ingvar D, Lassen N, Schurmann K (eds): Cerebral Blood Flow. Berlin Heidelberg, Springer-Verlag, 1969
1a. Agnoli A, Prencipe M, Priori A, Bozzao L, Gullotta C, Fieshchi C: Present status of the technique employing intravenous injection of 133-Xe for measuring regional cerebral blood flow. In: Cerebral Blood Flow, Pitman Medical and Scientific Publishing, 1970
2. Austin G, Haugen G, LaManna J, et al: Cortical oxidative metabolism during microanastomosis for cerebral ischemia. Presented at the American Physiological Society, Anaheim, 1976. In press.
3. Austin G, Haugen G, Schuler W: Transient ischemic attacks and metabolic aspects of their relief by microneurosurgical anastomosis. In Fein J, Reichman OH (eds): Microvascular Anastomosis for Cerebral Ischemia. New York, Springer-Verlag, 1977.
4. Austin G, Horn N, Rouhe S, et al: Description and early results of an intravenous radioisotope technique for measuring regional cerebral blood flow in man. Presented at the Fifth International Symposium on CBF. Eur Neurol 8:43, 1972
5. Austin G, Laffin D, Evans R, et al: Microcerebral anastomosis for the prevention of stroke. Proceedings of the International Symposium of Microneurosurgery, Kyoto, 1973, Tokyo, 1975, pp. 47–67
6. Austin G, Laffin D, Hayward W: Evaluation of fast component (gray matter) by 12 minute IV method using analog computer analysis. In Harper AM (ed): Blood Flow and Metabolism in the Brain. Edinburgh, Churchill Livingstone, 1976, pp. 8.25–8.29
7. Austin G, Laffin D, Hayward W: Physiological factors in the selection of patients for superficial temporal artery to middle cerebral anastomoses. Presented at the Society of University Surgeons, St. Louis, Missouri, February 1974. Surgery 75(6):861, 1974
8. Austin G, Laffin D, Hayward W: Cerebral blood flow in patients undergoing microanastomosis for modification or prevention of stroke. Presented at the 25th Anniversary Meeting of the Association of Clinical Scientists, Philadelphia, 1974. Ann Clin Lab Sci 5(4):229, 1975
9. Austin G, Laffin D, Rouhe S, et al: Intravenous isotope injection method of cerebral blood flow measurement. In Methodology II. New York, Springer-Verlag, 1975
10. Austin G, Schuler W, Haugen G, et al: Simulated transient ischemic attacks in cat and man. Presented at Third International Symposium on Microneurosurgery for Cerebral Ischemia, June 1976. In press

11. Chater N, Peters N: Neurosurgical microvascular bypass for stroke. West J Med 124:1, 1976

12. Cooper L, Steinberg D: Introduction to Methods of Optimization. Philadelphia, Saunders, 1970

13. Crawley JCW: An analogue computer for calculating blood perfusion rates. Biomed Eng 3:256, 1968

14. Crawley JCW, Veall N: Recent developments in the [133]xenon inhalation technique for cerebral flow. J Nucl Biol Med 19:205, 1975

15. Crowell RM: Electromagnetic flow studies of superficial temporal artery to middle cerebral branch artery bypass graft. Presented at the First International Symposium on Microneurosurgical Anastomoses for Cerebral Ischemia, Loma Linda, California. In Austin G (ed): Microneurosurgical Anastomoses for Cerebral Ischemia. Springfield, Ill, Thomas, 1976, pp. 116–124

16. Harper A, Glass H, Stephen J, et al: The measurement of the local blood flow in the cerebral cortex for the clearance of xenon. J. Neurol Neurosurg Psychiat 27:255, 1964

17. Harper AM: Autonomic control of cerebral blood flow. In Whisnat JP, Sandok BA (eds): Cerebral Vascular Diseases. New York, Grune & Stratton, 1975, pp 27–47

18. Hoedt-Rasmussen K, Sveinsdotter E, Lassen NA: Regional cerebral blood flow in man determined by the intra-arterial injection of a radioactive inert gas. Circ Res 18:237, 1966

19. Ingvar DH, Lassen NA: Methods for cerebral blood flow measurement in man. Br J Anaesth 27:216, 1965

20. Jobsis FF, LaManna J: Kinetic aspects of intracellular redox reactions. In vivo effects during and after hypoxia and ischemia. In Robin ED (ed): The Extrapulmonary Manifestations of Respiratory Diseases. 1976, in press

21. Kety SS: The physiology of the cerebral circulation in man. In McMichael J (ed): Proceedings of the Harvey Tercentenary Conference. Oxford, Blackwell, 1957, p 237

22. Kety SS: Measurement of local circulation within the brain by means of inert, diffusible tracers. Examination of the theory, assumptions, and possible sources of error. Acta Neurol Scand (Suppl) 14:20, 1965

23. Kety SS, Schmidt CF: Nitrous oxide method for quantitative determination of cerebral blood flow in man. J Clin Invest 27:476, 1948

24. Mallet BL, Veal N: Investigation of cerebral blood flow in hypertension, using radioactive-xenon inhalation and extracranial recording. Lancet 1:1081, 1963

25. McHenry L Jr, Jaffe M, Kawamura H, et al: I. Effect of papaverine on regional blood flow in focal vascular disease of the brain. N Engl J Med 282:1167, 1970

26. Mellor JC: Higher Mathematics for Students of Chemistry and Physics, 4th ed. New York, Dover, 1955

27. Nilsson B, Norberg K, Seisjo K: Biochemical events in cerebral ischaemia. Br J Anaesth 47:751, 1975

28. Obrist WD, Thompson HG, King CH, et al: Determination of regional cerebral blood flow by inhalation of [133]-xenon. Circ Res 20:124, 1967

29. Reichman O, Satovich W, Davis DO, et al: Collateral circulation to the middle cerebral artery, etc. In Avicenum G (ed): Proceedings

of the Fourth European Congress of Neurosurgery, 1971. Prague, Czechoslovakia Medical Press, 1972

30. Schmiedek P, Steinhoff H, Gratzl O, et al: rCBF measurements in patients treated for cerebral ischemia by extra-intracranial vascular anastomosis. Eur Neurol 6:354, 1971–1972

31. Schmiedek P, Steinhoff H, Gratzl O: Selection of patients for extra-intracranial arterial bypass surgery based on rCBF measurements. J. Neurosurg 44:303, 1976

32. Schuler W, Austin G, Laffin D, et al: Autoregulation of cerebral blood flow in patients with transient ischemic attacks. Presented at the Federation of Western Societies of Neurological Sciences, Santa Barbara, February, 1976. In Austin G (ed): Contemporary Aspects of Cerebrovascular Disease. Professional Information Library, Dallas, Texas. 1976, pp 215–219

33. Schuler W, Lichter E, Austin G: Autoregulation in patients with brain ischemia. Presented at the Sixth Annual Meeting of the Society for Neuroscience, Toronto, November 1976

34. Ueda, H, Hatano S, Molde T, Gondoaira T: Discussion on compartmental analysis of the human brain blood flow. Acta Neurol Scand 41(14):88, 1965

VI
CLINICAL RESULTS

23

Progression of middle cerebral artery stenosis to occlusion without symptoms following superficial temporary artery bypass: Case report[1]

Norman L. Chater and Philip R. Weinstein

A case of clinically silent progression of middle cerebral artery (MCA) stenosis to complete occlusion following superficial temporal artery to MCA anastomosis is presented. This case suggests the possible prophylactic benefit of collateral augmentation surgery.

Clinical History

A 54-year-old black female schoolteacher suffered two attacks of left hemiparesis and numbness lasting 48 to 72 hours. The second attack occurred while she was in Ralph K. Davies Medical Center under a regimen of anticoagulation therapy and restricted activity. Arteriograms at that time revealed an 80% stenosis of the right middle cerebral artery with no evidence on the arch studies of a proximal source for emboli. The hemiparesis resolved and a right superficial temporal artery bypass was performed without complications in February 1973. Arteriograms obtained 1 week postoperatively showed a patent and well-functioning bypass.

The patient has remained asymptomatic since then, without transient attacks of any kind. Follow-up arteriograms at 1 year, performed to evaluate the bypass, revealed that middle cerebral stenosis had progressed to complete occlusion without associated symptoms (Fig. 23.1). The middle cerebral artery beyond the occlusion now receives substantial blood flow through the bypass, as demonstrated by selective external carotid artery arteriogram. As expected, the diameter of the superficial temporal artery has enlarged (Fig. 23.2).

[1]Presented at the Second International Symposium on Microsurgical Anastomosis for Cerebral Ischemia, Chicago, June 22, 1974

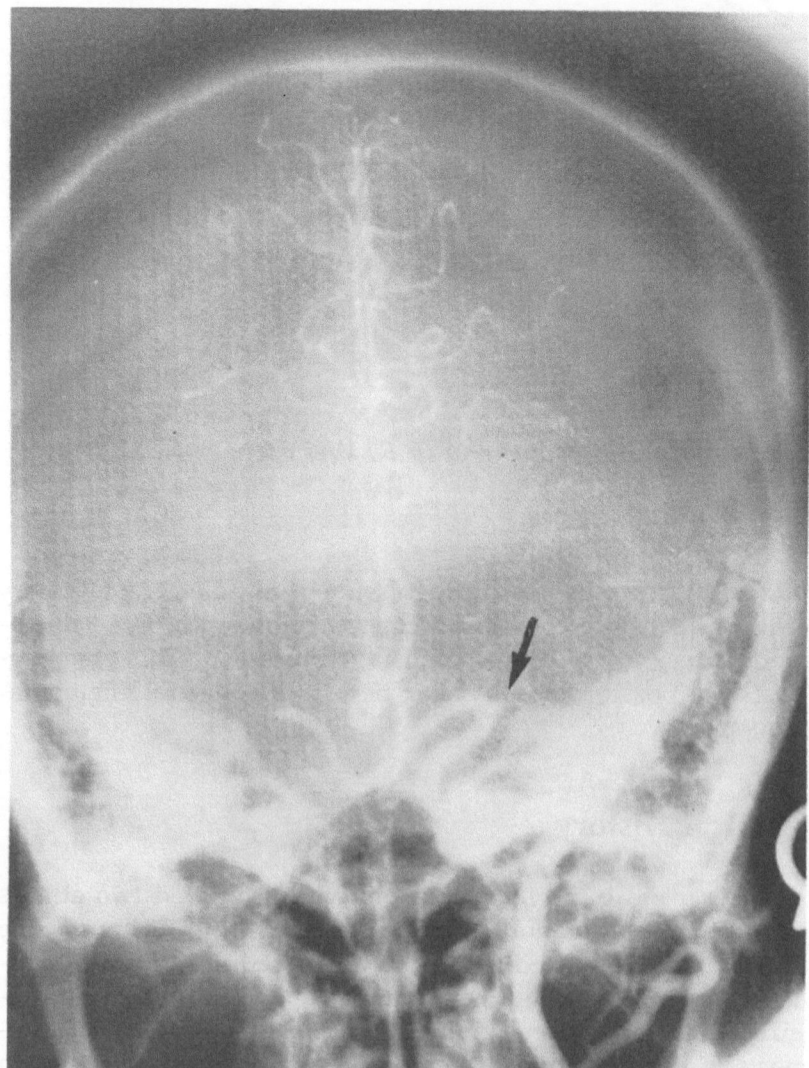

Fig. 23.1. Left internal carotid arteriogram showing progression to occlusion of the origin of the middle cerebral artery 1 year after superficial temporal artery bypass relieved intractable transient hemiparetic attacks.

Discussion

In the past several years there has been considerable interest in microsurgical cerebral revascularization. Many critical problems remain to be solved before the effectiveness of this operative approach can be established. Key issues to be resolved include long-term patency, effect on the quality of life, and, of greatest importance, protection against a completed stroke. Results may then be compared to the natural history of cerebrovascular disease and the anticipated incidence of fixed ischemic damage following transient ischemic warning attacks.

Recent reports have documented the low mortality and morbidity rates of this surgical procedure.(1) Relief of transient attacks has occurred in 80% of patients and quality of life seems

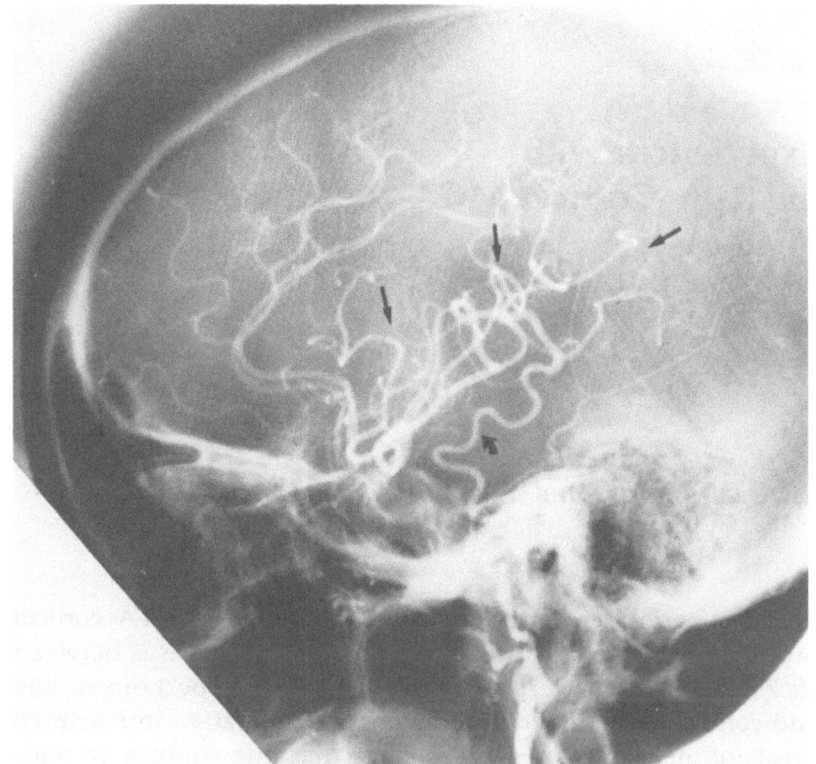

Fig. 23.2. Selective left external carotid arteriogram showing extensive perfusion of the middle cerebral artery branches distal to the occlusion through the bypass.

to be improved. In our study of 100 cases of cerebrovascular occlusive disease treated by extra- to intracranial bypass, the incidence of ipsilateral completed stroke (average follow-up, 18 months) was 2%; in one of these cases, the bypass was nonfunctioning. Other reports suggest that the anticipated incidence of completed stroke after transient ischemic attacks is much higher, and in the Mayo Clinic analysis after 2 years' follow-up it was 22%.(2)

Conclusion

Cases such as the one presented here provide furher presumptive evidence that extra- to intracranial bypass may prevent cerebral infarction in patients at high risk due to symptomatic preocclusive intracranial lesions.

REFERENCES

1. Chater N, Popp J: Microsurgical vascular bypass for occlusive cerebrovascular disease. Review of 100 cases. Surg Neurol 6:115, 1976
2. Whisnant J, Matsumoto N, Lila E: Transient cerebral ischemic attacks in Rochester, Minnesota, 1945–1969. Mayo Clin Proc 48:194, 1973

24

Experiences with
the STA–Cortical MCA anastomosis
in 46 cases

M. Gazi Yasargil and Yasuhiro Yonekawa

We have performed the superficial temporal artery (STA–cortical middle cerebral artery (MCA) anastomosis on 46 cases between 1967 and 1974. The purpose of this paper is to report our results and consider the data derived from intraoperative intraarterial pressure measurements. We believe that this study may reinforce the theoretical background for this type of operation.

Cases and Results

The clinical classification suggested by Dr. C. M. Fischer was used (personal communication, 1970). The results are listed in Table 24.1. In two cases the operation was performed as prophylaxis for cerebral ischemia in the surgical treatment of giant aneurysms (ophthalmic and middle cerebral). The group labeled "Others" in Table 24.1 includes patients with transient ischemic attacks (TIA) or reversible ischemic neurologic deficits (RIND), with minor or moderate neurologic deficits.

Table 24.2 lists the angiographically verified occlusive lesions in our cases. Middle cerebral occlusive disease occurred in only about 23% of the cases. A patient who suffers from TIA or RIND with or without a moderate neurologic deficit, and who demonstrates bilateral occlusion of the internal carotid artery, might be one of the best candidates for this operation.

Follow-up angiography was performed on 23 cases (Table 24.3) after at least 1 week had elapsed. Thus, the phase of vasospasm secondary to the operative procedure could be avoided. The overall patency rate was 80%. Neurologic improvement in the face of an occluded graft should be carefully evaluated.

The frequencies of the complication encountered are listed

Table 24.1. Categories and results (N = 46)

	Total cases	Improved	Unchanged	Worse
ICA				
TIA	5	3	—	2
Fixed neurologic				
deficit	8	7	—	1
Others	19	13	6	—
MCA				
TIA	—	—	—	—
Fixed neurologic				
deficit	5	2	3	—
Others	5	5	—	—
Miscellaneous				
Four-vessel	1	1	—	—
occlusion (TIA)				
Moyamoya	1	—	1	—
Aneurysm	2	—	2	—
Total	44(46)	31(71%)	10(22%)	3(7%)

Table 24.2. Angiographically verified lesions (N = 44)

	No. cases
One carotid	13 (occlusion: 6)
Both carotids	10 (bilateral occlusion: 2)
Both carotids and	7
vertebral(s)	
Middle cerebral	10 (occlusion: 6)
Other multiple	4

Table 24.3. Angiographic patency (N = 23)

	No. cases
Patent anastomosis	18(80%)
Persistent TIA	1
Stroke	1
Occluded anastomosis	5(20%)
Improvement	2

in Table 24.4. Marginal necrosis of the skin flap was one of the problems managed satisfactorily by conservative treatment. Epilepsy occurs in about 10% of cases soon after operation. In one case a single tiny perforating branch was coagulated to dissect a recipient cortical artery, but this was apparently enough to produce postoperative epilepsy. Postoperative subdural hematoma should be strictly avoided. A thin subdural hematoma was enough to cause persistent aphasia and severe

Table 24.4. Complications

	No. cases
Infection	
Skin flap	2
Systemic	1
Skin flap necrosis	5
Subdural hematoma	2
Epilepsy	5
Graft occlusion	5
Late stroke	2
Early death	2
Systemic infection	1
Stroke	1

hemiparesis in a case of TIA. A small hematoma might be sufficient to induce irreversible neurologic deficits in the presence of cerebral ischemia.

Measurement of Intraarterial Pressure of the STA and Cortical MCA

Methods and Results

A silastic tube filled with heparin solution is introduced into the distal and proximal parts of the cortical MCA through an elliptical opening which has been prepared for end-to-side anastomosis. The STA is similarly cannulated. The radial or brachial artery is punctured with an 18-gauge needle. The arteries are connected to a Statham model P23 transducer and pressure waves are recorded. After the measurement, the operative procedure for the STA–cortical MCA anastomosis is continued.

These measurements were performed on five cases (Fig. 24.1). "Normal" values are from the data of Bakay and Sweet.(1) From our results one might conclude that there is a greater pressure gradient between the STA and cortical MCA in cases with cerebrovascular occlusive disease than in cases without such disease.

Discussion

It is now well accepted that the extracranial-intracranial anastomosis using microsurgical technique offers new possibilities for the surgical treatment of cerebrovascular occlusive disease in cases which cannot be treated with conventional techniques of vascular surgery. Morbidity and mortality rates due to the

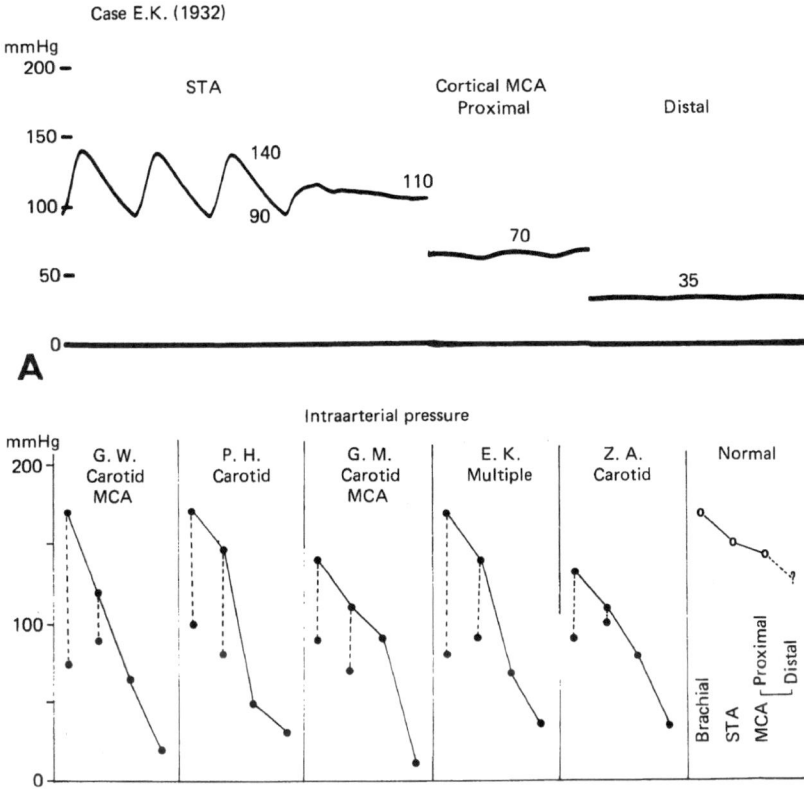

Case E.K. (1932)

Fig. 24.1. Recording of the intraarterial pressures in a case with multiple occlusive lesions. (b) Diagram of intraarterial pressures in five cases wth cerebrovascular occlusive disease.

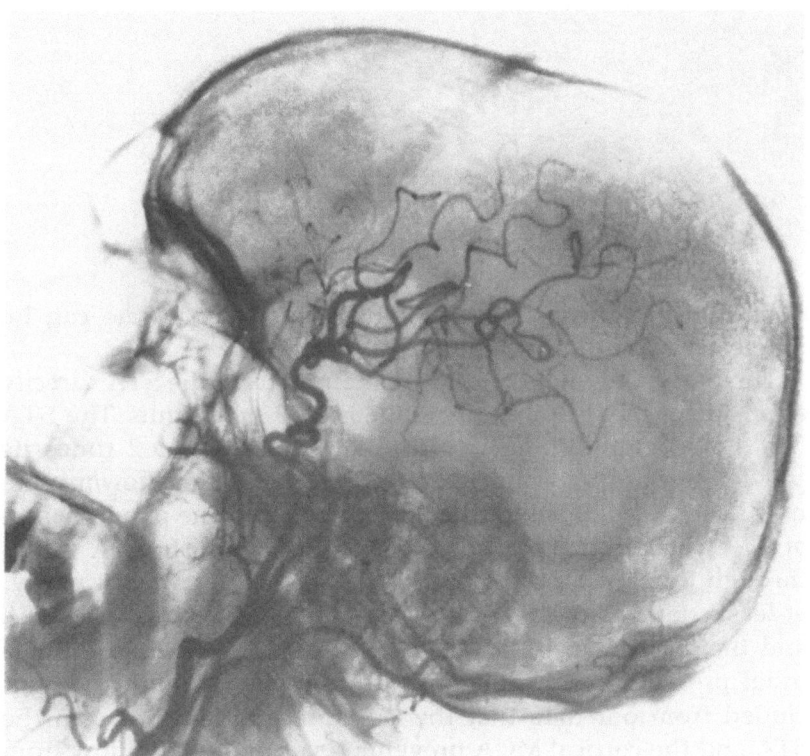

Fig. 24.2. Dilated STA that contributes entire filling of the MCA. Follow-up angiography 3 years after operation in a case with bilateral carotid occlusions.

Discussion

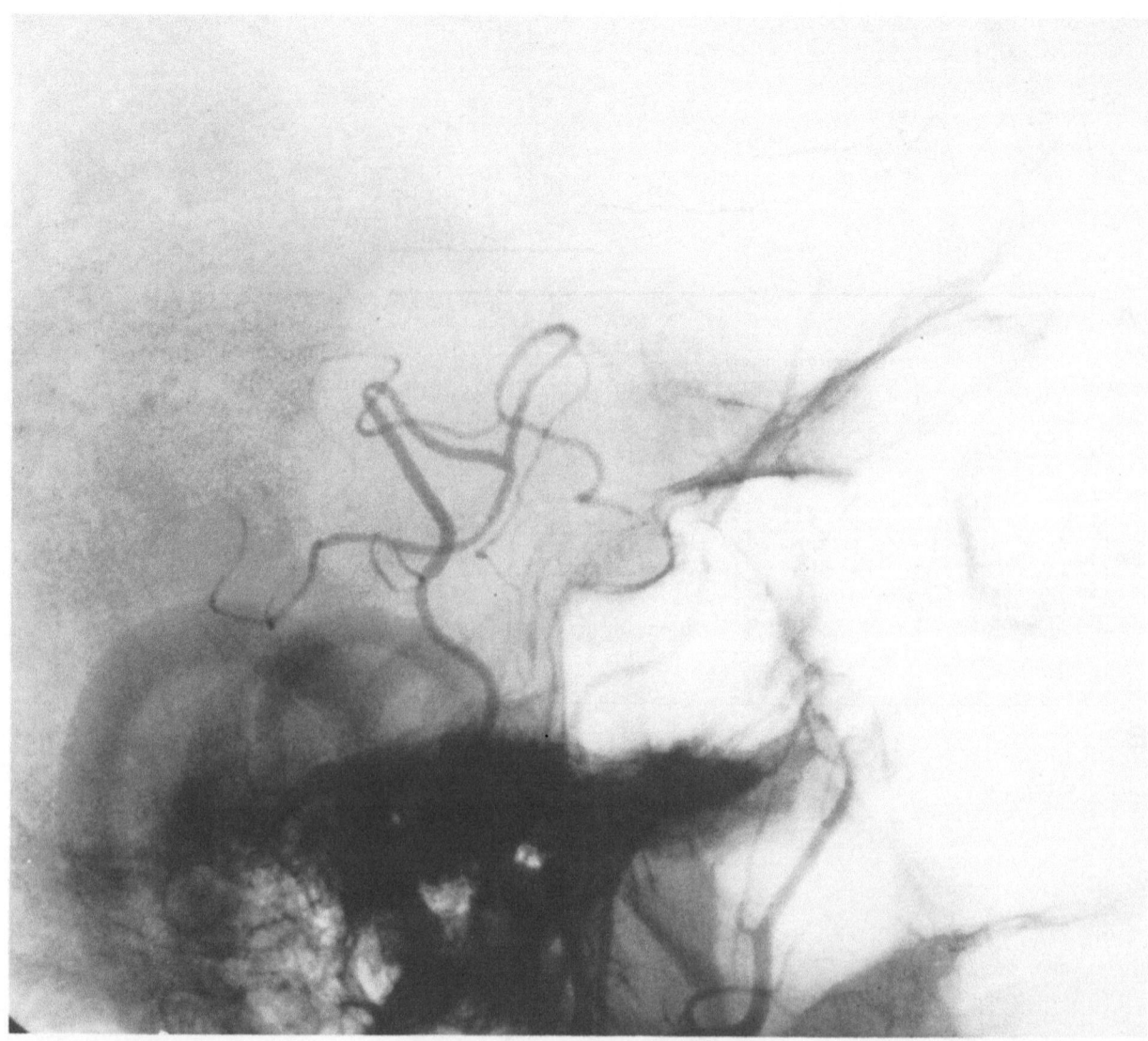

Fig. 24.3. Partial filling of the MCA through the STA in a case with siphon stenosis.

operation are small and acceptable. The patency rate can be increased by sufficient laboratory exercise.

The blood flow which can be obtained from the STA directly after operation is approximately 20 to 30 ml/minute. The STA has, however, the tendency to dilate up to 1.5 to 2 times its previous diameter, so that about 50 ml of blood flow/minute may later be available for the ischemic brain. The phenomenon of STA dilatation (Fig. 24.2), various degrees of MCA filling through the STA (Fig. 24.3, and the patency rate might partly, at least, depend upon the pressure gradient between the STA and the cortical MCA. Further measurement of these intraarterial pressures may elucidate these issues. It might be concluded from our data that the pressure gradient between the STA and the cortical MCA prevents reversal of blood flow from the intracranial to the extracranial circulation. Furthermore, the pressure gradient is larger in cases with occlusive disease than in cases without such disease.

Measurement of regional cerebral blood flow and the development of methods to detect a reversible neuronal injury due to ischemia may help us assess the precise indications for surgery.

REFERENCE

1. Bakay L, Sweet WH: Cervical and intracranial intraarterial pressure with and without vascular occlusion. Surg Gynecol Obstet 95:67, 1952

25

Clinical experiences
with STA–MCA anastomosis in 54 cases

Haruhiko Kikuchi and Jun Karaswaw

Since 1970 superficial temporal artery–middle cerebral artery (STA–MCA) anastomosis has been performed in 54 patients. These patients were randomized into six categories (Table 25.1). On the basis of this experience certain observations are pertinent. We have not noted a significant difference in the operative results when comparing patients with internal carotid lesions and patients with middle cerebral artery lesions. By far the best results were obtained when STA–MCA anastomosis was utilized as the treatment for patients suffering transient ischemic attacks with evidence of occlusive organic vascular lesions. We feel that patients with severe fixed neurologic deficits are not useful candidates for the procedure. The relationship of age to postoperative results is given in Table 25.2. We have not been able to relate the factor of age to a specific postoperative result. The duration from the onset of the first vascular insult to the time of surgery does not appear to be an important factor in postoperative prognosis (Table 25.3). The

Table 25.1. Location of lesion STA-MC anastomosis, 54 cases

Type of CVA	Location	Case	Clinical course	
			Improved	Unchanged
TIA	I. C.	3	3	0
	M. C.	3	3	0
Fixed deficits	I. C.	8	2	6
	M. C.	14	6	8
All others	I. C.	14	8	6
	M. C.	12	7	5
Total	I. C.	25	13	12
	M. C.	29	16	13

Table 25.2. Age distribution

Age	Case	Improved	Unchanged
10	1	1	0
20	3	2	1
30	9	4	5
40	12	5	7
50	15	9	6
60	12	7	5
70	2	1	1
Total	54	29	25

clinical syndrome is clearly the most important factor in deciding whether such operation may be useful.

Following the lead of Reichman's recent report we have attempted both suprasylvian selective anastomosis as well as double anastomoses. The latter method appears to be most indicated in patients with distal middle cerebral artery occlusion. Our criteria for selecting the recipient vessel were also influenced by the affected branch artery. The latter judgments were made by both angiographic and clinical findings.

STA suprasylvian anastomosis was performed in 11 cases. In seven of these cases clinical improvement was noted. The details of the angiographic findings and the cortical vessel to which anastomosis was performed are given in Table 25.4. Figures 25.1 to 25.3 are reproductions of arteriograms in which various vessels were used as recipient vessels successfully.

With experience and technical advance the patency rate of the anastomoses can be assured and is no longer the limiting factor in the successful microsurgical treatment of these patients. Selective grafting to suprasylvian vessels is now possible without fear of incurring a postoperative deficit from manipulation in this area. After establishing the STA–MCA circulation the anastomosis remained patent and hypertrophy of the superficial temporal artery was seen and is documented in one case in Figure 25.4. The indications for this operation still need to be developed further. Further methods need to be developed

Table 25.3. Time from first vascular accident to operation

	Case	Improved	Unchanged
<1M	5	4 (80%)	1 (20%)
<3M	9	7 (78%)	2 (22%)
<6M	11	5 (45%)	6 (55%)
<1Y	14	7 (50%)	7 (50%)
>1Y	15	6 (40%)	9 (60%)
	54	29	25

Table 25.4. Case of distal MC occlusion (11 cases)
7 cases improved clinically

Case	Age	Occluded Vessels	Host Vessels
T. S.	47	except angul. a.	roland. a., post. temp. a.
K. O.	46	except post. temp. a.	angul. a.
S. M.	57	except mid. temp. a.	angul. a., post. pariet. a.
M. I.	54	except post. temp. a.	roland. a., post. temp. a.
K. H.	38	post. temp. a.	post. temp. a.
M. A.	60	angul. a. & post. temp. a.	post. temp. a.
S. K.	45	except Aa. ascendentes	ant. pariet. a., post. temp. a.
S. O.	52	angul. a.	roland. a. — angul. a.
J. N.		Aa. ascendentes	ant. temp.
H. Y.	22	Aa. ascendentes — post.	ant. pariet. — post. temp.
	52	temp.	
K. J.	63	angul. a.	angul. a.

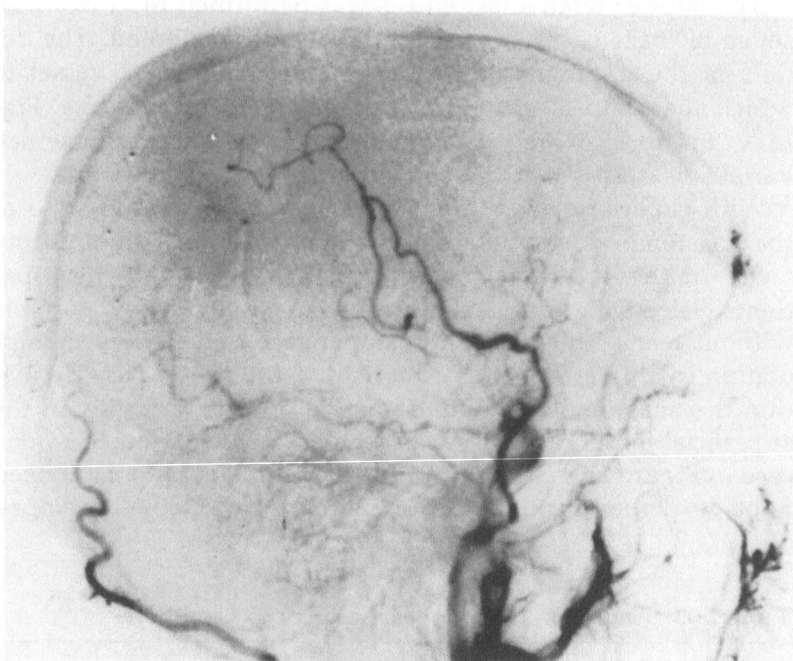

Fig. 25.1. STA-rolandic anastomosis.

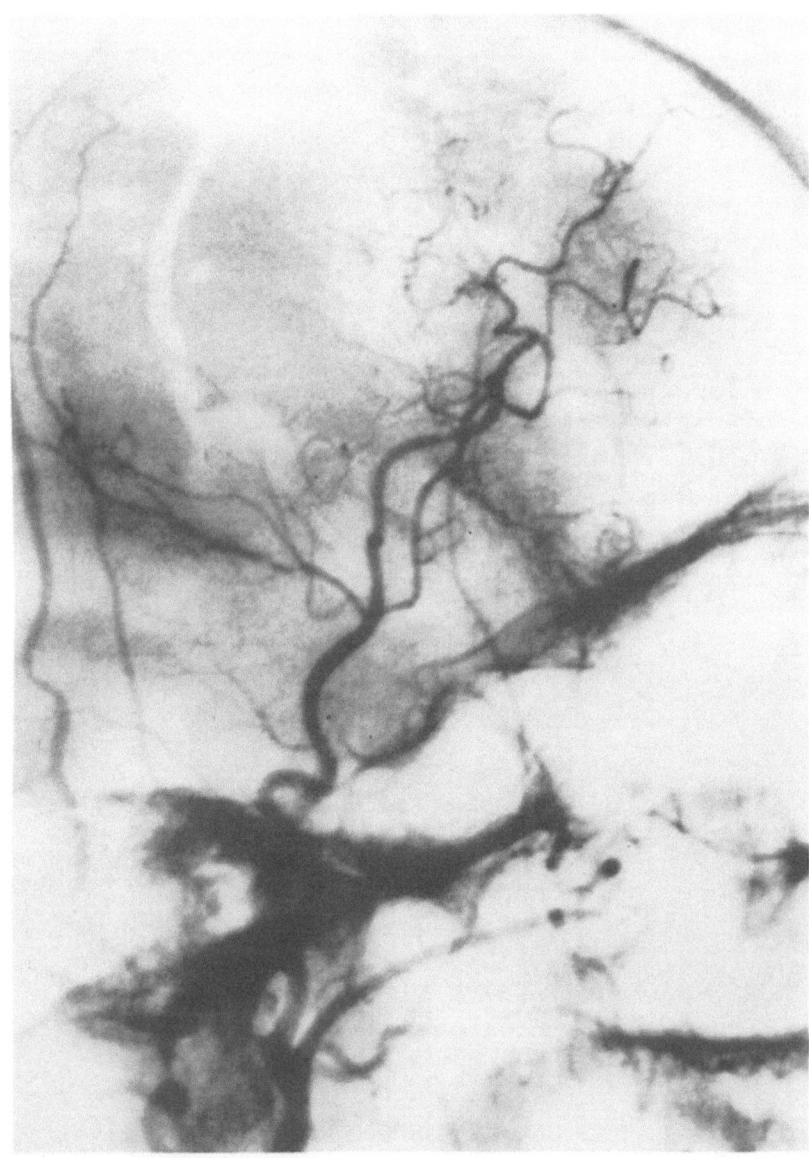

Fig. 25.2. STA-ascending anastomosis.

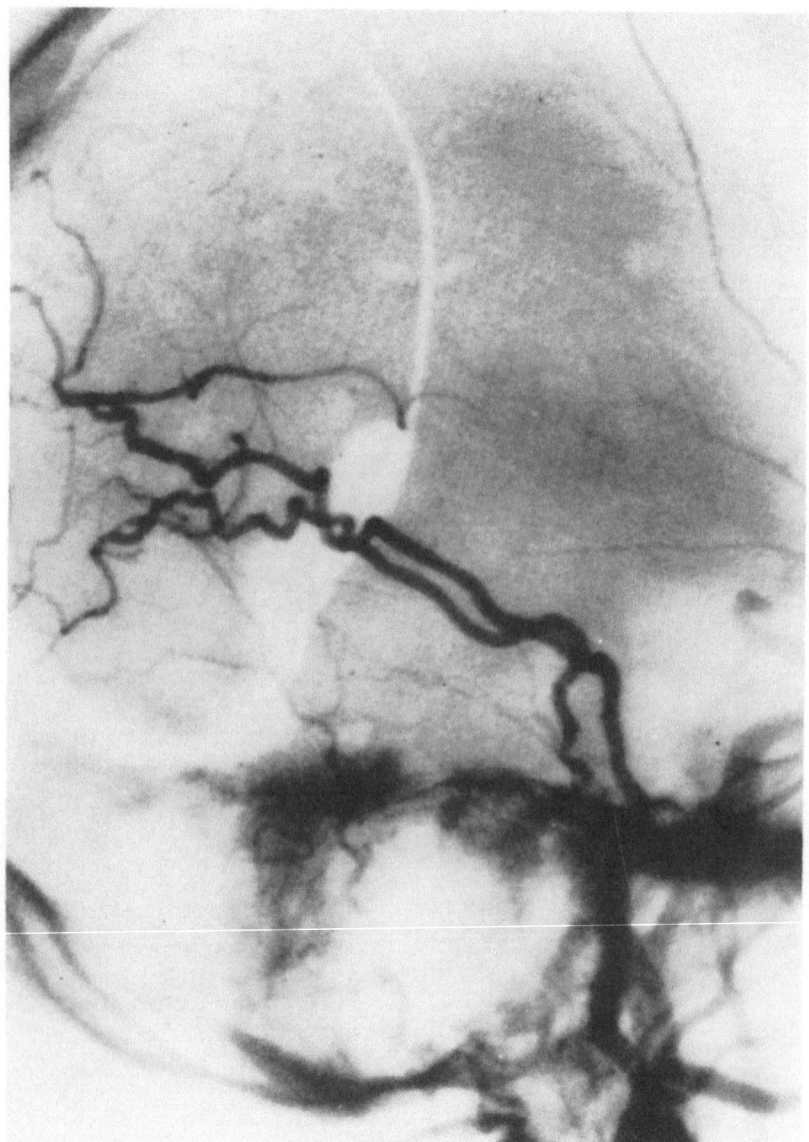

Fig. 25.3. STA-angular anastomosis.

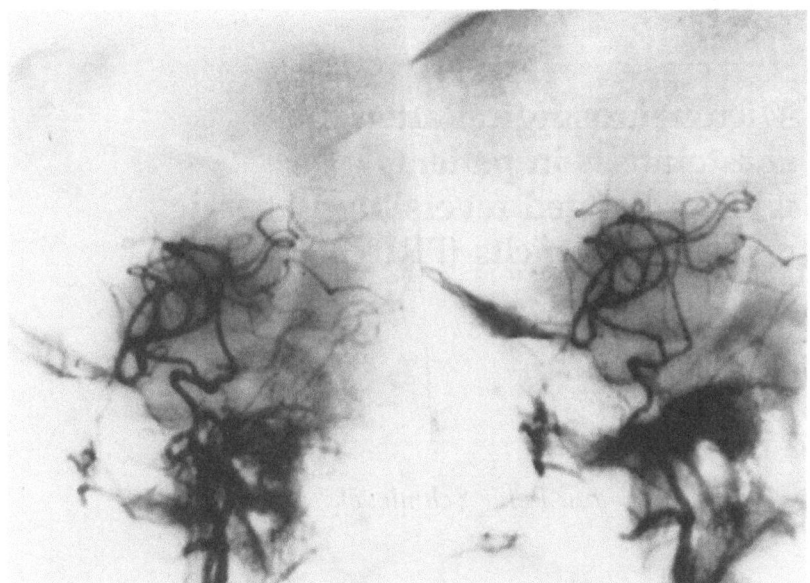

Fig. 25.4. Followup angiography.
Left: 3 weeks after surgery.
Right: 1 year after surgery.

to assess the reversibility of the changes in the affected area in cases of low perfusion. At present the indications and selection of patients for this operation are largely based on the clinical symptomatology coupled with the finding of an appropriate lesion on angiography.

26

Microneurosurgical arterial
anastomoses in patients
with prolonged reversible ischemic
neurologic deficits (PRIND)

Otmar Gratzl and Peter Schmiedek

During the first symposium on extracranial-intracranial anastomoses in Loma Linda, California,(1) there was almost general agreement that this operation should be performed as a prophylactic measure in patients with a history of transient ischemic attacks (TIA). That this clinical condition still represents the best indication is well supported by an up-to-date review of our own series including 62 operated cases. Those patients with episodes of focal cerebral dysfunction of vascular origin lasting for no longer than 24 hours do show the most promising postoperative results, according to a long-term follow-up study.

In order to analyze the therapeutic effect of the microneurosurgical anastomosis on brain blood flow a topical and quantitative evaluation has been carried out. For this purpose the data of clinical investigation, angiography, and measurement of regional cerebral blood flow (rCBF)—were collected and compared for the pre- and postoperative situation.

Examples of these studies on a 42-year-old customs officer are given in Figures 26.1 to 26.3. When this patient was admitted to our hospital he reported four typical episodes of left-sided hemiparesis with concomitant impairment of his sensory function. All of them had occurred during a 3-week period when he was on night duty. Angiography demonstrated a stenosis of the right middle cerebral artery (MCA) with a delayed and partly incomplete filling of the distal arterial branches. The ^{133}xenon flow study (Fig. 26.1) revealed an ischemic focus over the central and parietotemporal region. The mean hemispheric blood flow was reduced to approximately 65% of normal. Eight days postoperatively a normalization of rCBF within the ischemic region and a significant increase in mean hemispheric blood flow to more than 80% of normal were demonstrated

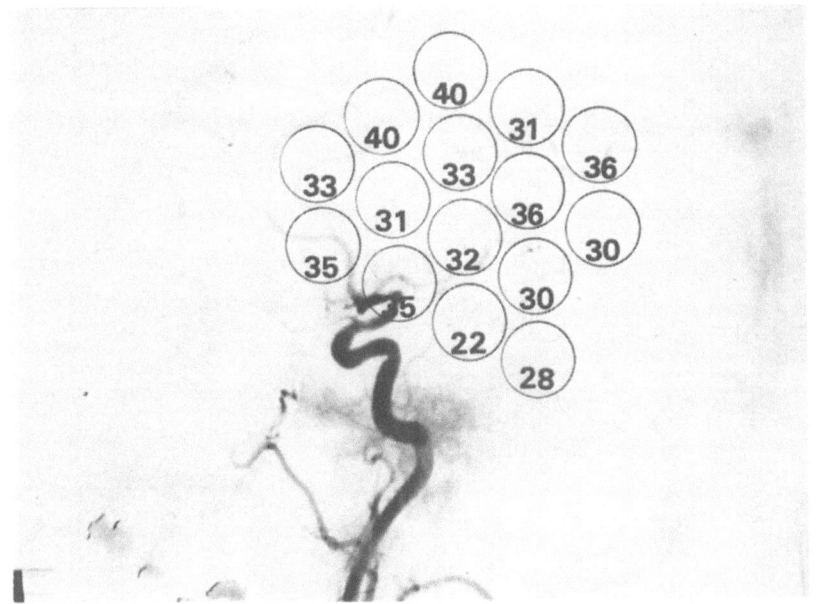

Fig. 26.1. Preoperative ^{133}Xe flow study revealing an ischemic focus over the central and parietotemporal region.

(Fig. 26.2). The external carotid artery angiogram gave good evidence of a functioning anastomosis supplying multiple branches of the MCA, especially the posterior temporal and angular arteries. On repeated study 8 months later the trunk of the MCA was occluded (Fig. 26.3), whereas the anastomosis was feeding the MCA territory quite sufficiently. This was concluded from his asymptomatic neurologic status and the CBF measurement, which was within normal limits. Enhancement of a stenosing vascular process following a bypass operation which changes the pressure-flow-regulation has been previ-

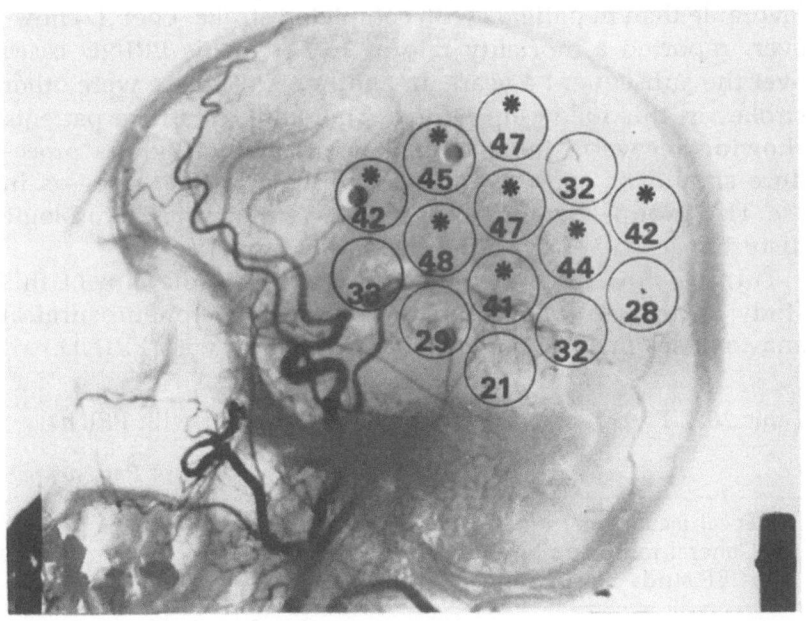

Fig. 26.2. Postoperative rCBF measurement demonstrating a normalization of flow within the formerly ischemic region.

Microneurosurgical Arterial Anastomoses

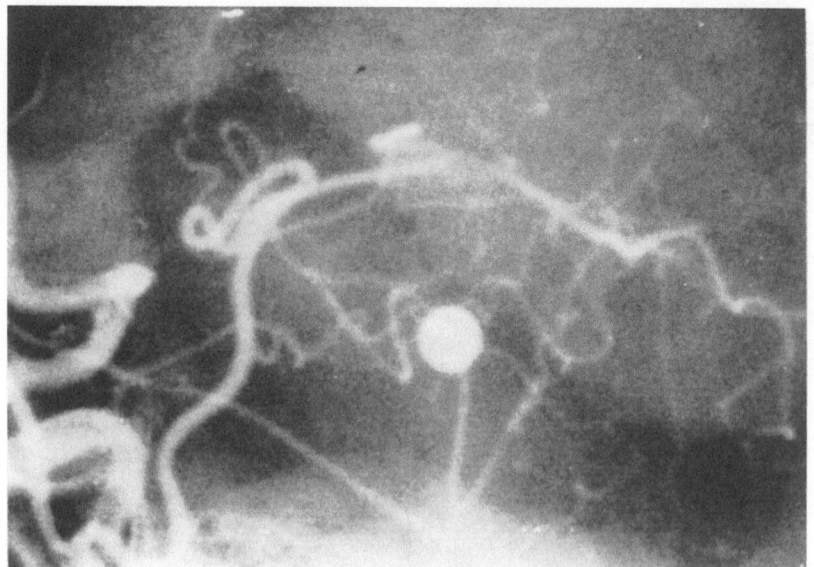

Fig. 26.3. Repeated postoperative angiographic study showing occlusion of the trunk of the middle cerebral artery.

ously reported in association with aortocoronary bypass surgery. As demonstrated by this example, there is no unfavorable influence of the vascular occlusion in those brains protected by a microsurgical anastomosis.

When dealing with ischemic neurologic deficits lasting for longer than 24 hours, the group of patients presenting with prolonged reversible ischemic neurologic deficits (PRIND) should be considered separately regarding prognosis. Neurologic symptoms in these cases are focal in nature, showing spontaneous restitution except for slight residual deficits such as decreased motor activity confined to one extremity, or minimal speech disturbances. The prognosis in these cases is more favorable than in patients with completed stroke. Loeb,(2) however, reported a mortality rate of 16.7% in his PRIND cases over the subsequent 4 years. In another 9.5% there were other strokes in this follow-up period. Therefore, in stroke patients showing recovery, the extracranial-intracranial bypass procedure should be considered as a prophylactic measure—as in the TIA group—because the patients with minor neurologic disturbances are endangered by further strokes.

Turning now from theory to practice, it is the aim of this study to analyze the therapeutic effect of microneurosurgical anastomoses in 13 of our patients presenting with PRIND.

Table 26.1. Properative rCBF findings in 13 patients with PRIND

	No. of Patients
Focal ischemia	4
General reduction + ischemic focus	7
rCBF study not performed	2

Table 26.2. Postoperative rCBF findings in 13 patients with PRIND

	No. of Patients
Function of bypass established	9
Improvement in rCBF	4

Table 26.3. Pre- and postoperative neurology in 13 patients with PRIND

	Hemiparesis	Dysphasia	Asymptomatic
Preoperative	11	2	—
Postoperative	7	2	4

Preoperative cerebral angiography either disclosed hemo-dynamically less significant extracranial or intracranial stenosis or, on the other hand, occlusion of vessels, preferably of multiple branches of the MCA, which was usually well compensated by natural collateral circulation. When regional cerebral blood flow was measured, however, brain regions with an insufficient blood supply could be detected in all cases (Table 26.1). These blood flow derangements were always locally confined. In four cases there was a focal decrease in CBF without any alteration of the nutritional blood flow of the remaining cerebral hemisphere. Eight days postoperatively the patency of the bypass could be demonstrated in all cases angiographically. When comparing pre- and postoperative CBF studies in these cases, there was a complete normalization of CBF in the region previously found to be ischemic and a significant increase in mean hemispheric blood flow in four patients (Table 26.2). The

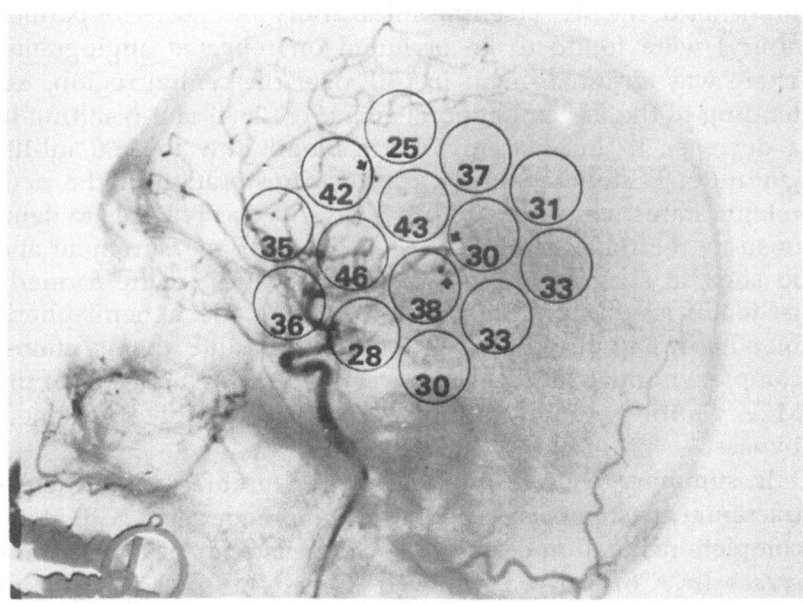

Fig. 26.4. Preoperative ^{133}Xe study. Impairment of CBF over central region extending to the parietotemporal area.

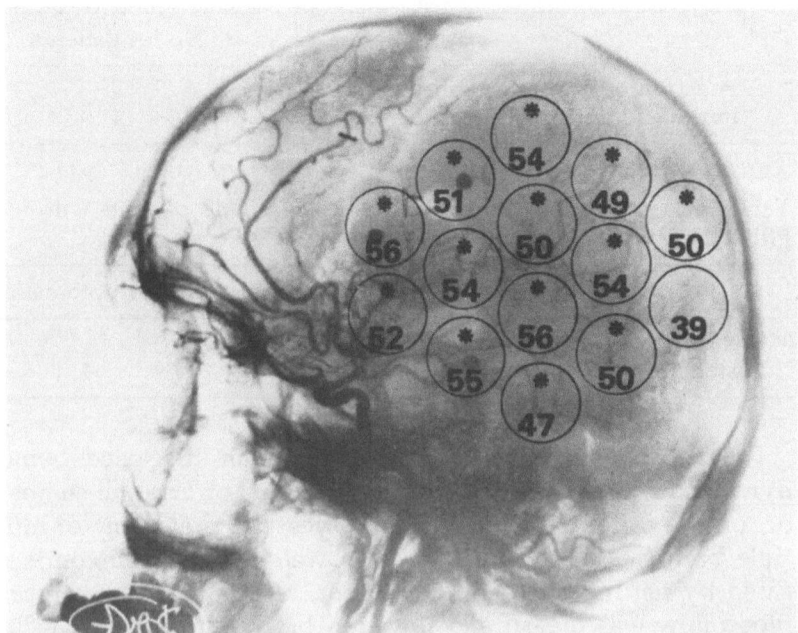

Fig. 26.5. Postoperative rCBF measurement demonstrating significant increase in the values in the formerly ischemic area.

neurologic findings correlated with the CBF studies (Table 26.3): complete restoration of neurologic deficits was seen within the early postoperative phase before dismissal from the hospital in those four patients presenting minor focal changes of CBF in their preoperative studies. Significant changes in either the clinical or the CBF findings were not seen during the later follow-up period which has now lasted up to 12 months.

The following case report illustrates these findings. A 50-year-old man presented with a mild paresis of his right arm after a stroke with incomplete recovery 6 months ago. Two branches of the MCA (central sulcal artery and posterior parietal artery) were found to be occluded on repeated angiograms. There was an impairment in CBF over the central region, extending to the parietotemporal area (Fig. 26.4) and resulting in a decrease in mean hemispheric blood flow to 36.0 ml/100 g/minute. Postoperatively, a complete restoration of the neurologic status was found within 8 days. It was possible to demonstrate the function of the bypass by rCBF measurement and to show a significant increase in the values in the formerly ischemic area (Fig. 26.5). The calculated mean hemispheric blood flow had increased to 48.0 ml/100 g/minute, that is, almost complete normalization. There was filling of all branches of the MCA via the common carotid artery and preferably by the new bypass.

In summary, by suitably locating the cerebral site of the extracranial anastomosis according to the preoperative rCBF data, complete restoration of neurologic deficits and a significant increase in rCBF can be achieved in patients presenting with PRIND and focal impairment of CBF. The results are not as favorable as in patients with TIA, but there is a clear difference when compared with cases with completed stroke, in whom a normalization of blood flow and neurologic status was never seen postoperatively. These results suggest an extension of the indications for this surgical procedure, which until now was recommended for use in cases with TIA: promising effects of the microneurosurgical bypass procedure may be obtained in certain patients with PRIND as well.

REFERENCES

1. Austin GM: Microneurosurgical Anastomoses for Cerebral Ischemia. Proceedings of the First International Symposium in Loma Linda, 1972. Springfield, Ill, Thomas, 1976
2. Loeb C: Cited by Meyer JS: Summary of the 6th Salzburg conference on cerebral vascular disease. Stroke 4:2, 1973

27

Review of experience
with 50 consecutive cases
of superficial temporal artery
to middle cerebral artery anastomosis
for treatment of
cerebrovascular occlusive disease

N. L. Chater, S. J. Peerless, and P. R. Weinstein

Introduction

The probable incidence of stroke in the United States is slightly less than 2 per 1000 population, but this rises sharply with advancing age. In Middlesex County, Connecticut, the adjusted incidence was 1.7 per 1000.(6) The President's Commission on Heart Disease, Cancer, and Stroke pointed out that stroke was the third leading cause of death, and in 1964 there were 2 million people alive who had suffered a stroke.(20) Statistics from the National Cooperative Study also substantiate the fact that the onset of a stroke occurs very frequently in the so-called "productive years," ie, below age 65.(7) Stroke is therefore the primary neurologic disease problem existing in North America at present.

After a completed stroke has occurred rehabilitation frequently has limited success,(10) and there is some question whether stroke intensive care units significantly change the death rate at this time.(13) The catastrophic extent of the problem is therefore apparent in terms of suffering and economic loss of human productivity. The key aim of stroke therapy, therefore, should be to prevent the onset of fixed ischemic damage to the brain and to improve the quality of life in patients suffering from subjective complaints and symptoms of cerebrovascular insufficiency.

Present Clues to the Natural History of Cerebral Vascular Disease

Clinical Presentation

Patients who have developed transient ischemic attacks (TIA) are reported to have an 18 to 60% chance of developing a completed stroke within a year.(1,9,17) A comprehensive study recently published from Rochester, Minnesota, reports an annual incidence of TIA of 0.31 in 1000 with a 20% chance of a completed stroke in 12 months.(21) Many of these strokes occurred shortly after the onset of the warning attacks.

A recent study from the University of California at Los Angeles revealed that of 123 consecutive patients presenting with transient cerebral vascular ischemic symptoms only, 19% had a completely occluded internal carotid artery as the cause of their "hemodynamic" cerebrovascular insufficiency. In a short follow-up period three patients of this particular subgroup (N = 23) suffered a completed stroke.(16) Computer analyses and follow-up of the natural history of patients suffering from internal carotid occlusion from the National Cooperative Study reveal that this is not a benign condition and the outlook is poor.(14) Similar depressing results have been reported by Hardy and his coworkers.(11)

Arteriographic Findings

In a series of 100 consecutive patients presenting with TIAs (or TIAs with a mild completed stroke), 33% of those studied by arteriography demonstrated significant obstructive lesions classified as "inaccessible or inoperable" by general vascular techniques.(12) Other arteriographic studies have reported 33% of obstructive lesions to be intracranial.(3)

Results of Joint Cerebrovascular Disease Study

Haas et al catalog cerebrovascular arteriographic lesions as accessible or inaccessible.(12)

Inaccessible Arteriographic investigations from the National Cooperative Study reveal 6% of the patients had purely inaccessible surgical lesions and an additional 33% demonstrated inaccessible lesions combined with accessible ones, the so-called "tandem lesion."(2) As cerebrovascular atherosclerotic disease is a multifocal entity, this is an expected finding.

Inoperable   An additional 16% of patients studied for cerebrovascular symptoms were shown to have old completed internal carotid occlusions which, at present, are not subjected to surgical exploration by vascular surgeons because of the low success rate in reopening the vessel.(2) However, vascular surgeons are also loathe to operate on an acute internal carotid occlusion because of the reported high incidence of precipitating a hemorrhagic infarct.(23)

Thus, some 22% of patients studied by arteriography may demonstrate "inoperable lesions" or inaccessible ones by present conventional surgical techniques.(2) This amounts to a significant number of individuals per year.

Surgical Technique

Using microvascular techniques, the superficial temporal artery (average diameter, 2 mm) is dissected free from the scalp and a small craniectomy is fashioned of sufficient size to expose a suitable cortical artery 1 mm in diameter or larger. Such a vessel may now be found with a high degree of reliability based on some 50 brain dissections. An end-to-side anastomosis between the superficial temporal artery and the appropriate cortical artery is then performed with the operating microscope, using microinstrumentation under × 16 to 25 magnification. In occasional cases the occipital artery has been employed with success when the superficial temporal artery is too small or has been obliterated due to previous surgery.

Suggested Present Indications for Microvascular Bypass Surgery

Lateralized Low Perfusion Syndromes

Symptoms
Symptoms depend on the vessel involved, usually the middle cerebral artery (MCA), and the functional collateral supply available; may be transient or progressive.

Types of Etiology
1. Old internal carotid occlusions with poor collaterals
2. Carotid siphon stenosis with poor collaterals
3. Middle cerebral stenosis with poor collaterals
   a. Atherosclerotc
   b. Vasculitis(15,18,19)
4. Middle cerebral occlusions with mild deficit
   a. Absent recanalization
   b. Poor collaterals

5. Vertebral basilar lesions with poor collaterals(5) (occipital artery employed)
6. Carotid aneurysms with poor collaterals (inoperable intracranially, but unable to occlude internal carotid artery without precipitating neurologic deficit)

Generalized Low Perfusion Syndromes (generalized cerebral ischemia)

Symptoms
1. May be persistent or intermittent
2. Impaired mentation
3. Ataxia
4. Visual dimming
5. Syncopal episodes
6. Postural vertigo
7. Lightheadedness on change of position
8. Transient motor, speech, or sensory deficits
9. Dementia

Types of Etiology
1. Multiple vessel occlusions
2. Multiple vessel inaccessible stenoses
3. Occlusion and stenosis with inadequate collaterals sufficient to permit repair of accessible stenotic artery

Complications

Complications were as follows:

1. Transient increase in CNS deficit: (10%)
2. Permanent increase in CNS deficit: (0%)
3. Scalp ischemia: (6%); no surgery required
4. Infection: (2%)
5. Intracranial hemorrhage: (2%); subdural hematoma
6. Graft stenosis: (6%)
7. Graft occlusion (STA smaller than 1 mm): (4%)
8. Operative deaths (within one week): (2%); stroke on opposite side
9. Early deaths (within 30 days): (6%)
   a. GI hemorrhage (chronic duodenal ulcer);
   b. Myocardial infarct;
   c. Myocardial infarct
10. Late stroke:
    a. With graft patent (0%)
    b. With graft occlusion (2%)
11. Late death (due to myocardial infarct) (2%)

Contraindications

The following contraindications are noted:
1. Severe longstanding neurological deficit
2. Marked hypertension with small vessel disease demonstrated by arteriography
3. Severe cardiovascular disease
4. Severe diabetes with diffuse peripheral vascular disease
5. Inadequate diameter of donor bypass artery (smaller than 1 mm)

Surgical Results

This microvascular bypass operative approach was developed by Professor M. G. Yasargil while perfecting microvascular neurosurgical techniques in Zurich, and in the laboratory of R. M. P. Donaghy in Burlington, Vermont, in 1966.(24,25)

In October 1967 the first microvascular superficial temporal artery bypass operations were attempted in Burlington and Zurich for the treatment of occlusive cerebrovascular disease.(22) One of the initial operations performed in Zurich was in a patient suffering from a bilateral internal carotid and unilateral vertebral occlusion with disabling transient ischemic attacks. This superficial temporal bypass has remained patent to date and continues to enlarge after 5 years, suggesting that long-term patency is feasible.(4) Stimulated by these technical operative successes, surgeons in various international centers have been performing this procedure in carefully selected cases of stroke. In 1971, Yasargil's 32 cases were reviewed by one of us (Chater) and the patency rate was found to be 66%, paralleling the incidence of significant clinical improvement.(4) At a recent international symposium it was documented that approximately 1350 cases had been performed to date worldwide.(8)

Based on these results we feel that in "hemodynamic" cerebrovascular insufficiency states, superficial temporal artery bypass may be a useful method to surgically produce an improved collateral supply in selected problems of occlusive cerebral vascular disease. Such a procedure at present appears to improve the quality of life in a significant number of patients. The natural history of TIAs and subsequent completed stroke is becoming relatively well known. Whether the operations will diminish the predicted incidence of fixed stroke and modify other aspects of the natural history of the disease requires further extensive study and analysis, but the present results appear promising.

A summary of the types of lesions and the results of surgery is given in Table 27.1. The results of bypass surgery is given in more detail in Tables 27.2 to 27.6.

Table 27.1. STA–MCA anastomosis

Type of Case	Number	Average Follow-up (months)	Patency (%)	Improvement (%)	Completed Stroke
Multiple occlusions (4 vessels)	2	43	100	100	—
Bilateral internal carotid occlusions	12	18	100	75	8% (1), side opposite to bypass
Multiple occlusions plus stenosis	9	31	100	80	12% (1), side opposite to bypass
Internal carotid occlusions	12	12	100	92	—
Siphon stenosis	9	20	88	88	12% (1), bypass nonfunctioning
Middle cerebral stenosis	4	16	100	100	—
Middle cerebral occlusion	2	12	50	50	50% recurrent hemiparesis, secondary to auricular fibrillation and emboli

Table 27.2. Current results of bypass operations:[a] Multiple Occlusions—4 Vessels

Patient	Symptoms Preoperative	Arteriograms Preoperative	Months Postoperative	Present Clinical Symptoms	Postoperative Arteriograms
Male, 55 years	Dementia, psychopathic depression Mute, akenetic One seizure	4-vessel occlusion BICO BVO	59 months bilateral STA–MCA bypass	Working as a timekeeper Drives a car	Jan 1974 both bypasses open Excellent cerebral perfusion
Male, 48 years	RIND both hemispheres TIAs both hemispheres Apraxia, memory loss, R-L disorientation	4-vessel occlusion BICO BVO	27 months bilateral STA–MCA bypass	No TIAs or RINDS Progressive improvement intellect 12 months. Drives car No apraxia No R-L disorientation	June 1973 both bypasses patent and enlarging

[a]Key for Tables 2 to 6: TIA, transient ischemic attacks (less than 24 hours); RIND, recovery but neurologic deficit lasting 23 hours; ICO, internal carotid occlusion; CCO, common carotid occlusion; BICO, bilateral internal carotid occlusion; STA, superficial temporal artery; MCA, middle cerebral artery, cortical branch; O, occipital artery, scalp; VS, vertebral stenosis; VO, vertebral occlusion; BS, basilar stenosis; SS, siphon stenosis; SO, siphon occlusion; MCS, middle cerebral stenosis, MCO, middle cerebral occlusion; R, right; L, left.

Table 27.3. Current results of bypass operations[a]: Bilateral Internal Carotid Occlusions

Patient	Symptoms Preoperative	Arteriograms Preoperative	Months Post-operative	Present Clinical Symptoms	Postoperative Arteriograms
Male, 47 years	TIAs both hemispheres; 3 L hemisphere; 1 R hemisphere	BICO	50 months bilateral STA–MCA bypass	No TIAs; working plywood mill	Both bypasses open with good cerebral perfusion
Male, 62 years	TIAs both hemispheres; 12 attacks; mild dementia; poor memory	BICO	37 months; 35 months bilateral STA–MCA bypass	? episodes brain stem ischemia; not working	Left bypass stenosed, right bypass good, July 1973
Male, 54 years	TIAs right hemisphere; attacks of confusion lasting hours	BICO	24 months; 23 months bilateral STA–MCA bypass	TIAs (× 2) R hemisphere postop 2 months; none since; no attacks of confusion	December 1973, both bypasses patent
Male, 59 years	Poor memory; episode ataxia; episode confusion	BICO	20 months; 10 months bilateral STA–MCA bypass	No attacks of confusion; slight memory improvement; episodes of ataxia less	Left bypass patent, right not studied, May 1973
Male, 55 years	Bilateral TIAs; 3 R hemisphere, 12 L hemisphere	BICO	19 months left STA–MCA bypass	No further TIAs left hemisphere; 4 TIAs right hemisphere; part-time work	Left bypass patent, February 1974
Male, 44 years	Left hemiparesis on head rotation with vertigo, memory loss	BICO, small vertebrals	15 months R STA–MCA bypass	No symptoms; working postal clerk	R bypass patent; February 1974; enlarging
Male, 67 years	TIAs left hemisphere; old mild infarct right hemisphere; mild dementia	BICO	15 months L STA–MCA bypass	Decreased TIA L hemisphere; less speech involvement; not working	L bypass patent (small), January 1974

Table 27.3. Current results of bypass operations[a]: Bilateral Internal Carotid Occlusions *(continued)*

Patient	Symptoms Preoperative	Arteriograms Preoperative	Months Post-operative	Present Clinical Symptoms	Postoperative Arteriograms
Male, 60 years	TIAs R hemisphere; no change by Dicumarol	BICO	13 months R STA–MCA bypass	Several mild TIAs R hemisphere; major infarct L hemisphere (own control)	R bypass open, December 1974
Male, 64 years	Memory loss; RIND 2 attacks both hemispheres; mild dementia	BICO	10 months left STA–MCA bypass	No change	No angiogram; bruit over anastomosis
Male	2 attacks; loss of consciousness no warning; EEG normal; no cardiac cause	BICO	6 months R STA–MCA bypass	No symptoms	Patent, enlarging anastomosis, January 1974
Male, 62 years	Right hemisphere TIAs with syncope and visual blurring	BICO	6 months R STA–MCA bypass	No symptoms; manager of motel	Patent enlarging bypass, January 1974
Male, 64 years	Progressive mental deterioration; RIND right hemisphere	BICO	5 months R STA–MCA bypass	Family reports intellectual improvement; no TIAs	Patent enlarging bypass, December 1973

[a]See Table 27.2 for legend.

Table 27.4. Current Results of Bypass Operations[a]: Multiple Occlusions and Stenoses

Patient	Symptoms Preoperative	Arteriograms Preoperative	Months Postoperative	Present Clinical Symptoms	Postoperative Arteriograms
Male, 58 years	TIA speech, R hand weak; multiple episodes up to 20-day; not improved on anticoagulants or platelet suppression	L carotid occluded; R carotid stenosed; severe intracranial carotid disease	53 months L STA–MCA/ anastomosis	Last TIA involving L hemisphere 2 months after procedure; had one episode of TIA involving R hemisphere; on Anturane and ASA	Anastomosis open, December 1973
Male, 51 years	2 TIAs L hemisphere; 1 RIND R hemisphere; dress apraxia; clumsy left arm	Left carotid occlusion; right carotid stenosis	51 months R STA–MCA anastomosis	Working as salesman; continued to have mild TIAs of R hemisphere until placed on platelet suppression; almost complete recovery of R parietal signs	Anastomosis patent, November 1973
Male, 55 years	3 TIAs R hemisphere; then multiple TIAs L hemisphere	Left carotid occluded; right carotid stenosis, mild	46 months L STA–MCA 2 vessels	Occasional TIAs involving R leg, weakness, and numbness; no further speech disorder; working as watchman; on platelet suppression	Anastomosis patent, November 1973
Male	1 RIND R hemisphere 1970; 3 TIAs L hemisphere; dysphasia and monocular blindness	R carotid occluded; tandem stenosis; L carotid severe in siphon	40 months L STA–MCA	No further TIAs; not working but active as a commodities speculator; on platelet suppression	Anastomosis patent, June 1972
Male, 65 years	Repeated attacks left sided hemiparesis and numbness	SS R (90%); L ICO	20 months R STA–MCA bypass	Asymptomatic	Anastomosis patent, February 1973

Table 27.4. Current Results of Bypass Operations[a]: Multiple Occlusions and Stenoses *(continued)*

Patient	Symptoms Preoperative	Arteriograms Preoperative	Months Postoperative	Present Clinical Symptoms	Postoperative Arteriograms
Male, 68 years	Attacks; marked dizziness; memory loss; speech slurring	CCO L; vertebral occusion L	15 months L STA–MCA bypass	No speech difficulty; rarely dizziness	Refused; not done; Doppler flow good
Male, 57 years	Poor memory; bilateral transient visual impairment; syncope × 3 (seizures)	R carotid stenosis; L carotid occlusion; L vertebral occlusion	18 months L STA–MCA bypass (2 vessels)	Memory slightly improved; has had 2 further episodes of visual difficulty in past 6 months; one further episode of syncope	1 vessel occluded, 1 patent and good caliber, January 1974
Male, 55 years	Alternating numbness, weakness of legs with dysphasia more marked on left	ICO R; ICS L (95%); cervical vertebral stenosis L	R STA–MCA bypass	Died 5 days postop from emboli to siphon from contralateral stenotic lesion in neck with occlusion of siphon (arteriographically proven)	Autopsy not obtained; bypass on R side patent by arteriography; patient died from left hemisphere infarction and swelling, showing no sign of left-sided weakness, suggesting bypass able to carry adequate flow
Male, 49 years	Multiple attacks R hemisphere; 1 attack right-sided weakness	BICO; basilar stenosis	5 months R STA–MCA bypass	Weakness left leg for 2 weeks postop, then clearing	Bypass patent and enlarging, February 1974

[a]See Table 27.2 for legend.

Table 27.5. Current Results of Bypass Operations[a]: Internal Carotid Occlusion

Patient	Symptoms Preoperative	Arteriograms Preoperative	Months Post-operative	Present Clinical Symptoms	Postoperative Arteriograms
Male, 66 years	Remote RIND L hemisphere; fluctuating dysphasia; clumsy arm with intermittent numbness	ICO L	22 months L STA–MCA bypass	Marked improvement in speech and arm function	Patent bypass, October 1973; fills most of MCA
Male, 55 years	Progressive astereognosis; numbness; weakness of left arm	ICO R hemisphere; filling through PCA only	20 months R STA–MCA bypass	Improvement in strength left arm; some astereognosis, but improved	Patent bypass; marked enlargement; suffered 2 myocardial infarcts with hypotension without stroke
Male, 62 years	Right progressive hemiparesis; 3 days stroke in evolution	ICO R	14 months R STA–MCA bypass	Progression arrested; moderate improvement hand function	Died MI 14 months; bypass patent at autopsy
Male, 69 years	Daily TIAs left hemisphere; dextran, dicumarol, aspirin	ICO L	14 months L STA–MCA bypass	No further TIAs	Bypass patent, January 1974, and enlarging
Female, 49 years	Nurse; recurrent TIAs, left hemisphere	ICO L	14 months L STA–MCA bypass	None; night supervisor, orthopedics ward	Patent bypass, October 1973
Male, 45 years	Right hemiparesis aphasia; wife-nurse	ICO L; poor crossover	14 months L STA-5MCA bypass	Marked recovery; slightly spastic leg; minimal dysphasia; working supervision card dealers	Patent bypass; STA has tripled in size; fills MCA plus anterior cerebral
Female, 57 years	Multiple attacks amaurosis, L; with TIAs L hemisphere	ICO L	13 months L STA–MCA bypass	No further TIAs; occasional mild blurring vision of left eye; housewife	Declined arteriogram; bypass open with Doppler ultrasound

Table 27.5. Current Results of Bypass Operations[a]: Internal Carotid Occlusion *(continued)*

Patient	Symptoms Preoperative	Arteriograms Preoperative	Months Post-operative	Present Clini-cal Symptoms	Postoperative Arteriograms
Male, 50 years	2 attacks RIND L hemi-sphere with recovery	ICO L	12 months L STA–MCA bypass	No symptoms; car salesman	Patent anasto-mosis, en-larging, Oc-tober 1973
Female, 58 years	Recurrent TIAs L hemi-sphere	ICO L	7 months L STA–MCA bypass	No symptoms; housewife; 6 hours dys-phasia, post-op	Declined arter-iogram; Doppler shows pat-ency
Male, 54 years	Recurrent TIAs L hemi-sphere	ICO L	6 months L STA–MCA bypass	One TIA, pos-top 4 weeks; none since	Bypass patent, enlarging
Male, 64 years	RIND with re-sidual dys-phasia, L hemisphere, 5 months	ICO L	5 months L STA–MCA bypass	Speech moder-ately im-proved; no TIAs	Bypass patent; left ascend-ing, frontal
Male, 67 years	TIAs, L hemi-sphere; re-current	ICO L	5 months L STA–MCA bypass	No symptoms; financier; 12 hours dys-phasia post-op	Bypass open to Doppler; se-vere heart disease; de-clined arter-iogram

[a]See Table 27.2 for legend.

Table 27.6. Current Results of Bypass Operations[a]: Siphon Stenosis

Patient	Symptoms Preoperative	Arteriograms Preoperative	Months Post-operative	Present Clini-cal Symptoms	Postoperative Arteriograms
Female, 38 years	1 TIA, L hemi-sphere	L carotid SS	51 months L STA–MCA bypass	No further TIAs; func-tioning as housewife and caring for 5 chil-dren; no neurologic deficits; no medications	Anastomosis patent, No-vember 1973
Male, 55 years	Repeated at-tacks left-sided hemi-paresis and numbness	SS 90%	25 months R STA–MCA bypass	Asymptomatic; working as optical sales-man	Patent 1 year postop

Table 27.6. Current Results of Bypass Operations*a*: Siphon Stenosis *(continued)*

Patient	Symptoms Preoperative	Arteriograms Preoperative	Months Post-operative	Present Clinical Symptoms	Postoperative Arteriograms
Male, 42 years	RIND R hemisphere; 2 TIAs R hemisphere	R carotid stenosis in siphon; L carotid and vertebrals OK	22 months R STA–MCA bypass	No further episodes of RIND or TIA; on platelet suppression	Anastomosis patent, February 1974
Male, 63 years	Memory loss, attacks of progressive weakness right side with ataxia	SS L 60%	18 months L STA–MCA bypass	3 months post-op completed right side stroke secondary to carotid siphon occlusion	Nonfunctionary bypass, technical reason; cortical artery 0.07 mm in diameter
Female, 61 years	Dizziness on changes of position; severe numbness right arm and face with weakness	SS L 70%	14 months L STA–MCA bypass	Asymptomatic	Scheduled (not done); Doppler flow excellent
Female, 58 years	4 months mild completed stroke with clumsiness of right hand, pain, numbness of right arm; dizziness, fluctuating dysphasia	SS L 80%	13 months L STA–MCA bypass	No subjective complaints; improvement of function of right arm and hand; typing	Declined; Doppler flow excellent
Male, 69 years	Recurrent dizziness, numbness, and weakness left arm and hand; severe diabetes	SS R 80%	13 months R STA–MCA bypass	Minimal subjective complaints; no findings neurologically	Declined because of diabetes; Doppler flow excellent

Table 27.6. Current Results of Bypass Operation[a]: Siphon Stenosis *(continued)*

Patient	Symptoms Preoperative	Arteriograms Preoperative	Months Post-operative	Present Clinical Symptoms	Postoperative Arteriograms
Male, 46 years	Blind R eye abrupt; RIND R hemisphere, clearing at time of operation	Right carotid occlusion at siphon and up to posterior communicating artery	13 months R STA–MCA bypass	Complete recovery of hemisphere function; improved vision in R eye, central retinal artery occluded; on platelet suppression	No arteriogram; hand bruit over anastomosis
Male, 73 years	One RIND R hemisphere	R SS 70%	7 months R STA–MCA bypass	Asymptomatic; postop subdural hygroma drained through 2 burr holes	Patent bypass, January 1974

[a]See Table 27.2 for legend.

REFERENCES

1. Acheson J, Hutchison EC: Observations on the natural history of transient cerebral ischaemia. Lancet 2:871, 1964
2. Blaisdell WF, Clauss RH, Galbraith JG, et al: Joint study on extracranial arterial occlusion. IV. A review of surgical considerations. JAMA 209:12, 1969
3. Blaisdell WF, Hall AD, Thomas AM, et al: Cerebrovascular occlusive disease, experience with panarteriography in 300 consecutive cases. Calif Med 5:321, 1965
4. Chater NL, Yasargil MG: Results of temporal artery bypass procedures in the treatment of cerebrovascular disease. Presented at Congress of Neurological Surgeons, Miami, Florida, October 1971
5. Devivi DC: Vertebrobasilar occlusive disease in children. Arch Neurol 26:278, 1972
6. Eisenberg H, Morrison JT, Sullivan P, et al: Cerebrovascular accidents. Incidence and survival rates in a defined population. Middlesex County, Connecticut. JAMA 189:883, 1964
7. Fields WS, North RR, Hass WK, et al: Joint study of extracranial arterial occlusion as the cause of stroke. JAMA 203:955, 1968
8. First International Symposium Microneurosurgical Anastomosis for Cerebral Ischemia, Loma Linda, California, June 1973 (ed. G.M. Austin) Springfield, Ill, 1976
9. Friedman GD, Wilson WS, Mosier JM, et al: Transient ischemic attacks in a community. JAMA 210:1428, 1969

10. Gordon EE, Kohn KH: Evaluation of rehabilitation methods in the hemiplegic patient. J Chronic Dis 19:3, 1966
11. Hardy WG, Lindner DW, Thomas LM, et al: Anticipated clinical course in carotid artery occlusion. Arch Neurol: 7:74-86, 1962
12. Hass WK, Fields WS, North RR, et al: Joint study of extracranial arterial occlusion. II. Arteriography, techniques, sites, and complications. JAMA 203:961, 1968
13. Kennedy FB, Pozen TJ, Gabelman EH, et al: Stroke intensive care. An appraisal. Am. Heart J 80:188, 1970
14. Lemak N: Personal communication. National Computer Analysis. Joint Study Computer Analysis and Followup. Houston, Texas, February 1974
15. Levine J, Swanson PD: Non-atherosclerotic causes of stroke. Ann Intern Med 70:807, 1969
16. Machleder H, Barker W: Stroke on the wrong side. Arch Surg 105:943, 1972
17. Marshall J: The natural history of transient ischaemic cerebrovascular attacks. Q J Med 33:309, 1964
18. Senevirante BIB, Ameratunga B: Strokes in young adults. Br Med J 2:791, 1972
19. Tavares J: Multiple progressive intracranial arterial occlusions. A syndrome in children and young adults. Am J Roentgenol 106:235, 1969
20. The President's Commission on Heart Disease, Cancer, and Stroke. Washington DC, USGPO, 1964
21. Whisnant J, Matsumoto N, Lila E: Transient cerebral ischemic attacks in Rochester, Minnesota. Mayo Clinic Proc 48:194, 1973
22. Wylie EJ, Ehrenfeld WK: Extracranial Occlusive Cerebrovascular Disease. Diagnosis and Management. Philadelphia, Saunders, 1970, p 231
23. Wylie EJ, Hein JD, Adams JE: Intracranial hemorrhage following revascularization for treatment of acute stroke. J Neurosurg 21:202, 1964
24. Yasargil MG: Microsurgery Applied to Neurosurgery. Stuttgart, Thieme, 1969
25. Yasargil MG, Krayenbuhl JA, Jacobson JH II: Microneurosurgical arterial reconstruction. Surgery 1:221, 1970

VII
OTHER APPLICATIONS

28

Microvascular anastomosis and carotid artery ligation for fibromuscular hyperplasia and carotid artery aneurysm

Harry W. Stephens, Jr.

Fibromuscular hyperplasia is a characteristic dysplasia of the walls of medium- and small-sized arteries, reported initially in young adult females with the clinical picture of ischemic hypertension. The changes of fibromuscular hyperplasia have been observed in renal, celiac, superior mesenteric, inferior mesenteric, external iliac, and internal carotid arteries.(2,6) The first histologically verified case of fibromuscular hyperplasia involving an extracranial segment of the internal carotid artery in a patient with stroke was reported(1) in a 34-year-old female by Connett and Lansche in 1965. Since that time further cases have been described including bilateral involvement of the internal carotid arteries or involvement of carotid and vertebral arteries.(2,3,4)

McCormack(8) identified four distinguishing pathologic features in these vessels: (1) intimal fibroplasia; (2) medial fibroplasia, usually with mural microaneurysms; (3) subadventitial fibroplasia, often involving the external elastic membrane; and (4) genuine fibromuscular hyperplasia with segmental concentric stenosis produced by cuffs of hyperplastic smooth muscle and collagen fibers.

The pathognomonic angiographic appearance of fibromuscular hyperplasia is characterized by notching and aneurysmal outpouchings of the arterial lumen giving the familiar "string of pearls" appearance.

It is evident that fibromuscular hyperplasia involving multiple arteries is being recognized with increasing frequency and that common etiologic factors are responsible for both the extracranial and intracranial forms of the arterial dysplasia.

In general, patients presenting with T.I.A. secondary to an internal carotid artery lesion carry a poor prognosis. Many of these patients are affected by stroke of varying degree during the acute phase of the disease. Experience has shown that endarterectomy of accessible internal carotid lesions provides symptomatic relief with possible prevention of subsequent stroke. Direct surgical treatment of a lesion not lending itself to endarterectomy was first reported by Connett and Lansche.(1) The lesion, confined to the proximal half of the internal carotid artery, was successfully resected and replaced with autogenous saphenous vein. Morris et al(9) performed intraoperative graduated dilatation of the internal carotid artery in a selected series of eight patients having fibromuscular dysplasia. These patients had internal carotid lesions extending to the carotid foramen. Arteriographic studies performed 2 weeks to 4 years after graduated dilatation showed no recurrent stenosis in five of these arteries. This therapy appears to be lasting in nature for a select group of patients. No operative deaths or permanent neurologic deficits were attributed to the procedure, and no recurrent neurologic symptoms were observed during the postoperative period.

Unfortunately, there are certain lesions of the internal carotid artery which are technically inoperable either because of the location or extent of the lesion. Examples are lesions extending intracranially or totally occluding the extracranial segment of the internal carotid artery. Studies conducted by Whisnant et al(10) in a series of 198 patients showed that the probability of stroke in untreated patients having T.I.A.s was about 20% during the 6-month period after an initial T.I.A. There was a significant decrease in the incidence of stroke subsequent to the first month following the initial T.I.A., but long-term follow-up showed that there was no significant difference in survival time between patients treated with anticoagulants and untreated patients. A disadvantage of anticoagulation therapy is the associated morbidity and mortality resulting from complications of hemorrhage.(10)

Lesions located intracranially and not accessible to either endarterectomy, autogenous vein replacement, or graduated dilatation can be by-passed with a shunt. A microsurgical anastomosis of the superficial temporal artery (STA) or the occipital artery (OA) to cortical branches of the middle cerebral artery (MCA) will bypass lesions of the internal carotid artery and provide blood flow to the ischemic cerebral hemisphere. Patency of the external carotid artery is required for success of the shunting technique and endarterectomy and/or replacement of segments of diseased external carotid artery may be considered in addition to the by-pass procedure.

Angiographic documentation of internal carotid stenosis progressing to total occlusion, along with the increasing flow through a functioning shunt, is one indication that the shunt can in fact provide sufficient flow to prevent stroke. Percutaneous compression of the carotid artery,(7) intraoperative in-

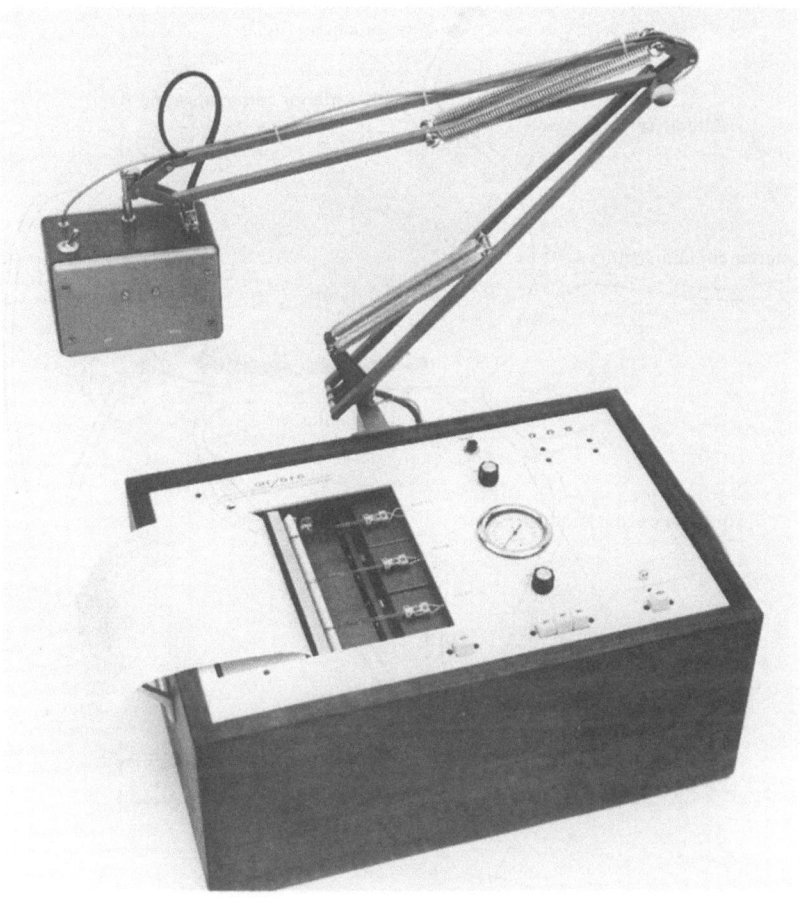

Fig. 28.1. Ocular pneumoplethysmography (OPG) console containing recorder, electronic components, and pneumatic components used for noninvasive recording of intraocular pressure. The OPG reflects intracranial internal carotid artery pressure and can evaluate the adequacy of collateral hemispheric blood pressure. (Courtesy of W. Gee, M.D.)

travascular pressure measurements, and ocular pneumoplethysmography(5) (OPG) have all been used to assess the safety of carotid ligation. These techniques provided a method of determining the pressure of both ipsilateral hemisphere blood pressure (IHBP) and collateral hemispheric blood pressure (CHBP) to within an accuracy of ± 5 mmHg (Figs. 28.1 to 28.3). The OPG has been used during surgery for comparison of ophthalmic artery pressure before and after shunting and has been applied to predict the safety of occlusive procedures performed in patients exhibiting CHBP above 50 mmHg. Patients with an OPG reading below 50 mmHg were either allowed to develop IHBP above 50 mmHg or underwent a bypass graft to the hemisphere to bring the IHBP above 50 mmHg. The internal carotid artery was then occluded without danger of neurologic complications.

Case Studies

The following cases are presented to illustrate clinical situations in which the extracranial–intracranial bypass protected the ip-

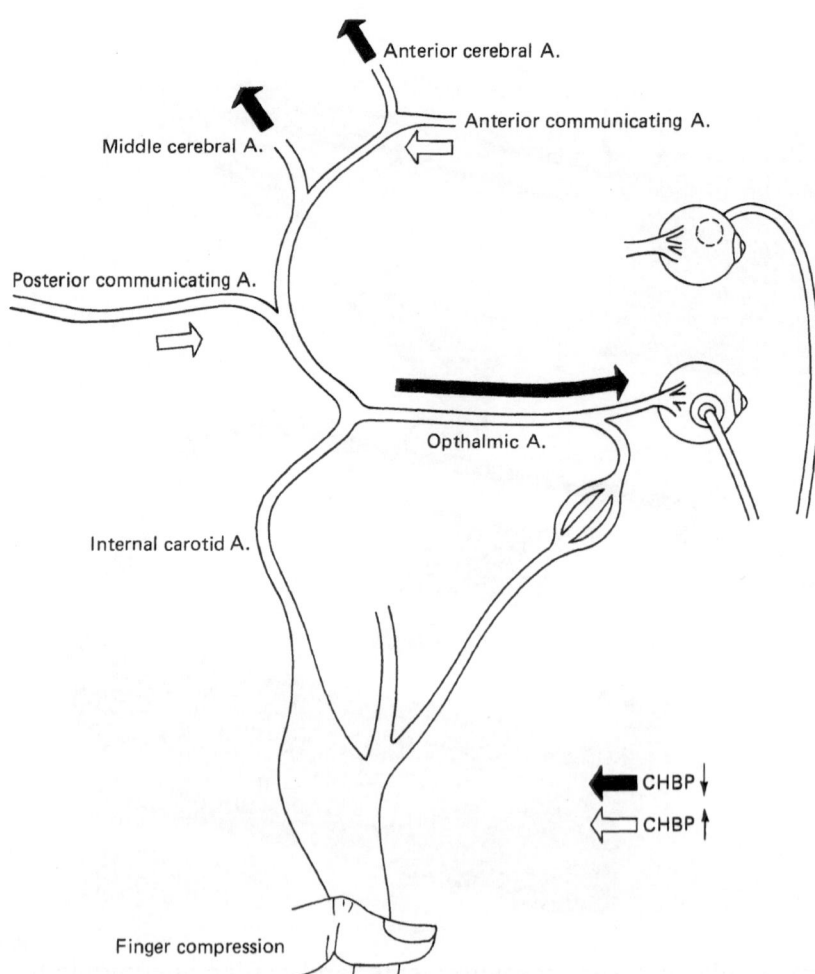

Fig. 28.2. Diagram representing the collateral hemispheric blood pressure (CHBP) with carotid artery compression. Open arrows indicate pathways which increase collateral hemispheric blood pressure. Dark arrows indicate pathways which decrease collateral hemispheric blood pressure. (Courtesy of W. Gee, M.D.)

Labels in figure:
Anterior cerebral A.
Anterior communicating A.
Middle cerebral A.
Posterior communicating A.
Opthalmic A.
Internal carotid A.
CHBP ↓
CHBP ↑
Finger compression

silateral hemisphere from the sequelae of internal carotid occlusion.

Case 1

A 43-year-old white female was seen September, 1973. She complained of sudden onset of blurring of vision in her right eye. There was associated numbness and weakness of her left upper and lower extremities. These symptoms lasted for several hours without any neurologic sequelae. Several transient ischemic attacks occurred during the ensuing days. There was no family history of cerebrovascular disease.

She also had a bruit in the neck on the right side. An arch study with selective four vessel catheterization demonstrated 75% stenosis of the right internal carotid artery from the carotid bifurcation to 3 cm below the internal carotid siphon (Figs.

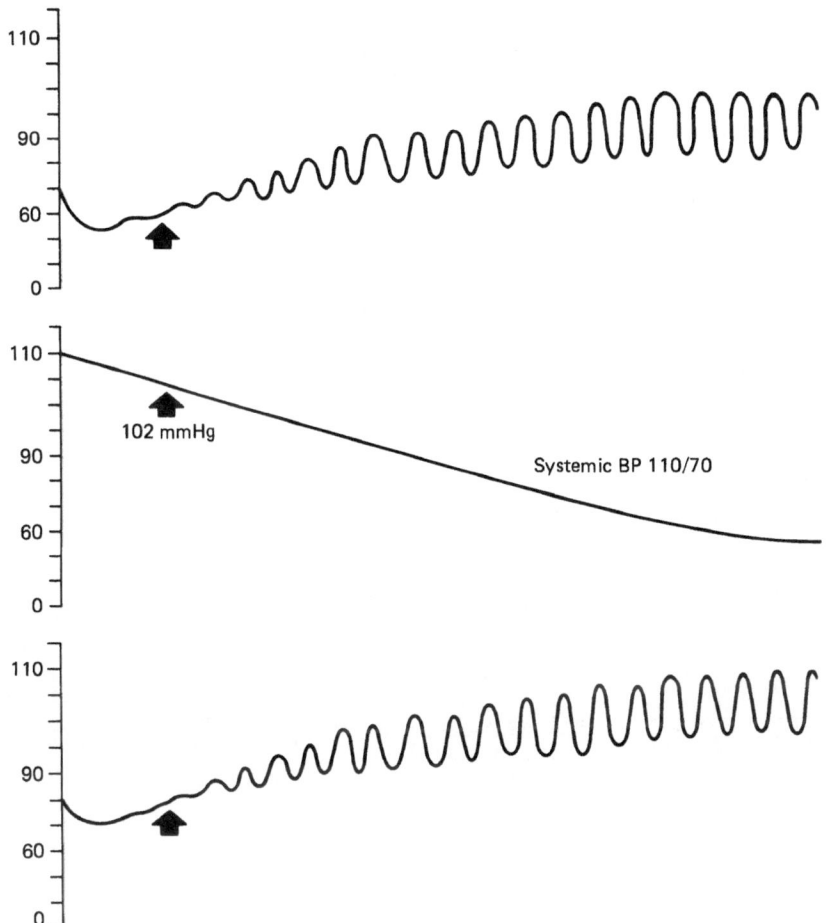

Fig. 28.3. OPG with normal ophthalmic evaluation. *Middle tracing:* Vacuum decrement from 110 to 0 mmHg blood pressure. *Upper tracing:* OPG right eye. Onset of pulsations at 102 mmHg blood pressure. *Lower tracing:* OPG left eye. Onset of pulsations at 102 mmHg blood pressure.

28.4a,b). The lesion was deemed inoperable and the patient was placed on anticoagulants. Despite anticoagulation, the patient experienced transient cerebral ischemic attacks followed by a stroke. She had a complete recovery from the stroke except for a residual paresthesia of her face.

On November 12, 1973, a superficial temporal artery (2 mm) to angular (1.8 mm) and opercular (1.5 mm) branches of the right middle cerebral artery anastomosis was performed. The patient was discharged from the hospital on the seventh postoperative day.

During the ensuing month, she experienced two transient ischemic attacks of lesser severity.

An angiogram was performed 6 weeks following the initial surgery (Fig. 28.5b). The study demonstrated a functioning superficial temporal artery to middle cerebral artery anastomosis at the angular and opercular sites. A 75% internal carotid artery stenosis was demonstrated again.

Transient ischemic symptoms of dizziness, blurring vision, and tingling of the left arm were reproduced by a 10-second

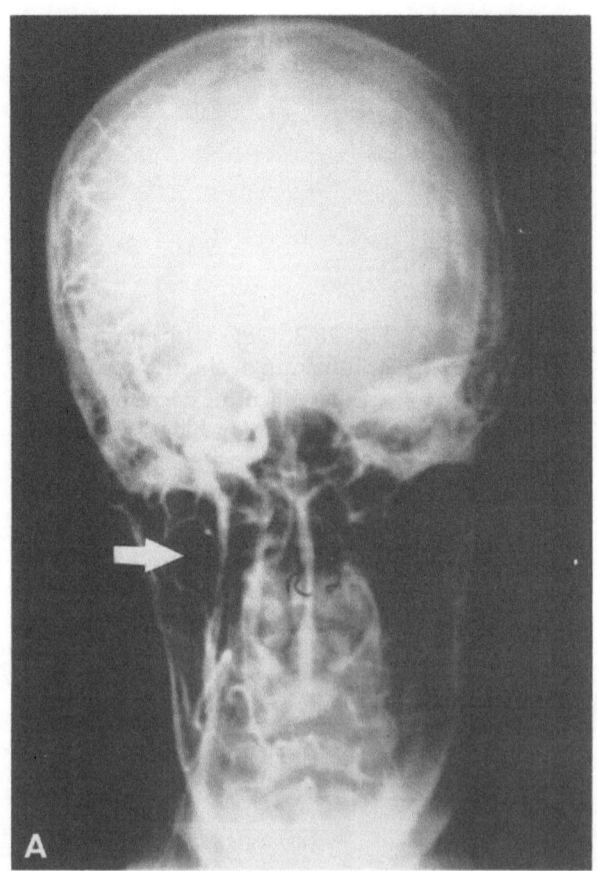

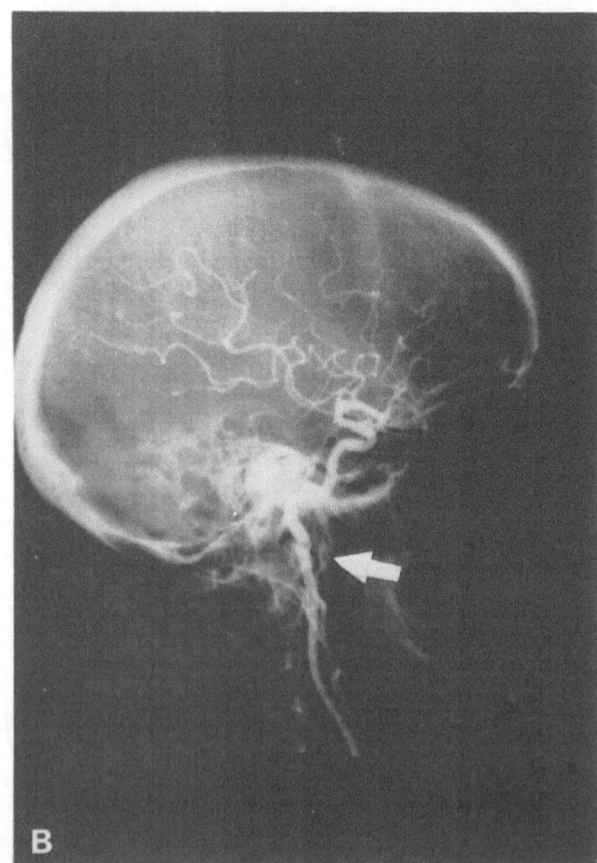

Fig. 28.4. Case 1. AP (a) and lateral (b) views of angiogram. Demonstrates inoperable carotid stenosis (arrows).

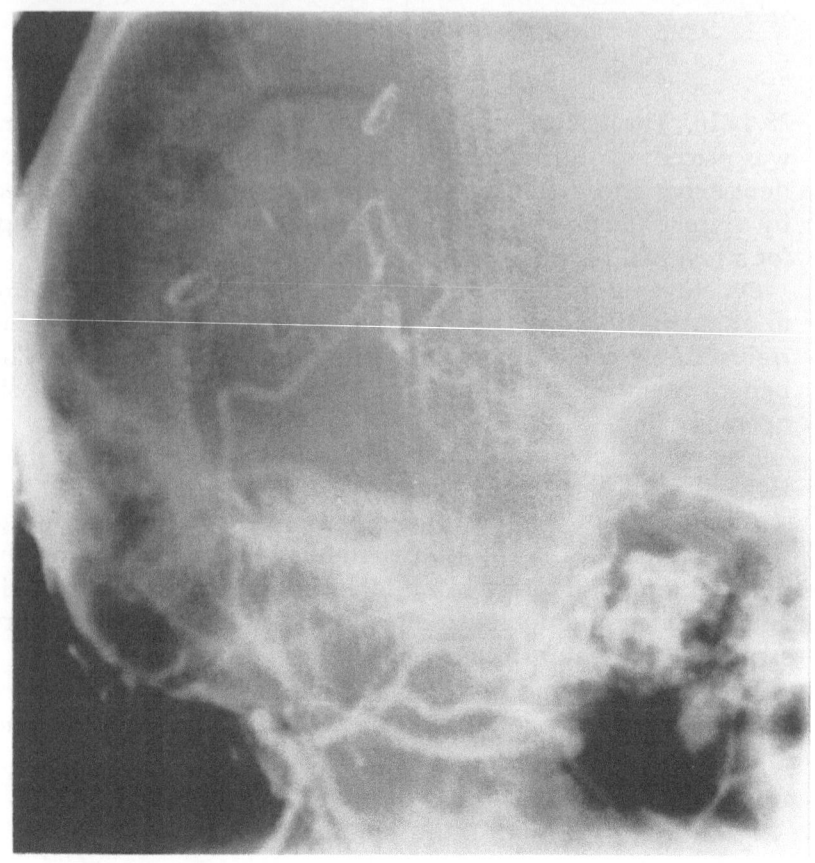

Fig. 28.5. Postoperative angiogram (oblique view). Demonstrates functioning STA–MCA shunt. The patient continued to have occasional transient ischemic attacks.

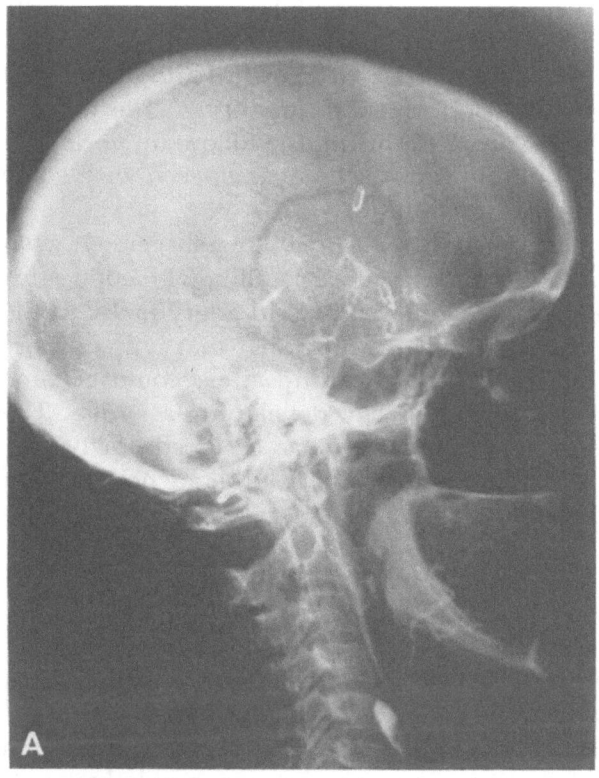 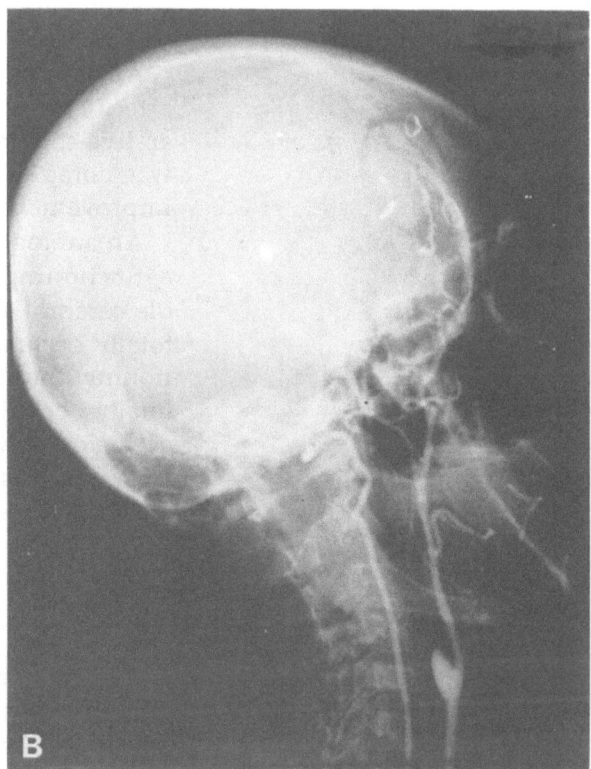

digital compression of the right superficial temporal artery over the zygoma.

Six weeks after the initial surgery a Selverstone carotid clamp was placed on the right internal carotid artery 1 cm above the bifurcation. The vessel was gradually occluded over the next 48 hrs. Following total occlusion, the vessel was ligated (Fig. 28.6a,b). Sections of the artery suggested fibromuscular hyperplasia. She was discharged on the third postoperative day. Presently, she is free of any symptoms and attending normal duties as a nurse.

Fig. 28.6. Case 1. Lateral (a) and oblique (b) views of angiogram. Demonstrates functioning STA–MCA shunt and occluded carotid artery. Patient is free of transient ischemic attacks.

Case 2

A 53-year-old white male was treated in June, 1972. He suffered from a transient ischemic attack affecting his speech and his right arm. He was left with a slight residual paresis of the right upper extremity and dysphasia that was noted to be progressing. Diabetes was well-controlled and he had mild hypertension.

Angiography of the cerebral vessels showed total occlusion of the right internal carotid artery and an inoperable 75% stenosis of the left internal carotid artery. Perfusion of the brain was by vertebral arteries with delayed filling of the left middle cerebral artery.

A left superficial temporal artery to a cortical middle cerebral artery anastomosis was performed in July, 1972. The postoperative course was uneventful. During the follow-up period he was noted to have definite improvement in speech with some improvement in motor function.

An angiogram performed 3 weeks following surgery showed a functioning STA–MCA shunt with early filling of the left middle cerebral artery. The left internal carotid artery had become totally occluded. This patient demonstrated that with a functioning shunt a diseased internal carotid artery could become totally occluded without necessarily developing a stroke. The occlusion of the internal carotid artery had occurred slowly over a 3-week period and demonstrated that deliberate occlusion of a diseased vessel could be safely considered.

Case 3

A 24-year-old white male had a sudden onset of right upper arm weakness with aphasia that gradually resolved over a 24-hr period. Angiography demonstrated an inoperable aneurysm of the left internal carotid artery. Ocular pneumoplethysmography (OPG) with alternate carotid compression to determine collateral hemispheric blood pressure demonstrated that the carotid stump pressure was below the minimum of 50 mmHg CHBP (Fig. 28.7). This suggested that internal carotid artery ligation could not be predicted as safe. A left superficial temporal artery to angular branch of the left middle cerebral artery anastomosis was performed. Intraoperative OPG's demonstrated a CHBP of 92 mmHg reflecting the internal carotid artery stump pressure (Fig. 28.8). Acute ligation of the internal carotid artery was done and the patient recovered with no neurologic deficit and has had no TIA's.

This case demonstrates that elective carotid artery occlusion can be carried out safely if the known CHBP is above 50 mmHg.

Conclusion

We have observed certain patients with occasional TIA's persisting after a functioning STA–MCA shunt has been established. These TIA's ceased when the diseased internal carotid artery became totally occluded. With both of these facts in mind, a combined technique was performed in a 43-year-old female patient suffering TIA's from an inoperable fibromuscular dysplasia lesion of the internal carotid artery. The patient had a STA–MCA shunt performed, but when the TIA's did not

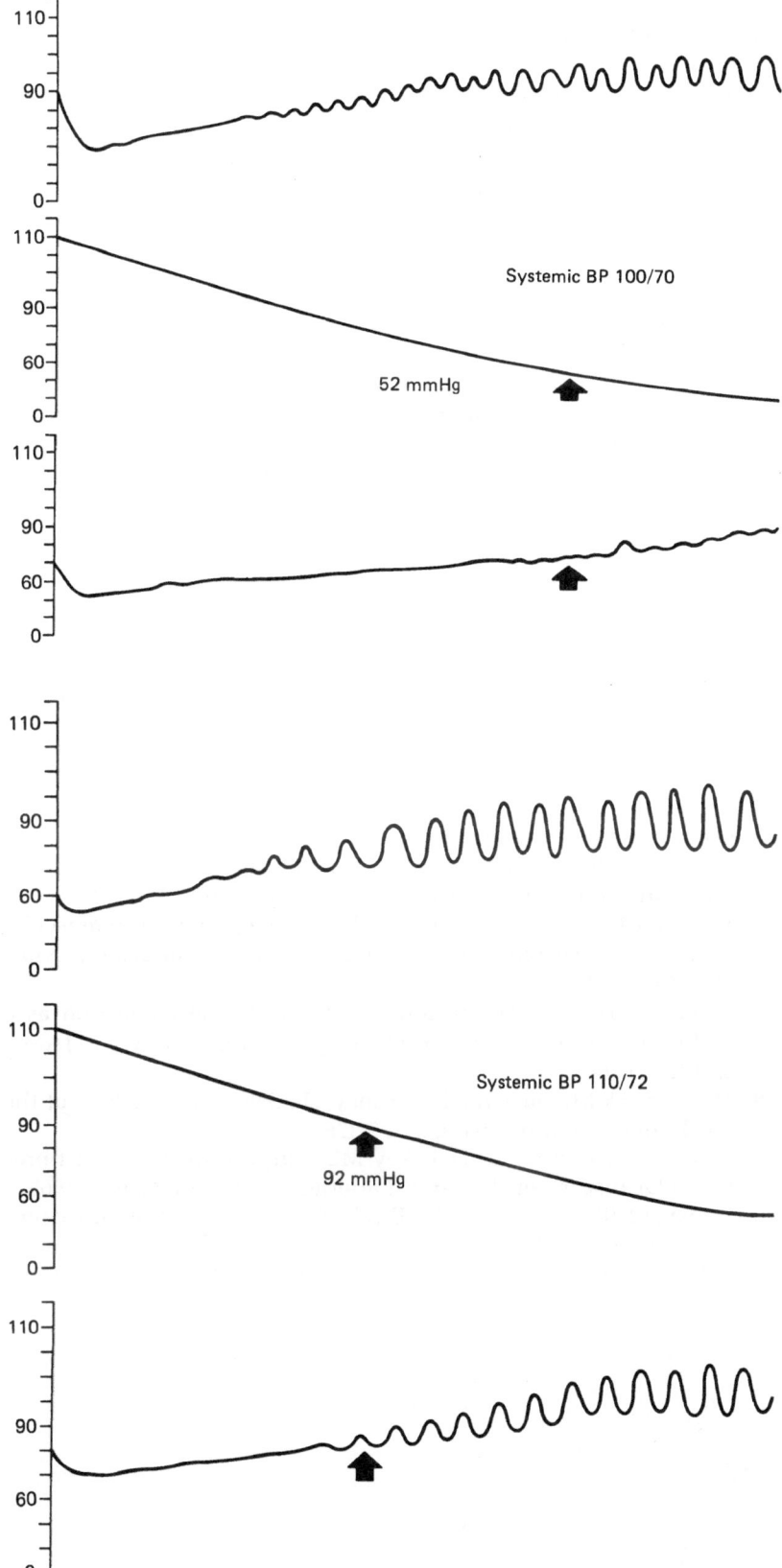

Fig. 28.7. Case 3. OPG with left carotid artery compressed. Preoperative evaluation. *Middle tracing:* Vacuum decrement from 110 to 0 mmHg blood pressure. *Upper tracing:* OPG right eye. Onset of pulsations at 96 mmHg blood pressure. *Lower tracing:* OPG left eye. Onset of pulsations at 52 mmHg blood pressure.

Fig. 28.8. Case 3. OPG with left carotid artery ligation and functioning STA–MCA shunt. *Middle tracing:* vacuum decrement from 110 to 0 mmHg blood pressure. *Upper tracing:* OPG right eye. Onset of pulsations at 96 mmHg blood pressure. *Lower tracing:* OPG left eye. Onset of pulsations at 92 mmHg blood pressure.

Conclusion

315

cease completely, her diseased internal carotid artery was gradually occluded over a period of several days with a Selverstone clamp. The patient became free from further TIA's and was able to carry out her normal duties.

OPG can be employed to demonstrate acceptable CHBP as evidence that a diseased internal carotid artery can be ligated safely in preference to gradual occlusion by carotid clamp.

ACKNOWLEDGMENTS

This work was encouraged and supported by Robert M. Jaeger, M.D., Department of Neurological Surgery, and Harry Kaupp, M.D., Department of Vascular Surgery. The financial aid of Mr. Leonard Pool provided the necessary equipment.

REFERENCES

1. Connett MC, Lansche JM: Fibromuscular hyperplasis of the internal carotid artery. Report of a case. Ann Surg 162:59, 1965
2. Ehrenfeld WK, Stoney RJ, Wyler EF: Fibromuscular hyperplasia in the internal carotid artery. Arch Surg 95:284, 1967
3. Ennis JT, Bateson EM: Fibromuscular dysplasia of the internal carotid arteries—a report of three cases. J Radiol 43:452, 1970
4. Galligioni, F, Iraci G, Marin G: Fibromuscular hyperplasia of the extracranial internal carotid artery. J Neurosurg 34:647, 1971
5. Gee W, Smith CA, Hinsen CE, et al: Ocular pneumoplethysmography in carotid artery disease. Med Instrument 8:1, 1974
6. Harrison EG, Hunt JC, Bernatz PE: Morphology of fibromuscular dysplasia of the renal artery in renovascular hypertension. Am J Med 45:97, 1967
7. Matas R: Testing the efficiency of the collateral circulation as a preliminary to the occlusion of the great surgical arteries. JAMA 63:1441, 1914
8. McCormack LJ, Dustan HP, Meaney TF: Selected pathology of the renal artery. Semin Roentgenol 2:126, 1963
9. Morris GC, Lechter A, DeBakey ME: Surgical treatment of fibromuscular disease of the carotid arteries. Arch Surg 96:636, 1968
10. Whisnant JP, Matsumoto N, Elveback L: The effect of anticoagulant therapy on the prognosis of patients with transient cerebral ischemic attacks in a community. Mayo Clin Proc 48:844, 1973

Index

Ocular pressure, measurement of, 118
Ocular pulse, carotid artery and, 117
ODM, *see* Ophthalmodynamometry
Omentum, transplantation of in brain
    revascularization, 195–198
Ophthalmodynamometry, ocular pressure
    measurement by, 118–119
Otic artery, persistent, 144
Oxidative metabolism
  ATP and, 60
  in cerebral ischemia, 59–83
  electron-transport systems and, 63–64
  in focal ischemic insufficiency, 66–67
  glycolysis rate and, 60–62
  zone of infarction and, 73
Oxidative phosphorylation, 64–65
Oxygen, transport and delivery of, 59–60
Oxygen availability, as stroke factor, 241
Oxygen extraction, in medial cortical tissue, 72

Pancreatitis, atherosclerosis and, 106
Patency
  angiographic and histologic, 32–33
  blood flow and, in arterial vein grafts to basilar
    artery, 27–34
  by electromagnetic flow technique, 33
  prostaglandin E_1 and, 45–53
  small vessel, 45–53
PCA, *see* Posterior cerebral artery
Pco_2, arterial, 70
Penetrating vessels, anatomy of in stroke, 3–4
Penicillin, in cerebral ischemia risk, 115
Persistent hypoglossal artery, anastomosis of, 144
Persistent otic atery, anastomosis of, 144
PFK, *see* 6-Phosphofructokinase
PGE_1, *see* Prostaglandin E_1
pH, arterial, 59
Phosphates, high-energy, 60
  6-Phosohofructokinase
  glycolysis and, 61
  kinetic parameters of, 62
Phosphoenolypyruvate, conversion of to
    pyruvate, 63
Phospholipoprotein, 45–46
Phosphorylation, oxidative, 64–65
Pial window, blood flow measurements through,
    67–68
PICA, *see* Posterior inferior cerebellar artery
Platelet aggregation
  ADP and, 52
  collagen and, 52
  PGE_1 and, 48
Platelet factor III, 45–46
Platelet stimulation, factors in, 45

Plethysmography, ocular, 117–130
Po_2 values, tissue hypoxia and, 60
Polyarteritis, in cerebral ischemia, 114
Polycythemia vera, 114
  as risk factor, 108
  treatment of, 116
Postanastomosis
  collateral, 151–152
  prostaglandin E_1 and, 49
Posterior cerebral artery
  calcarine or parietooccipital branch of, 24
  occlusion of, 137
Posterior circulation
  anatomical studies of in occipital artery bypass,
    23–25
  recipient vessel sites for, 24
Posterior-inferior cerebellar artery,
    tonsillohemispheric branch of, 24
Preanastomosis, collateral, 148–151
Preoperative angiographic visualization, 145–146,
    see also Angiography
PRIND, *see* Prolonged reversible ischemic
    neurologic deficits
Progressive systemic sclerosis, in cerebral
    ischemia, 114
Prolonged reversible ischemic neurologic deficits
  microneurosurgical arterial anastomoses in,
    284–289
  in TIA, 211–212
Prostaglandin E_1
  effect of in small vessel patency, 45–53
  postanastomosis effects and, 49
Prostaglandins
  adenylcyclase activity and, 47
  ADP and, 47–48
  cyclic-AMP and, 47
  defined, 46
  discovery of, 46
Pulmonary syndrome, in cerebral ischemia, 113
Pyruvate kinase
  catalytic action of, 63
  glycolysis and, 61

Radiophosphorus, in polycythemia vera, 116
Rat
  aorta of, 40
  common carotid artery in, 36–39, 41
rCBF, *see* Regional cerebral blood flow
Recipient vessels, in posterior circulation anatomy
    studies, 24–25
Reduced nicotinamide-adenine dinucleotide, *see*
    NADH
Regional cerebral blood flow, 167
  analog computer analysis of, 255–256